Springer Series on Child and Family Studies

Series Editor

Nirbhay N. Singh, Medical College of Georgia, Augusta University, Augusta, GA, USA

The Springer Series on Child and Family Studies addresses fundamental psychological, educational, social, and related issues within the context of child and family research. Volumes published in this series examine clinical topics with an additional focus on epidemiological, developmental, and life span issues. Leading scholars explore such factors as race and immigration, parenting, and the effects of war and violence on military families and unite a vast literature into a comprehensive series of related research volumes.

Laura Nabors • Jessica Dym Bartlett
Editors

Family Engagement in Mental Health Interventions for Young Children

Springer

Editors
Laura Nabors
College of Education, Criminal Justice
Human Services, and Information
Technology
University of Cincinnati
Cincinnati, OH, USA

Jessica Dym Bartlett
Thriving Together, LLC
West Newton, MA, USA

ISSN 2570-0421 ISSN 2570-043X (electronic)
Springer Series on Child and Family Studies
ISBN 978-3-031-47916-8 ISBN 978-3-031-47917-5 (eBook)
https://doi.org/10.1007/978-3-031-47917-5

This Springer imprint is published by the registered company Springer Nature Switzerland AG
The registered company address is: Gewerbestrasse 11, 6330 Cham, Switzerland

Paper in this product is recyclable.

Preface

This book, entitled *Family Engagement in Mental Health Interventions for Young Children*, focuses on effective and equitable approaches to family engagement in mental health interventions for young children, from infancy to early elementary school (birth to 8 years of age). Young children can and do experience mental health problems and, as a population, are exposed to multiple adversities that increase their risk for developing mental disorders (Dalsgaard et al., 2020). In our view, this book adds to the literature by concentrating on the critical nature of family engagement in the context of reviewing evidence-based treatments and promising interventions and their impact on outcomes for children and families participating in mental health services. The chapter authors take a critical look at the evidence on engaging families from diverse racial, ethnic, and socioeconomic backgrounds. They also present key data on evidence-based interventions to improve the engagement of families with children who have special needs, highlighting interventions for autism spectrum disorder and children with chronic illnesses. Additionally, chapters review family engagement interventions for young children who have experienced trauma, providing critical information to guide practitioners and researchers on maximizing family engagement to help children heal. Another chapter presents innovative policies, theory, and research on the importance of engaging families in young children's mental health treatment as part of a larger systems of care to promote the well-being of young children and their families.

The chapters in this volume also highlight inequities in access to infant and early childhood mental health treatment and to equitable outcomes among families living in poverty and families of color, along with strategies to reduce disparities. The orientation of each chapter is to present and guide research in the field and its translation into effective policy and practice to promote young children's psychological well-being. Within this orientation, authors highlight the importance of diverse family perspectives on family engagement in mental health interventions for their young children (Posey-Maddox & Haley-Lock, 2020). They also emphasize the importance of culturally adapted care to successfully engage families with diverse beliefs, values, and preferences related to the treatment of mental disorders in early childhood (Vasileva et al., 2021). In addition, chapters highlight the importance of relationship-based, two-generation (or multi-generation), trauma-informed, and culturally grounded services.

The organization of this book highlights the importance of developmentally appropriate approaches with an emphasis on equity in engaging families in mental health treatment, including meeting treatment needs and engagement approaches that are appropriate for families with young children (ages birth to 8 years) across a wide range of interventions to promote infant and early childhood mental health (IECMH). An emphasis on young children's development is essential to supporting their long-term well-being, as young children have unique developmental needs and their experiences with caregivers and in the world play a significant role in shaping their rapidly developing brains and relatedly, their social and emotional functioning. Moreover, at this young age, parents and other primary caregivers are critical to the success of mental health interventions, making this an important arena to discuss family engagement (Copple & Bredekamp, 2009; Sprenger, 2008).

D. W. Winnicott (1960) famously asserted that the infant (young child) must be considered within the context of maternal (family) care. Thus, to be effective, treatment of early childhood disorders must include a child's primary caregivers. It is also essential to account for the influence of the broader ecology in which young children and their families are embedded, by identifying and addressing social determinants of health that influence parenting quality and the family's ability to engage and remain in services for their young children (e.g., McKay & Bannon, 2004). Of course, a contemporary understanding of "maternal care" must be expanded to include all parents and caregivers, including fathers, same-sex parents, resource (foster) parents and kinship caregivers, adoptive parents, and other primary caregivers. That is, to be effective, mental health practitioners and programs need to engage a broad range of families in positive, respectful, and culturally and linguistically responsive partnerships that support each family's progress toward their goals (U.S. Department of Health and Human Services, Administration for Children and Families, Office of Head Start, National Center on Parent, Family, and Community Engagement, 2018). Relatedly, authors discuss the importance of incorporating lived experience into all levels of decision-making in young children's mental health care to help providers and programs better understand and integrate the perspective of individuals with first-hand knowledge of mental health and parenting challenges, who can help guide decisions that affect families receiving services (National Center on Substance Abuse and Child Welfare, n.d.).

In addition, this book presents a broad array of areas for research on family engagement, including but not limited to: family-centered care, relationship-based care, two-generation interventions, trauma-informed care, equitable care, factors influencing engagement to therapist recommendations, and research on client-centered (in this case child- and family-centered) change processes (King et al., 2014). However, the most effective strategies for family engagement may vary across cultural, developmental, and linguistic contexts (Fehrer & Tognozzi, 2018; Halgunseth, 2009). This book offers an in-depth look at family engagement across different theoretical orientations, contexts, conditions for the child, cultures, and-family members, which we believe will be helpful to researchers, policymakers, and practitioners alike. Our aim is to review the latest research and key concepts in different areas and offer recommendations for future work to support mental health and health professionals' efforts to enhance family engagement in mental health treatment for young children.

Taken together, the chapters in this book offer a critical analysis of extant research on family engagement in mental health treatment for young children (birth – 8 years) and their families and how it applies to future research, policy, and practice. The authors of each chapter emphasize a particular age group, service setting, or approach, including interventions for infants and toddlers, preschoolers, and school-age children; children with disabilities and chronic illness; children who have experienced trauma; fathers; systems of care; and equity. The final chapter briefly synthesizes their work and other literature to date on effective family engagement practices, identifies lines of inquiry warranting further attention, and offers suggestions for future research, policy, and practice.

Cincinnati, OH, USA Laura Nabors
West Newton, MA, USA Jessica Dym Bartlett

References

Copple, C., & Bredekamp, S. (2009). *Developmentally appropriate practice in early childhood programs serving children from birth through age 8*. National Association for the Education of Young Children. ERIC Number: ED510265.

Dalsgaard, S., Thorsteinsson, E., Trabjerg, B. B., Schullehner, J., Plana-Ripoll, O., Brikell, I., Wimberley, T., Thygesen, M., Madsen, K. B., Timmerman, A., Schendel, D., McGrath, J. J., Mortensen, P. B., & Pedersen, C. B. (2020). Incidence rates and cumulative incidences of the full spectrum of diagnosed mental disorders in childhood and adolescence. *JAMA Psychiatry, 77*(2), 155–164. https://doi.org/10.1001/jamapsychiatry.2019.3523

Fehrer, K., & Tognozzi, N. (2018). Cultural & linguistic responsiveness and meaningful family engagement: Why it matters in early education (4 pages). Early Child Language and Development Institute: *John W. Gardner Center for Youth and Their Communities*. Stanford University. ERIC Number: ED594175.

Halgunseth, L. (2009). Family engagement, diverse families, and early childhood. *Young Children, 64*(5), 56–58 (see www.naeyc.org/files/naeyc/file/ecprofessional/EDF_Literature%20Review.pdf for the full report)

King, G., Currie, M., & Petersen, P. (2014). Child and parent engagement in the mental health intervention process: A motivational framework. *Child and Adolescent Mental Health, 19*(1), 2–8. https://doi.org/10.1111/camh.12015

McKay, M. M., & Bannon Jr., W. M. (2004). Engaging families in child mental health services. *Child and Adolescent Psychiatric Clinics, 13*(4), 905–921. https://doi.org/10.1016/j.chc.2004.04.001

National Center on Substance Abuse and Child Welfare. (n.d.). *Engaging parents and youth with lived experience: Strengthening collaborative policy and practice initiatives for families with mental health and substance use disorders*. Children's Bureau, Administration for Children and Families & the Substance Abuse and Mental Health Service Administration. https://ncsacw.acf.hhs.gov/files/live-experience.pdf

Posey-Maddox, L., & Haley-Lock, A. (2020). One size does not fit all: Understanding parent engagement in the contexts of work, family, and public schooling. *Urban Education, 55*(5), 671–698. https://doi.org/10.1016/j.ecresq.2020.05.006

Sprenger, M. (Ed.). (2008). *The developing brain: Birth to age eight*. Corwin Press.

U.S. Department of Health and Human Services, Administration for Children and Families, Office of Head Start, National Center on Parent, Family, and Community Engagement (2018). *Key indicators of high-quality family engagement for Quality Rating Improvement Systems*. https://childcareta.acf.hhs.gov/sites/default/files/public/indicators-final-508.pdf

Vasileva, M., Graf, R. K., Reinelt, T., Petermann, U., & Petermann, F. (2021). Research review: A meta-analysis of the international prevalence and comorbidity of mental disorders in children between 1 and 7 years. *Journal of Child Psychology and Psychiatry, 62*(4), 372–381. https://doi.org/10.1111/jcpp.13261

Winnicott, D. W. (1960). The theory of the parent-infant relationship. *International Journal of Psycho-Analysis, 41*, 585–595.

Contents

Chapter 1
Family Engagement in Mental Health Interventions for Infants and Toddlers

Abigail Palmer Molina

It is important to first understand what is meant by "mental health" for infants and toddlers before discussing the wide variety of programs and interventions that seek to engage families and support mental health for young children. Infant and early childhood mental health (IECMH) has been defined as the "young child's capacity to experience, regulate, and express emotions, form close and secure relationships, and explore the environment and learn—all in the context of family, community, and culture" (Zero to Three Infant Mental Health Taskforce Steering Committee, 2001). IECMH takes a holistic view of a child's well-being and is therefore focused on health promotion across a continuum, rather than just diagnosing and treating deficits.

A closely related concept is the idea of "early relational health" (ERH), which has emerged more recently in health and public health discourse (Willis & Eddy, 2022). ERH is defined as a "foundational, culturally embedded and developing of positive, responsive, and reciprocal interactions from birth that nurture and build emotional connections between caregivers, infants, and young children and result in emerging confidence, competence, and emotional well-being for all" (Willis & Eddy, 2022, p. 364). Both of these definitions are influenced by attachment theory, which asserts that (a) young children have an innate need to develop close emotional bonds with one or more primary caregivers, and (b) the quality of these bonds during the early years of life has a strong influence on the child's emotional health and relationships over the lifespan (Bowlby et al., 1992). Therefore, both definitions emphasize the importance of the relationship between infants toddlers and their caregivers as a key building block for children's well-being, exploration, learning, and growth. As such, IECMH is inextricably linked to the quality of young

A. Palmer Molina (✉)
Erikson Institute, Chicago, IL, USA
e-mail: apalmermolina@erikson.edu

L. Nabors, J. D. Bartlett (eds.), *Family Engagement in Mental Health Interventions for Young Children*, Springer Series on Child and Family Studies,
https://doi.org/10.1007/978-3-031-47917-5_1

children's attachment to their caregivers, which also influences other aspects of well-being in the early years, including physical, cognitive, and language development. Furthermore, interventions designed to promote the mental health of children from birth to 3 must also focus on the well-being of their caregivers, families, and communities.

Mental Health Interventions

Considering this broad definition of "mental health" for infants and toddlers, it comes as no surprise that there is a wide array of programs and interventions that target and promote mental health among our youngest children. In fact, IECMH focuses not only on treating mental health concerns but on promoting mental health for all children and preventing the development of future mental health problems. First, there are several formal evidence-based mental health therapies that directly target mental health concerns among infants and toddlers. Second, there are many other services that promote IECMH in nontraditional mental health settings, like home visiting, early care and education, health care, and child welfare. As such, IECMH intervention is inherently interdisciplinary.

Family Engagement

Across multiple intervention types and settings, IECMH practitioners support young children by partnering with their caregivers and family. Although IECMH intervention has historically focused on working with the dyad—namely, the mother-child relationship—recent efforts have focused on broadening this perspective to engage all important caregivers in a young child's life. For example, cross-cultural attachment research shows that a child's overall sense of emotional security can result from integrating multiple attachment relationships (Otto & Keller, 2014), defined as relationships with caregivers[1] with whom a child consistently seeks comfort and proximity (Bowlby et al., 1992). Calls to move beyond the mother-infant dyad help crystalize the importance of family engagement within any program or effort aimed at supporting the mental health of infants and toddlers. Families should not be viewed as barriers or as an afterthought but as the first place to begin when seeking to support a young child, since they are the key to promoting child well-being (Shonkoff & Fisher, 2013). The concept of family "engagement" moves beyond mere involvement or participation and emphasizes that clinicians and

[1] "Caregiver" refers to anyone who regularly takes care of a child, including parents, early childhood educators, etc.

practitioners should aim to help caregivers feel accepted, valued, and seen, since research shows that children's symptoms and functioning improve in mental health treatment when their caregivers are engaged (Haine-Schlagel & Walsh, 2015). It is also important to understand what types of support the families of young children want and need, and how they vary for different groups of families, so that intervention is most effective.

Mental Health Problems in Infancy and Toddlerhood

Infants and toddlers can experience mental health issues like regulatory problems (e.g., sleeping and feeding issues, attachment difficulties; externalizing behaviors like aggression and defiance; internalizing issues like depression and anxiety; and posttraumatic stress symptoms Izett et al., 2021). These challenges can impact many other aspects of the child's development, and related behavioral difficulties can also result in suspension and expulsion from early care and education centers (Gilliam et al., 2016). Factors that precipitate IECMH problems include child risk factors like health problems and a difficult temperament; family risk factors like insensitive parenting, parental mental health concerns, and family violence; and societal and community risk factors like poverty, lack of resources, and racism (Berry et al., 2021; Izett et al., 2021). Research shows that 16–18% of children between the ages of 1 and 5 years old experience mental health problems (von Klitzing et al., 2015). If left untreated, mental health concerns in infancy and early childhood can have lasting impacts on mental, cognitive, physical, and social functioning in childhood, adolescence, and adulthood (Izett et al., 2021).

Mental Health Interventions for Infants and Young Children

This section provides an overview of IECMH interventions for infants, toddlers, and their families, with a focus on the breadth of approaches across the prevention-intervention continuum. It describes evidence-informed and evidence-based approaches that provide direct therapy intervention, as well as IECMH approaches provided in nontraditional mental health settings like health care, home visiting, early care and education, and child welfare.

Evidence-Based Mental Health Interventions for Infants and Young Children

Evidence-based interventions (EBIs) are typically defined as interventions that have evidence from rigorous research studies to show their effectiveness (Miller et al., 2005). Traditionally, research evidence has been defined using a hierarchy in which randomized controlled trials (RCTs) are considered the highest level. In RCTs, participants are randomized to a treatment condition. However, there is some debate about what truly makes an intervention "evidence-based," and for whom an intervention is evidence-based. Conducting rigorous studies like RCTs requires significant resources, and therefore the research base typically advantages Western, White ways of thinking at the expense of other communities and ways of knowing, particularly for historically and currently marginalized groups (Adams et al., 2009). Furthermore, many EBIs have not been extensively studied with marginalized groups. So, while the next section of the chapter discusses EBIs, it will also consider the limitations of EBIs, and discuss promising evidence-informed interventions (i.e., those that may have research support from studies using less rigorous research designs).

There are several evidence-based and evidence-informed mental health interventions for infants and toddlers. In this chapter, the EBIs Child-Parent Psychotherapy, Attachment and Biobehavioral Catch-Up, and Parent-Child Interaction Therapy will be reviewed, as well as Circle of Security, Interaction Guidance, Video Interaction Guidance, and Watch, Wait, and Wonder, which are evidence-informed. Key details for each intervention are presented in Table 1.1. Family engagement is emphasized in each model, but in very different ways as described below.

In Child-Parent Psychotherapy (CPP), treatment begins by building a relationship with the caregiver during the assessment and engagement phase, before treatment shifts to focus on intervening with the caregiver and child together (Lieberman & Van Horn, 2015). This phase typically lasts for at least 4–6 sessions, though it can sometimes last longer based on caregiver needs. CPP provides time not only to develop trust and rapport with the caregiver, but also to assess the caregiver's mental health and trauma history and help the caregiver process difficulties or reactions that impact their ability to respond to their young child. CPP is an EBI that is particularly attuned to the needs of caregivers and the potential impact of the caregiver's history on the parent-child relationship and, ultimately, the child (Lieberman & Van Horn, 2015). RCTs of CPP have been conducted with racially and ethnically diverse families, showing effectiveness in improving maternal representations, maternal distress, and children's behavioral problems (Lieberman et al., 1991, 2006; Toth et al., 2002), establishing it as an evidence-based treatment. Although CPP emphasizes caregiver engagement, particularly by providing caregivers with individual sessions and addressing caregiver mental health issues, there is some evidence that retention in the yearlong intervention is a challenge (Guild et al., 2021). This highlights the importance of considering how to better promote family engagement in CPP.

In Attachment and Biobehavioral Catch-Up (ABC), home visitors meet weekly with families for 10 weeks and target parenting to improve sensitive and nurturing behaviors (Dozier & Bernard, 2019). They also coach caregivers to follow their child's lead and reduce harsh and frightening parental behavior. In the final weeks of the model, caregivers are guided to think about their own early relational experiences growing up and how these relate to current parenting issues. ABC is an evidence-based treatment that has demonstrated efficacy in several clinical trials,

Table 1.1 Evidence-based and evidence-informed mental health interventions for infants and toddlers

Name of intervention	Age range	Brief description	Qualifications of providers
Child-Parent Psychotherapy (CPP), Lieberman and Van Horn (2015)	Prenatal–5 years	Intensive, psychodynamic intervention focused on promoting healthy attachment between caregiver and child	Master's level or higher mental health professional
Attachment and Biobehavioral Catch-Up (ABC), Dozier and Bernard (2019)	Infancy version: 6–24 months; Toddler version: 24–36 months	Short-term, manualized home visiting program that addresses attachment difficulties by improving parenting behaviors	No educational level requirement for parent coaches
Parent-Child Interaction Therapy (PCIT), Eyberg et al. (1995)	2–8 years	Structured behavioral intervention that provides intensive parent coaching sessions, developed for children exhibiting behavioral problems	Master's level or higher mental health professional
Infant and Early Childhood Mental Health Consultation (IECMHC)	Birth–5 years	Capacity-building intervention that helps early childhood practitioners and families build their reflective capacity and foster children's social emotional development	Mental health professionals, varies by region and setting
Circle of Security (COS), Powell et al. (2014)	Birth–5 years	Intervention provided in a group or individual format to help caregivers understand their child's cues and alternating needs for safety/comfort and exploration	COS-Parenting can be provided by anyone with 4-day training, COS-Intensive by master's level or higher licensed mental health clinician
Interaction Guidance (IG)-Geneva Model, McDonough (2004)	Birth–5 years	Short-term, family systems intervention that promotes nurturing relationships between infants and caregivers	Professionals trained in IG (speech therapists, therapists, pediatricians)
Video Interaction Guidance (VIG), Kennedy et al. (2010)	Birth–12 years	Short-term intervention that uses video feedback to build on family strengths and promote sensitive and nurturing parenting	Mental health therapists, physicians, nurses, etc. trained as VIG "guiders"
Watch, Wait, and Wonder (WWW), Lojkasek et al. (2008)	Birth–4 years	Unstructured intervention that uses infant-led play to promote attachment between child and caregiver	Mental health therapists

Note: Additional information about intervention adaptations for different populations, settings, and age ranges is included in the text and showed positive impacts on children's attachment, biological regulation, impulse control, language, and brain development, as well as on parental sensitivity and parental brain activity (Dozier & Bernard, 2019; Grube & Liming, 2018; O'Byrne et al., 2023). ABC has been tested with racially and ethnically diverse families, particularly Black families, and found to be effective (Grube & Liming, 2018; O'Byrne et al., 2023). ABC shows rates of attrition similar to other interventions in community-based settings. One analysis found that caregivers who dropped out of treatment showed similar improvements in parenting behavior as those who completed treatment (Caron et al., 2016).

Parent-Child Interaction Therapy (PCIT) is an intensive evidence-based parent coaching intervention that has been well-supported by empirical evidence (Eyberg et al., 1995; Thomas et al., 2017). PCIT includes two phases of treatment; first, caregivers are coached in relationship-building skills, and then they are coached in setting appropriate limits using direct commands and implementing consequences like time-out. An adaptation of PCIT, PCIT-Toddler (PCIT-T), is more appropriate for younger children because it emphasizes attachment-based principles and developing self-regulation (Girard et al., 2018). In PCIT-T, caregivers are coached in the "CARES" model, which stands for Come in, Assist, Reassure, Emotional Validation, and Soothe when their toddlers are experiencing strong emotions. Caregivers are also coached to discern the underlying reasons for the child's behavior, rather than ignoring those behaviors like in traditional PCIT. Studies examining the effectiveness of the child-directed portion of PCIT-T show significant improvements in parenting skills, parental emotional availability and mental health, attachment security, and child behavior (Kohlhoff et al., 2020, 2021; Kohlhoff & Morgan, 2014), and adaptations of PCIT for children aged 12–24 months have been shown to be as effective as PCIT for older children (Phillips & Mychailyszyn, 2022). Although rates of attrition from community-based PCIT vary from 12 to 67%, one study found a large effect size for families who completed just four PCIT sessions, although gains were still greatest for families who completed treatment (Lieneman et al., 2019). Additionally, PC-CARE is a promising seven-session intervention that has been adapted to address the barriers that families often experience when participating in PCIT (Hawk et al., 2022). PCIT has also been adapted for specific cultural groups, including "Honoring Children, Making Relatives," which incorporates the teachings and practices of American Indian and Native Alaskan communities (BigFoot & Funderburk, 2018) and *Guiando a Ninos Activos* (Guiding Active Children) for Mexican American families, which includes the incorporation of culturally specific values and the incorporation of extended family members (McCabe & Yeh, 2009). These adaptations would benefit from additional testing.

Circle of Security (COS)-Parenting aims to promote the parent-child attachment relationship and caregiver reflective capacity, or the caregiver's ability to understand their own thoughts and feelings, as well as those of the child (Powell et al., 2014). COS includes an intensive version and a shorter parenting program. The goal in any COS intervention is to teach caregivers about two important functions they serve, namely, acting a "safe haven" when a child is distressed and acting as a "secure base" when the child is ready to explore. Caregivers are taught how to understand children's cues, primarily by using video clips of child-caregiver interactions. COS also encourages caregivers to process their own early childhood relationships and identify how these experiences may cloud their ability to understand their child's needs. A COS adaptation for infants includes four individual sessions provided to the caregiver-child dyad in a home-based setting (Cassidy et al., 2011). One meta-analysis showed that COS was effective in improving children's attachment security and the quality of caregiving, and also reducing caregiver depression (Yaholkoski et al., 2016), though RCTs have shown fewer impacts on parenting behavior and child functioning (Cassidy et al., 2011, 2017; Ramsauer et al., 2020). Two of these RCTs included predominantly ethnic minority samples (Cassidy et al., 2011, 2017). Maxwell et al. (2021) and found that COS-Parenting practitioners and parents reported some limitations of the program, including that some concepts are difficult to understand, self-reflection is challenging, and some parents would prefer more concrete strategies. Importantly, although COS predominantly focuses on the relationship between the primary caregiver and the child, adaptations have broadened this focus to include co-parenting partners, like early education teachers (Powell et al., 2014).

The Interaction Guidance (IG)-Geneva Model conceptualizes the interactions between infant and caregiver as reflecting the representational worlds of both parties, as well as the family's structure (McDonough, 2004). In this model, primary caregivers are encouraged to involve a "co-parenting partner," which could include a grandparent, friend, parent, sibling, or other relative of the child. Clinical work in IG begins with engaging the family and then using video to reflect on family interactions, and weekly sessions are typically held for 10–12 weeks. The IG therapist begins by asking family members to play with the infant or young child as they would at home for a short time, and these interactions are recorded. Subsequently, the family reviews the recording, and the therapist elicits their reflections and responses about what they see. The therapist also highlights strengths in terms of how the caregivers respond to the child's needs. Importantly, IG provides time for the caregivers to reflect on their reactions to the video, and the developers note that this often allows for a discussion of how past experiences impact current caregiving interactions (McDonough, 2004). Studies have demonstrated the efficacy of IG in improving interactions between caregivers and children and maternal representations of the child (Madigan et al., 2006; Robert-Tissot et al., 1996), though more rigorous studies are needed to establish a strong evidence base, particularly those that include racially and ethnically diverse populations.

In the Video Interaction Guidance (VIG)-UK intervention, a clinician first engages the caregiver in identifying goals for treatment, which are referred to as "helping questions" (Kennedy et al., 2010). Then, interactions between the child and caregiver are filmed, and the clinician selects moments showing positive interactions to review with the client. Then, the client and practitioner watch these clips together and reflect on what the family is doing well together to reach their goals. A recent meta-analysis found that VIG demonstrated increased attunement and attachment in the parent-child relationship up to 20-month post-intervention (Dodsworth et al., 2021), though additional RCTs are needed that include diverse samples.

Watch, Wait, and Wonder (WWW) is an evidence-informed psychotherapeutic approach that uses child-led play to help caregivers become more responsive and attuned to their children's experiences (Lojkasek et al., 2008). In contrast to some of the other models discussed above, the focus in WWW is on the child as an active agent or "initiator," rather than focusing on the caregiver's experiences and behaviors as the port of entry for intervention (Cohen et al., 1999). During sessions, the caregiver is first instructed to put themselves in close physical proximity to the infant and follows the infant's activity and behavior as they play. In the second half of the therapy session, the therapist asks the caregiver to share their experiences and reflections of the play session. Caregiver and therapist then work together to identify the child's relational needs and work through any problems or challenges that arose. In one study, WWW decreased maternal depression, improved infant cognitive development and emotion regulation, and improved infant-mother attachment security (Cohen et al., 2002). However, to date no RCTs have been conducted. Additional research is needed to determine whether WWW is effective in engaging and retaining families.

IECMH Interventions in Nontraditional Mental Health Settings

As the IECMH field grows, it has become clear that IECMH interventions must move beyond traditional mental health treatment settings to reach young children and families where they are, including other systems like early care and education, home visiting, pediatrics, and child welfare. This shift reflects the changing focus from intervention to prevention of child mental health problems and overall promotion of well-being, since promotion and prevention efforts are more successful and cost-effective than intervening once symptoms worsen (Izett et al., 2021). This shift places an increased emphasis on the importance of engaging families across settings so that their children can benefit from services.

One promising evidence-informed approach is infant and early childhood mental health consultation (IECMHC), a capacity-building intervention that began in early care and education and has since been adopted in home visiting and other fields. In IECMHC, mental health professionals partner with early childhood practitioners and families to build their reflective capacity[2] and foster children's positive social emotional development (Center of Excellence in Infant and Early Childhood Mental Health Consultation, 2020a). IECMH consultants provide a warm and supportive stance that allows early childhood professionals to reflect on their interactions with young children and families and improve their skills. IECMHC has been implemented in a range of settings, including early childhood education, home visiting,

[2] Reflective capacity refers to the caregiver's ability to understand their own thoughts and feelings, as well as those of the child (Powell et al., 2014).

head start, early intervention for children with disabilities, child welfare, and healthcare systems.

The Center of Excellence for IECMHC has put forward a theory of change that asserts that IECMHC positively impacts child and family outcomes and program outcomes and reduces disparities by way of staff members' active engagement in the consultative relationship and participation in IECMHC activities (Tidus et al., 2022). Although there is a range of IECMHC approaches in different settings, there is some consensus on the essential activities of IECMH consultants. Activities that consultants commonly engage in include developing shared goals with their consultee, discussing how to establish rapport and trust with families, sharing knowledge about how to support the mental health of very young children, promoting the consultee's ability to reflect on their interactions with families, promoting the consultee's ability to engage in self-care activities, and deepening consultees' understanding of equity and the influence of cultural differences, bias, and discrimination (Center of Excellence in Infant and Early Childhood Mental Health Consultation, 2022).

Research on the effectiveness of IECMHC has predominantly focused on the early care and education sector, in which IECMH consultants partner with early childhood teachers to help provide support in addressing children with emotional and behavioral difficulties in the educational setting. In this setting, IECMHC has been found to reduce children's behavioral problems and expulsion risk (Silver et al., 2023). However, only one RCT has been conducted, and though it found that IECMHC reduced ratings of children's hyperactivity, restlessness, externalizing behaviors, and problem behaviors, it did not reduce the likelihood of expulsion (Gilliam et al., 2016). IECMHC in early care and education settings can also improve teacher outcomes like job stress, knowledge, efficacy, and competence, family outcomes like fewer days missed at work to address childcare issues, as well as program outcomes like reductions in staff turnover and improvements in classroom climate (Center of Excellence in Infant and Early Childhood Mental Health Consultation, 2020b; Silver et al., 2023).

IECMHC in home visiting has also been found to be a promising strategy. Under the federal Maternal, Infant, and Early Childhood Home Visiting (MIECHV) program, there are currently 18 evidence-based home visiting models in the USA, including Parents as Teachers, Nurse-Family Partnership, Family Connects, Child First, and Healthy Families America, among others (National Home Visiting Resource Center, 2022). Although evidence shows that some children who receive home visiting services exhibit fewer emotional and behavioral problems later in life, home visiting services alone are often not enough to effectively prevent and treat these issues (Peacock et al., 2013). Embedding IECMHC in home visiting aims to address IECMH concerns before they worsen, and has been found to improve home visitors' knowledge of children's social emotional development and mental health (Lambarth & Green, 2019). One study also showed that providing IECMHC in home visiting significantly improved home visitor responsiveness to families (Burkhardt et al., 2022), showing that IECMHC may be a key factor that can help improve family engagement in home visiting programs generally. Furthermore, home visitors who received IECMHC promoted higher parenting self-efficacy, positive parenting behavior, and responsive-parent child reactions compared to those who did not receive IECMHC (Burkhardt et al., 2022).

There has also been an increasing interest in embedding IECMHC within healthcare settings, particularly in pediatrics. This is because most young children will interact with the pediatric health system and because caregivers and families typically seek out and trust information from their pediatrician, factors which help facilitate family engagement. Healthy Steps for Young Children (HS) is an example of a program embedded within primary care that provides developmental and social-emotional support to infants, toddlers, and their families. Families in HS are seen by both a primary care physician and a developmental specialist, who is trained in child development and well-being and the importance of the caregiver-child relationship. A national evaluation of HS across 15 sites in the USA found that the program improved child well-being, including perceptual, physical, and motor development, as well as child social emotional development. HS also improved family health and provider satisfaction (Guyer et al., 2003).

Strategies to Improve Family Engagement in Interventions for Infants and Toddlers

There are several strategies that promote family engagement in mental health interventions for infants and toddlers. Some are components of the evidence-based and evidence-informed mental health treatments described above, and others include other therapeutic or systems-level innovations. Namely, these strategies and innovations include the following: (a) centering the importance of the child's attachment relationship(s), (b) using in-the-moment feedback with families, (c) capitalizing on strengths, (d) providing time for caregiver reflective work, (e) providing time for practitioner reflective work, and (f) integrating IECMH services with other systems, settings, and disciplines.

Focus on Relationships

Interventions with infants and toddlers typically center the importance of the child's attachment relationships (McLuckie et al., 2019). As Winnicott (1960) famously said, "there is no such thing as an infant," asserting that young children cannot be understood in isolation because they are deeply embedded in their relationships and sociocultural context. All of the targeted intervention approaches discussed above include a focus on the importance of the attachment relationship between the young child and their caregiver. Although this focus is emphasized in many models and approaches, important caregivers like fathers, grandparents, and fictive kin are often left out of IECMH approaches. Additionally, any intervention focused on infancy and toddlerhood must recognize that caregiver and family well-being affects the well-being of the young child and should therefore provide holistic family support (Shonkoff & Fisher, 2013). For example, studies show that economic pressure resulting from poverty can lead to parental psychological distress, impeding parenting and leading to children's social emotional difficulties (Masarik & Conger, 2017). Holistic family support could include supports focused on the family's basic needs, such as housing, food, etc. and the caregiver's mental health.

In-The-Moment Feedback

Next, it is important to consider in-the-moment feedback, or observations and reflections clinicians provide to caregivers as they engage with their child. Although there is a diverse array of targeted IECMH interventions, many of these interventions focus on providing in-the-moment feedback to increase attunement and positive caregiver-child interactions. For example, Attachment and Biobehavioral Catch-Up, Child-Parent Psychotherapy, Parent-Child Interaction Therapy-Toddler, and Watch, Wait, and Wonder provide real-time feedback during sessions in which the family is present in the room. In ABC, the focus is on the caregiver's behavior (Dozier & Bernard, 2019), whereas in CPP and PCIT-T, feedback might focus on the child's behavior or the parent's behavior (Eyberg et al., 1995; Lieberman & Van Horn, 2015), and in CPP practitioners may also focus on interpreting feelings and experiences or providing reflective developmental guidance (Lieberman & Van Horn, 2015). In WWW, the focus is on the child's behavior as the port of entry (Lojkasek et al., 2008). Typically, feedback is provided by first asking the caregiver to reflect and notice an interaction, prompting them to engage in the moment.

Video Feedback

Several mental health interventions use video to capture the organic, spontaneous interactions between caregivers and children in order to subsequently process these interactions and identify areas of strength and growth. These interventions include Circle of Security (Powell et al., 2014), Interaction Guidance (McDonough, 2004), Video Interaction Guidance (Kennedy et al., 2010), and Attachment and Biobehavioral Catch-Up (Dozier & Bernard, 2019), among others. Utilizing video feedback has been conceptualized as helping to facilitate the therapeutic relationship between the practitioner and the family, promote parental reflective functioning, and facilitate the processing of emotional and physiological reactions (Steele et al., 2014). Importantly, interventions that use in-the-moment feedback invite the caregiver-child relational dynamic into the space, literally or figuratively, and help caregivers become more present and mindful of these moments, which can improve their attunement to their child.

Strengths-Based Approaches

Many of the IECMH approaches focus on highlighting or emphasizing the family's strengths and the strengths in the caregiver-child relationship(s). IECMH is grounded in a strength-based perspective (Walsh et al., 2021) and is as interested in understanding what is working as it is in what might not be working in family relationships. Although specific evidence-based and evidence-informed interventions differ in their emphasis on strengths, most models recognize the strengths inherent in the family and caregiver-child relationships and focus on helping families notice these strengths and build upon them. For example, in the Video Interaction Guidance (VIG) intervention, the practitioner focuses exclusively on positive moments and moments of connection when working with the caregiver and young child (Kennedy et al., 2010). This approach recognizes what the caregiver is already doing well, which may help promote their engagement and the overall effectiveness of services.

Reflective Work

As mentioned previously in this section, many IECMH interventions promote caregiver reflective functioning, which refers to the caregiver's ability to understand their own thoughts and feelings, as well as those of the child (Powell et al., 2014). Models and programs differ in the space allowed for this processing, but many models explicitly address the impact of the caregiver's own early life experiences. For example, Child-Parent Psychotherapy (Lieberman & Van Horn, 2015), Attachment and Biobehavioral Catch-Up (Dozier & Bernard, 2019), Circle of Security (Powell et al., 2014), and Interaction Guidance (McDonough, 2004) provide time for caregivers to make connections between their own upbringing and their current relationship with their child, although models vary in the intensity of this focus. In CPP, this connection is made explicit where there is a discussion of both "ghosts" and "angels" in the nursery, referring to positive and negative early life experiences that may impact the way caregivers see and interpret their child's behaviors and needs (Fraiberg et al., 2018). Similarly, in Circle of Security, preconscious defenses that operate in the parent-child relationship are referred to as "shark music," and caregivers are coached to identify when their own shark music is playing, so to speak, and how to challenge this music so it does not obscure their ability to see and attune to their child (Powell et al., 2014).

Similarly, it is important for practitioners working in the IECMH field to engage in their own reflective work. Reflective practice is a central focus of IECMH and a core competency in training programs and across practice settings. Reflective practice has been defined as the capacity for self-awareness, curiosity, and critical thinking and the ability to utilize this reflective process to guide decision-making in the moment (Ringel, 2003). Ideally, IECMH practitioners should participate in regular reflective supervision to process interactions with families and understand their reactions, particularly those that might be impeding their ability to engage with a family. Reflective supervision in IECMH differs from regular clinical supervision and is defined as "the shared exploration of the emotional content of work with infants/toddlers and parents…within the context of a trusting supervisory relationship" (Weatherston & Tableman, 2015, p. 370). The "Facilitating Attuned Interactions" (FAN) is one approach that helps operationalize reflective practice by matching four core processes to the kind of interaction the caregiver is most able to use in the moment (Gilkerson & Imberger, 2016). For example, is the caregiver focused on their feelings, or are they ready to problem-solve or even try out a new behavior? This approach can be used as a reflective tool to promote family engagement within any IECMH intervention, and it has also been adapted to support reflective practice and facilitate reflective supervision for clinicians.

Interdisciplinary Approach

Lastly, IECMH is, by its very nature, an interdisciplinary field, and integration improves both child and family well-being (Shonkoff & Fisher, 2013). This includes integration between IECMH and other disciplines and settings, as well as integration across siloed "parent" and "child" services. For example, as discussed above, the majority of IECMH services provided in the USA are provided in nontraditional settings, rather than primary mental health settings. These include settings like home visiting, health services, early care and education, and child welfare, among others. Although attempts at integration have grown in recent years, the USA still lacks a coordinated early childhood system, and IECMH services are not fully integrated into many early childhood service systems (Walter et al., 2019), not to mention adult-focused service systems. Examples of innovative interdisciplinary IECMH approaches include Minding the Baby, in which a social worker and nurse are paired together, and Project BRIGHT (Building Resilience Through Intervention), which provides a relationship-based intervention for caregivers with substance use disorders within substance use treatment programs (Paris et al., 2017).

Critical Issues Related to Social Justice

Caregiver and family engagement is of paramount importance in promoting IECMH, but often families face many barriers to engaging in services. This is particularly true for marginalized families and families of color. For example, studies show that negative attitudes toward mental health, concerns about the relevance and acceptability of the intervention, caregiver mental health issues, a lack of culturally appropriate services, a weak alliance between the caregiver and provider, lack of culturally relevant services, and stressors like poverty, unemployment, transportation, insurance issues, racism and discrimination, and lack of child care can all negatively impact engagement in mental health interventions for children (Finan et al., 2018; Skale et al., 2020; Waid & Kelly, 2020). Furthermore, child and family services remain largely siloed, and it is often difficult for families to participate in child service sectors (Shonkoff & Fisher, 2013). Two-generation and whole-family approaches aim to change this dynamic, which are defined as approaches that build family well-being by intentionally and simultaneously working with children and the adults in their lives together (Ascend at the Aspen Institute, 2023). However, structural and financial barriers frequently prevent child-serving sectors from fully embracing the wide range of needs of families (Shonkoff & Fisher, 2013).

The Diversity-Informed Tenets for Work with Infants, Children and Families (2018) provide a foundational framework for all IECMH intervention as well as important guidelines for promoting family engagement, particularly for oppressed and marginalized groups (Irving Harris Foundation). For example, the Tenets emphasize the importance of honoring diverse family structures and encourage the IECMH field to "counter the historical bias toward idealizing (and conversely blaming) biological mothers while overlooking the critical child-rearing contributions of other parents and caregivers" (Irving Harris Foundation, 2018, p. 1). Similarly, Stern et al. (2021) have called for researchers and practitioners to recognize and measure the multiple sources of emotional support that young Black children benefit from, including support from fathers, mentors, grandparents, spiritual community members, and fictive kin (i.e., social ties not based on blood or marriage). Similarly, the Tenets include a focus on acknowledging privilege and combatting discrimination, recognizing and respecting nondominant bodies of knowledge, and engaging with families in their preferred language (Irving Harris Foundation, 2018), all of which may promote family engagement.

Although more work needs to be done to operationalize these principles within IECMH interventions, one notable exemplar is the Early Relational Health Conversations (ERH-C) approach. Specialists within the Healthy Steps model developed ERH-C to engage African American families in conversations about the importance of early caregiving relationships, and the approach may be applicable to other groups impacted by structural racism (Charlot-Swilley et al., 2022; Condon et al., 2022). ERH-C emphasizes eight components, including preparing and entering the ERH-C space, accessing strength and knowledge in a healing-centered space, pausing and co-creating, storytelling, witnessing, mutual reflection, affirming, and claiming their relationship narrative, and mutual insight. The ERH-C approach can be implemented in both targeted IECMH interventions and IECMH support embedded in nontraditional mental health systems like home visiting, early childhood education, and child welfare. To date, there are no outcome studies of ERH-C, so future research should investigate the impact of ERH-C on both family engagement and child outcomes.

Directions for Future Research, Policy, and Practice

Research

First, the IECMH field would benefit from a more robust research base that examines how family engagement shapes outcomes for infants, toddlers, and their families within mental health interventions to better inform practice on the ground. Second, studies should explore the needs of diverse families, particularly in terms of aspects of identity like socioeconomic status, gender, sexual orientation, cultural background, ability, and race. This would help IECMH practitioners more effectively engage caregivers from different backgrounds. Third, research should test not only existing IECMH interventions with families of diverse backgrounds but also privilege emerging IECMH intervention approaches from non-Western viewpoints, which would center the needs and perspectives of families. Fourth, there should be increased openness to nondominant ways of knowing as providing evidence of effectiveness (e.g., moving beyond the RCT). We need more qualitative and mixed methods work on families' experiences to inform intervention development, testing, and implementation so that our evidence-based interventions are most effective for infants and toddlers. Furthermore, research studies should include advisory boards that allow caregivers to actively co-construct intervention development, implementation, and testing (DuBois et al., 2011). The field as whole needs to move beyond traditional research designs to truly honor family voice and address the structural barriers related to engaging communities as partners in research (DuBois et al., 2011). Lastly, although there has been a growing call for anti-racist and anti-oppressive practice across the helping professions (Gebhard et al., 2022; Haeny et al., 2021), more research is needed about how to infuse these approaches within existing IECMH models and across the IECMH intervention continuum.

Policy

There are a number of policy changes that would support the spread of IECMH interventions and promote family engagement in services. First, sustainable financing is needed for a comprehensive, integrated IECMH system for infants, toddlers, and their families, and services need to be conceptualized as supporting the whole family, rather than just the identified client of the child (Kaminski et al., 2022; Zeanah et al., 2005). Two-generation and whole-family approaches align with IECMH values and can help ensure that families get the resources they need (Shonkoff & Fisher, 2013). Although many of the above models emphasize a two-generation approach, impact can be limited by structural factors like policies and funding requirements in local communities (Kaminski et al., 2022; Zeanah et al., 2005). Critical policy changes needed include increasing reimbursement rates for evidence-based IECMH services, allowing Medicaid billing for IECMH and adult mental health services across adult and child settings and practitioner roles, removing the requirement for a mental health diagnosis to bill for services, and allocating funding for capacity building within the IECMH field broadly (Margolis et al., 2020; Zeanah et al., 2005). All of these changes would promote the ability of families to access and engage in services more easily.

Practice

There are several areas for growth in IECMH practice and workforce development. First, all practitioners should engage in ongoing reflective supervision to overcome potential barriers to engaging families. Second, the Diversity-Informed Tenets (Irving Harris Foundation, 2018) provide a series of values to anchor IECMH work, but all IECMH practitioners should have the opportunity to be trained to utilize the tenets. Science suggests that the tenets should be operationalized within existing IECMH interventions that are widely disseminated to ensure that they are put into practice. For example, across the board IECMH interventions need to actively involve all important caregivers. In recent years there have been increasing calls for a focus on father involvement, but a recent review found that there is a striking lack of paternal engagement in IECMH interventions (McLuckie et al., 2019). Most IECMH models covered in this chapter focus on the mother-child dyad, overlooking family dynamics that influence infant and toddler mental health. Furthermore, academic programs that train many IECMH practitioners, including social work, marriage and family therapy, and psychology programs, can incorporate training on IECMH interventions and family engagement into their degree programs, and ongoing professional development should be provided on family engagement for the current workforce. Professional development should be provided within the work setting as well as by national training and technical assistance centers.

References

Adams, K. B., Matto, H. C., & LeCroy, C. W. (2009). Limitations of evidence-based practice for social work education: Unpacking the complexity. *Journal of Social Work Education, 45*(2), 165–186. https://doi.org/10.5175/JSWE.2009.200700105

Ascend at the Aspen Institute. (2023). *Whole family approaches to economic mobility: A funder's guide to supporting multigenerational policy and practice*. https://wholefamilyguide.org/about-this-toolkit/

Berry, O. O., Londoño Tobón, A., & Njoroge, W. F. (2021). Social determinants of health: The impact of racism on early childhood mental health. *Current Psychiatry Reports, 23*, 1–10. https://doi.org/10.1007/s11920-021-01240-0

BigFoot, D. S., & Funderburk, B. (2018). Cultural enhancement of PCIT for American Indian families: Honoring children, making relatives. In L. N. Niec (Ed.), *Handbook of Parent-Child Interaction Therapy: Innovations and applications for research and practice* (pp. 235–251). Springer Nature, Switzerland AG. https://doi.org/10.1007/978-3-319-97698-3_15

Bowlby, J., Ainsworth, M., & Bretherton, I. (1992). The origins of attachment theory. *Developmental Psychology, 28*(28), 759–775. https://doi.org/10.1037/0012-1649.28.5.759

Burkhardt, T., Huang, L. A., Herriott, A., Pacheco-Applegate, A., & Spielberger, J. (2022). Strengthening home visitor practice through an embedded model of infant and early childhood mental health consultation. *Prevention Science, 24*(1), 105–114. https://doi.org/10.1007/s11121-022-01461-6

Caron, E., Weston-Lee, P., Haggerty, D., & Dozier, M. (2016). Community implementation outcomes of Attachment and Biobehavioral Catch-up. *Child Abuse & Neglect, 53*, 128–137. https://doi.org/10.1016/j.chiabu.2015.11.010

Cassidy, J., Woodhouse, S. S., Sherman, L. J., Stupica, B., & Lejuez, C. W. (2011). Enhancing infant attachment security: An examination of treatment efficacy and differential susceptibility. *Development and Psychopathology, 23*(1), 131–148. https://doi.org/10.1017/S0954579410000696

Cassidy, J., Brett, B. E., Gross, J. T., Stern, J. A., Martin, D. R., Mohr, J. J., & Woodhouse, S. S. (2017). Circle of Security–Parenting: A randomized controlled trial in Head Start. *Development and Psychopathology, 29*(2), 651–673. https://doi.org/10.1017/S0954579417000244

Center of Excellence in Infant and Early Childhood Mental Health Consultation. (2020a). *Status of the evidence for infant and early childhood mental health consultation*. https://www.iecmhc.org/wp-content/uploads/2020/12/CoE-Evidence-Synthesis.pdf

Center of Excellence in Infant and Early Childhood Mental Health Consultation. (2020b). *Consultation competencies*. https://www.samhsa.gov/early-childhood-mental-health-programs/center-of-excellence-iecmh

Center of Excellence in Infant and Early Childhood Mental Health Consultation. (2022). *The essential activities of infant and early childhood mental health consultation: Guidance for the field from a consensus-building study*. https://www.iecmhc.org/documents/CoE-Delphi-Report-120822.pdf

Charlot-Swilley, D., Condon, M., & Rahman, T. (2022). At the feet of storytellers: Implications for practicing early relational health conversations. *Infant Mental Health Journal, 43*(3), 373–389. https://doi.org/10.1002/imhj.21981

Cohen, N. J., Muir, E., Lojkasek, M., Muir, R., Parker, C. J., Barwick, M., & Brown, M. (1999). Watch, wait, and wonder: Testing the effectiveness of a new approach to mother-infant psychotherapy. *Infant Mental Health Journal, 20*(4), 429–451. https://doi.org/10.1002/(SICI)1097-0355(199924)20:4<429::AID-IMHJ5>3.0.CO;2-Q

Cohen, N. J., Lojkasek, M., Muir, E., Muir, R., & Parker, C. J. (2002). Six-month follow-up of two mother-infant psychotherapies: Convergence of therapeutic outcomes. *Infant Mental Health Journal, 23*(4), 361–380. https://doi.org/10.1002/imhj.10023

Condon, M., Charlot-Swilley, D., & Rahman, T. (2022). At the feet of storytellers: Equity in early relational health conversations. *Infant Mental Health Journal, 43*(3), 390–409. https://doi.org/10.1002/imhj.21979

Dodsworth, E., Kelly, C., & Bond, C. (2021). Video Interaction Guidance with families: A systematic review of the research. *Educational and Child Psychology, 38*(3), 48–61. https://doi.org/10.53841/bpsecp.2021.38.3.48

Dozier, M., & Bernard, K. (2019). *Coaching parents of vulnerable infants: The Attachment and Biobehavioral Catch-up approach*. The Guilford Press.

DuBois, J. M., Bailey-Burch, B., Bustillos, D., Campbell, J., Cottler, L., Fisher, C. B., Hadley, W. B., Hoop, J. G., Roberts, L., Salter, E. K., Sieber, J. E., & Stevenson, R. D. (2011). Ethical issues in mental health research: The case for community engagement. *Current Opinion in Psychiatry, 24*(3), 208–214. https://doi.org/10.1097/YCO.0b013e3283459422

Eyberg, S. M., Boggs, S. R., & Algina, J. (1995). Parent-child interaction therapy: A psychosocial model for the treatment of young children with conduct problem behavior and their families. *Psychopharmacology Bulletin, 31*(1), 83–91.

Finan, S. J., Swierzbiolek, B., Priest, N., Warren, N., & Yap, M. (2018). Parental engagement in preventive parenting programs for child mental health: A systematic review of predictors and strategies to increase engagement. *PeerJ, 6*, e4676. https://doi.org/10.7717/peerj.4676

Fraiberg, S., Adelson, E., & Shapiro, V. (2018). Ghosts in the nursery: A psychoanalytic approach to the problems of impaired infant–mother relationships. In J. Raphael-Leff (Ed.), *Parent-infant psychodynamics* (pp. 87–117). Routledge.

Gebhard, A., McLean, S., & Denis, V. S. (Eds.). (2022). *White benevolence: Racism and colonial violence in the helping professions*. Fernwood Publishing.

Gilkerson, L., & Imberger, J. (2016). Strengthening reflective capacity in skilled home visitors. *Zero to Three, 37*(2), 46–53.

Gilliam, W. S., Maupin, A. N., & Reyes, C. R. (2016). Early childhood mental health consultation: Results of a statewide random-controlled evaluation. *Journal of the American Academy of Child & Adolescent Psychiatry, 55*(9), 754–761. https://doi.org/10.1016/j.jaac.2016.06.006

Girard, E. I., Wallace, N. M., Kohlhoff, J. R., Morgan, S. S. J., & McNeil, C. B. (2018). *Parent-Child Interaction Therapy with toddlers: Improving attachment and emotion regulation*. Springer Nature, Switzerland AG.

Grube, W. A., & Liming, K. W. (2018). Attachment and Biobehavioral Catch-up: A systematic review. *Infant Mental Health Journal, 39*(6), 656–673. https://doi.org/10.1002/imhj.21745

Guild, D. J., Alto, M. E., Handley, E. D., Rogosch, F., Cicchetti, D., & Toth, S. L. (2021). Attachment and affect between mothers with depression and their children: Longitudinal outcomes of Child Parent Psychotherapy. *Research on Child and Adolescent Psychopathology, 49*(5), 563–577. https://doi.org/10.1007/s10802-020-00681-0

Guyer, B., Barth, M., Bishai, D., Clark, B., Burkom, D., Genevro, J., Hou, W., Huang, K.-Y., Hughart, N., Jones, S., McLearn, K. T., Miller, T., Minkovitz, C., Scharfstein, D., Stacy, H., Strobino, D., & Tang, C. (2003). *Healthy steps: The first three years. The healthy steps for young children program national valuation*. https://ztt-healthysteps.s3.amazonaws.com/documents/139/attachments/2003_HS_National_Evaluation_Report.pdf?1539967824

Haeny, A. M., Holmes, S. C., & Williams, M. T. (2021). Applying anti-racism to clinical care and research. *JAMA Psychiatry, 78*(11), 1187–1188. https://doi.org/10.1001/jamapsychiatry.2021.2329

Haine-Schlagel, R., & Walsh, N. E. (2015). A review of parent participation engagement in child and family mental health treatment. *Clinical Child and Family Psychology Review, 18*(2), 133–150. https://doi.org/10.1007/s10567-015-0182-x

Hawk, B. N., Timmer, S. G., Armendariz, L. A. F., Boys, D. K., & Urquiza, A. J. (2022). Improving children's behavior in seven sessions: A randomized controlled trial of Parent-Child Care (PC-CARE) for children aged 2–10 years. *Child Psychiatry*. https://doi.org/10.1007/s10578-022-01406-8

Irving Harris Foundation. (2018). *Diversity-informed tenets for work with infants, children and families*. https://diversityinformedtenets.org

Izett, E., Rooney, R., Prescott, S. L., De Palma, M., & McDevitt, M. (2021). Prevention of mental health difficulties for children aged 0–3 years: A review. *Frontiers in Psychology, 11*, 500361. https://doi.org/10.3389/fpsyg.2020.500361

Kaminski, J. W., Robinson, L. R., Hutchins, H. J., Newsome, K. B., & Barry, C. M. (2022). Evidence base review of couple-and family-based psychosocial interventions to promote infant and early childhood mental health, 2010–2019. *Journal of Marital and Family Therapy, 48*(1), 23–55. https://doi.org/10.1111/jmft.12570

Kennedy, H., Landor, M., & Todd, L. (2010). Video Interaction Guidance as a method to promote secure attachment. *Educational and Child Psychology, 27*(3), 59–72. https://doi.org/10.53841/bpsecp.2010.27.3.59

Kohlhoff, J., & Morgan, S. (2014). Parent-Child Interaction Therapy for toddlers: A pilot study. *Child & Family Behavior Therapy, 36*(2), 121–139. https://doi.org/10.1080/07317107.2014.910733

Kohlhoff, J., Morgan, S., Briggs, N., Egan, R., & Niec, L. (2020). Parent–Child Interaction Therapy with Toddlers in a community-based setting: Improvements in parenting behavior, emotional availability, child behavior, and attachment. *Infant Mental Health Journal, 41*(4), 543–562. https://doi.org/10.1002/imhj.21864

Kohlhoff, J., Morgan, S., Briggs, N., Egan, R., & Niec, L. (2021). Parent–Child Interaction Therapy with Toddlers: A community-based randomized controlled trial with children aged 14-24 months. *Journal of Clinical Child & Adolescent Psychology, 50*(3), 411–426. https://doi.org/10.1080/15374416.2020.1723599

Lambarth, C. H., & Green, B. L. (2019). Exploring a model for infant and early childhood mental health consultation in early childhood home visiting. *Infant Mental Health Journal, 40*(6), 874–888. https://doi.org/10.1002/imhj.21818

Lieberman, A., & Van Horn, P. (2015). *Don't hit my mommy! A manual for Child-Parent Psychotherapy with young children exposed to violence and other trauma* (2nd ed.). National Center for Clinical Infant Programs.

Lieberman, A., Weston, D. R., & Pawl, J. H. (1991). Preventive intervention and outcome with anxiously attached dyads. *Child Development, 62*(1), 199–209.

Lieberman, A. F., Ghosh Ippen, C., & Van Horn, P. (2006). Child-Parent Psychotherapy: 6-month follow-up of a randomized controlled trial. *Journal of the American Academy of Child & Adolescent Psychiatry, 45*(8), 913–918. https://doi.org/10.1097/01.chi.0000222784.03735.92

Lieneman, C. C., Quetsch, L. B., Theodorou, L. L., Newton, K. A., & McNeil, C. B. (2019). Reconceptualizing attrition in parent–child interaction therapy: "Dropouts" demonstrate impressive improvements. *Psychology Research and Behavior Management, 12*, 543–555. https://doi.org/10.2147/PRBM.S207370

Lojkasek, M., Muir, E., & Cohen, N. J. (2008). Watch, Wait, and Wonder: Infants as agents of change in a play-based approach to mother-infant psychotherapy. In *Play therapy for very young children*. Rowman & Littlefield Publishers, Inc.

Madigan, S., Hawkins, E., Goldberg, S., & Benoit, D. (2006). Reduction of disrupted caregiver behavior using modified Interaction Guidance. *Infant Mental Health Journal, 27*(5), 509–527. https://doi.org/10.1002/imhj.20102

Margolis, K., Briscoe, A., & Tracey, J. (2020). *Babies don't go to the doctor by themselves: Innovating a dyadic behavioral health payment model to serve the youngest primary care patients and their families*. Zero to Three. https://cachildrenstrust.org/wp-content/uploads/2020/05/Dyadic_final_May2020.pdf

Masarik, A. S., & Conger, R. D. (2017). Stress and child development: A review of the family stress model. *Current Opinion in Psychology, 13*, 85–90. https://doi.org/10.1016/j.copsyc.2016.05.008

Maxwell, A., Reay, R. E., Huber, A., Hawkins, E., Woolnough, E., & McMahon, C. (2021). Parent and practitioner perspectives on Circle of Security Parenting (COS-P): A qualitative study. *Infant Mental Health Journal, 42*(3), 452–468. https://doi.org/10.1002/imhj.21916

McCabe, K., & Yeh, M. (2009). Parent–Child Interaction Therapy for Mexican Americans: A randomized clinical trial. *Journal of Clinical Child & Adolescent Psychology, 38*(5), 753–759. https://doi.org/10.1080/15374410903103544

McDonough, S. C. (2004). Interaction Guidance: Promoting and nurturing the caregiver relationship. In *Treating parent-infant relationship problems: Strategies for intervention* (pp. 79–96). The Guilford Press.

McLuckie, A., Landers, A. L., Curran, J. A., Cann, R., Carrese, D. H., Nolan, A., Corrigan, K., & Carrey, N. J. (2019). A scoping review of mental health prevention and intervention initiatives for infants and preschoolers at risk for socio-emotional difficulties. *Systematic Reviews, 8*(1), 183. https://doi.org/10.1186/s13643-019-1043-3

Miller, W. R., Zweben, J., & Johnson, W. R. (2005). Evidence-based treatment: Why, what, where, when, and how? *Journal of Substance Abuse Treatment, 29*(4), 267–276. https://doi.org/10.1016/j.jsat.2005.08.003

National Home Visiting Resource Center. (2022). *2022 home visiting yearbook*. James Bell Associates and the Urban Institute. https://nhvrc.org/yearbook/2022-yearbook/

O'Byrne, E., McCusker, C., & McSweeney, S. (2023). The impact of the "Attachment and Biobehavioural Catch-Up" program on attachment related parent behavior: A systematic review. *Infant Mental Health Journal, 44*(1), 76–91. https://doi.org/10.1002/imhj.22025

Otto, H., & Keller, H. (2014). *Different faces of attachment: Cultural variations on a universal human need*. Cambridge University Press.

Paris, R., Sommer, A., & Marron, B. (2017). Project BRIGHT: An attachment-based intervention for mothers with substance use disorders and their young children. In *Motherhood in the face of trauma*. Springer International Publishing.

Peacock, S., Konrad, S., Watson, E., Nickel, D., & Muhajarine, N. (2013). Effectiveness of home visiting programs on child outcomes: A systematic review. *BMC Public Health, 13*(17). https://doi.org/10.1186/1471-2458-13-17

Phillips, S. T., & Mychailyszyn, M. P. (2022). Parent-Child Interaction Therapy for preschool aged youth: A meta-analysis of developmental specificity. *Child & Youth Care Forum, 52*(2), 267–284. https://doi.org/10.1007/s10566-022-09694-w

Powell, B., Cooper, G., Hoffman, K., & Marvin, B. (2014). *The Circle of Security Intervention: Enhancing attachment in early parent-child relationships*. The Guilford Press.

Ramsauer, B., Mühlhan, C., Lotzin, A., Achtergarde, S., Mueller, J., Krink, S., Tharner, A., Becker-Stoll, F., Nolte, T., & Romer, G. (2020). Randomized controlled trial of the Circle of Security-Intensive intervention for mothers with postpartum depression: Maternal unresolved attachment moderates changes in sensitivity. *Attachment & Human Development, 22*(6), 705–726. https://doi.org/10.1080/14616734.2019.1689406

Ringel, S. (2003). The reflective self. *Journal of Teaching in Social Work, 23*(3–4), 15–28. https://doi.org/10.1300/J067v23n03_03

Robert-Tissot, C., Cramer, B., Stern, D. N., Serpa, S. R., Bachmann, J.-P., Palacio-Espasa, F., Knauer, D., De Muralt, M., Berney, C., & Mendiguren, G. (1996). Outcome evaluation in brief mother-infant psychotherapies: Report on 75 cases. *Infant Mental Health Journal, 17*(2), 97–114. https://doi.org/10.1002/(SICI)1097-0355(199622)17:2<97::AID-IMHJ1>3.0.CO;2-Y

Shonkoff, J. P., & Fisher, P. A. (2013). Rethinking evidence-based practice and two-generation programs to create the future of early childhood policy. *Development and Psychopathology, 25*, 1635–1653. https://doi.org/10.1017/S0954579413000813

Silver, H. C., Davis Schoch, A. E., Loomis, A. M., Park, C. E., & Zinsser, K. M. (2023). Updating the evidence: A systematic review of a decade of Infant and Early Childhood Mental Health Consultation (IECMHC) research. *Infant Mental Health Journal, 44*(1), 5–26. https://doi.org/10.1002/imhj.22033

Skale, G., Perez, H., & Williams, M. E. (2020). Factors influencing implementation of evidence-based mental health interventions for infants and young children. *The Journal of Behavioral Health Services & Research, 47*(4), 493–508. https://doi.org/10.1007/s11414-020-09694-5

Steele, M., Steele, H., Bate, J., Knafo, H., Kinsey, M., Bonuck, K., Meisner, P., & Murphy, A. (2014). Looking from the outside in: The use of video in attachment-based interventions. *Attachment & Human Development, 16*(4), 402–415. https://doi.org/10.1080/14616734.2014.912491

Stern, J. A., Barbarin, O., & Cassidy, J. (2021). Working toward anti-racist perspectives in attachment theory, research, and practice. *Attachment and Human Development, 24*(3), 392–422. https://doi.org/10.1080/14616734.2021.1976933

Thomas, R., Abell, B., Webb, H. J., Avdagic, E., & Zimmer-Gembeck, M. J. (2017). Parent-Child Interaction Therapy: A meta-analysis. *Pediatrics, 140*(3), e20170352. https://doi.org/10.1542/peds.2017-0352

Tidus, K. M., Schoch, A. E. D., Perry, D. F., Rabinovitz, L., & Horen, N. M. (2022). The evidence base for how and why infant and early childhood mental health consultation works. *NHSA Dialog, 25*(2), 1–22.

Toth, S. L., Maughan, A., Manly, J. T., Spagnola, M., & Cicchetti, D. (2002). The relative efficacy of two interventions in altering maltreated preschool children's representational models: Implications for attachment theory. *Development and Psychopathology, 14*(4), 877–908. https://doi.org/10.1017/S095457940200411X

von Klitzing, K., Döhnert, M., Kroll, M., & Grube, M. (2015). Mental disorders in early childhood. *Deutsches Ärzteblatt International, 112*, 375–386. https://doi.org/10.3238/arztebl.2015.0375

Waid, J., & Kelly, M. (2020). Supporting family engagement with child and adolescent mental health services: A scoping review. *Health & Social Care in the Community, 28*(5), 1333–1342. https://doi.org/10.1111/hsc.12947

Walsh, T. B., Paris, R., Ribaudo, J., & Gilkerson, L. (2021). Locating infant and early childhood mental health at the heart of social work. *Social Work, 66*(3), 187–196. https://doi.org/10.1093/sw/swab022

Walter, A. W., Yuan, Y., Morocho, C., & Thekkedath, R. (2019). Facilitators and barriers to family engagement and retention of young children in mental health care: A qualitative study of caregivers' perspectives. *Social Work in Mental Health, 17*(2), 173–196. https://doi.org/10.1080/15332985.2018.1517402

Weatherston, D. J., & Tableman, B. (2015). *Infant mental health home visiting: Supporting competencies/reducing risks* (3rd ed.). Michigan Association for Infant Mental Health.

Willis, D. W., & Eddy, J. M. (2022). Early relational health: Innovations in child health for promotion, screening, and research. *Infant Mental Health Journal, 43*(3), 361–372. https://doi.org/10.1002/imhj.21980

Winnicott, D. W. (1960). The theory of the parent-infant relationship. *The International Journal of Psychoanalysis, 41*, 585–595.

Yaholkoski, A., Hurl, K., & Theule, J. (2016). Efficacy of the Circle of Security intervention: A meta-analysis. *Journal of Infant, Child, and Adolescent Psychotherapy, 15*(2), 95–103. https://doi.org/10.1080/15289168.2016.1163161

Zeanah, P. D., Stafford, B. S., Nagle, G. A., & Rice, T. (2005). *Addressing social-emotional development and infant mental health in early childhood systems.* National Center for Infant and Early Childhood Health Policy. https://files.eric.ed.gov/fulltext/ED496853.pdf

Zero to Three Infant Mental Health Taskforce Steering Committee. (2001). *Definition of infant mental health.* https://www.ecmhc.org/IMH/defining-imh.html

Chapter 2
Family Engagement in Mental Health Treatment for Young Children

Jessica Dym Bartlett, Laura Nabors, and Alexandria Chase

Introduction

Mental health is a key determinant of individual development and well-being over the life course (Substance Abuse and Mental Health Services Administration [SAMHSA], 2014). The foundation for lifelong mental health is laid in early childhood, when young children's experiences with parents, family, and the broader environment have considerable influence on young children's rapidly developing brain (National Scientific Council on the Developing Child, 2007). Indeed, a strong and growing body of research demonstrates that "…the origins of disease are often found among developmental and biological disruptions occurring during the early years of life" (Shonkoff et al., 2009, p. 2252). Disturbances in children's relationships with their parents and other primary caregivers, such as child abuse and neglect and parental mental illness, have particular salience to early childhood mental health. Thus, engaging family members and other important adults in early identification and treatment of social, emotional, and behavioral challenges is essential to promoting positive mental health outcomes for children over the lifespan (Haine-Schlagel & Walsh, 2015; Ingolsby, 2010).

Young children can and do have mental health difficulties that can become more severe disorders when left untreated. However, despite the fact that the majority of

J. D. Bartlett (✉)
Thriving Together, LLC, West Newton, MA, USA
e-mail: jess@wearethrivingtogether.com

L. Nabors
School of Human Services, College of Education, Criminal Justice, Human Services, and Information Technology, University of Cincinnati, Cincinnati, OH, USA

A. Chase
Oberlin College, Oberlin, OH, USA

L. Nabors, J. D. Bartlett (eds.), *Family Engagement in Mental Health Interventions for Young Children*, Springer Series on Child and Family Studies,
https://doi.org/10.1007/978-3-031-47917-5_2

mental health disorders have their origins in childhood, children's mental health – especially young children's mental health – has often been overlooked. Perhaps this is due, in part, to pervasive myths that young children are "resilient" and relatively unaffected by trauma and adversity, or due to limited public awareness that mental health challenges can emerge very early in life. In fact, an estimated one in five children, age 6 or younger, has a diagnosable mental health disorder (Vasileva et al., 2021). In turn, young children are at elevated risk for developmental and behavioral challenges; compromised stress response and immune systems; difficulties learning; poor physical and psychological health; and increased need for services later in life (Shonkoff et al., 2009). Advances in neuroscience, epigenetics, and the behavioral sciences have elucidated the processes underlying these associations, including how early child-rearing environments influence the developing brain; how genes and environmental conditions interact to influence development; how epigenetic and metabolic processes affect children's response to adversity; and how young children's relationships with their caregivers influence these processes (Boyce et al., 2021).

The current chapter reviews extant research on family engagement in the treatment of early childhood mental health disorders using an ecological lens that recognizes the influence of parent-child relationships, family, and broader developmental contexts on the social and emotional well-being of preschool children (i.e., mental health). Specifically, this chapter focuses specifically on how early trauma influences parenting quality and family functioning, which in turn affect young children's mental health (Bronfenbrenner & Morris, 2006; Cicchetti & Valentino, 2006). We discuss the impact of mental health challenges on preschool-age children (3–6 years), their families, and on mental health providers, highlighting socioeconomic, racial, and ethnic inequities in early childhood mental health and related services. We describe promising, evidence-based treatments, and we identify central limitations of extant knowledge and offer recommendations for research, policy, and practice in early childhood mental health.

Early Childhood Mental Health

Early childhood mental health (ECMH), often referred to as infant and early childhood mental health (IECMH) to be inclusive of infants and toddlers, is more than the absence of psychological disorders. Rather, it represents the young child's developing social and emotional skills, including the ability to form healthy relationships with adults and peers, as well as to express and manage the full spectrum of human emotions (World Health Organization [WHO], 2022; Zero to Three, 2017, 2023). ECMH also represents the continuum of services, from promotion to prevention to treatment, which are needed to support young children's development, prevent mental health problems from emerging, and address social and emotional challenges before they become more serious disorders (Zero to Three, 2017, 2023).

A young child's risk for developing a mental or behavioral disorder depends in part on biological predispositions, but the environments in which children are embedded also exert a particularly strong influence (National Scientific Council on the Developing Child, 2004, 2023). For example, the quality of care children receive from their parents and other primary caregivers (i.e., biological, foster, and adoptive parents, foster and kinship caregivers, extended family, and others who care for the child on a regular basis) is one of the most salient factors influencing young children's mental health (National Academies of Science, Engineering, and Medicine, 2016). In the USA, common mental health disorders diagnosed in children ages 3 and older include depression, anxiety, and trauma/post-traumatic stress disorder (PTSD) (von Klitzing et al., 2015). Manifestations of ECMH challenges, including young children's level of distress, behavior, and overall adjustment, vary among children and families (WHO, 2022). Preschoolers' mental health also varies in relation to the nature of their experiences in the world, such as the type, severity, and chronicity of exposure to trauma (National Child Traumatic Stress Network [NCTSN], n.d.). In situations of extreme stress (e.g., separation from biological parents and placement into foster care or orphanages), young children may develop reactive attachment disorder (RAD), though the overall prevalence is low (one percent) (von Klitzing et al., 2015). Behaviors commonly observed during the preschool years that may indicate early trauma or another mental health condition include repeated reenactment of traumatic events or situations in play; avoidance of or extreme separation anxiety in absence of caregivers; compulsive behaviors (e.g., repeated handwashing or use of the same words or phrases); severe tantrums; withdrawal from or disinterest in social interactions; difficulties socializing with peers; highly aggressive or impulsive behavior; limited language development or communication; regression after achievement of developmental milestones (e.g., using the toilet, sleeping independently); and high levels of fear and anxiety (Zero to Three, 2017).

There is widespread consensus that the etiology of early mental health disorders is multidetermined – the product of a combination of biological and environmental forces (Swanson & Wadhwa, 2008). A young child's risk for developing a mental or behavioral disorder depends in part on biological predispositions, but the environments in which children are embedded exert a particularly strong influence (National Scientific Council on the Developing Child, 2004, 2023). The early years are a sensitive period in which prolonged periods of severe stress, unmitigated by positive experiences, can result in harmful impacts on early brain development (Birnie & Baram, 2022). Deficits related to ECMH problems can persist into young adulthood, with a trajectory of continuing educational, mental, and physical problems (Schlack et al., 2021). Treatment for mental health problems during this formative stage has been found to ameliorate many negative developmental outcomes and ensure more positive mental health for future generations (Kieling et al., 2011).

Inequities in Early Childhood Mental Health

Rates of ECMH disorders are especially high among historically impoverished and marginalized families (Jones et al., 2019). Poverty is an especially pernicious risk factor for poor childhood mental health, with particularly high rates of ECMH disorders observed among young children residing in low-income families (Zach et al., 2016). Children living in poverty are two to three times more likely to have a diagnosable mental health condition than those who live in financially secure families (Reiss, 2013).

Conversely, residing in positive caregiving environments has been found to reduce behavioral, social, and emotional problems, and increase family resilience to adversity and trauma (Council on the Developing Child, 2023). Racial and ethnic disparities in ECMH impede child and family well-being (Annie E. Casey Foundation, 2022). For example, children who are Native American, Black, and Latinx have higher rates of mental health challenges compared to their White peers (Annie E. Casey Foundation, 2022; Zach et al., 2016). These minoritized populations also have less access to high-quality treatment (across settings) due to factors such as structural racism, limited service availability, lack of insurance coverage, stigma, incongruence between the treatment approach and family culture, and language barriers (Rodgers et al., 2022).

The COVID-19 pandemic exacerbated mental health problems among young children and their families, as well as related racial and ethnic disparities in mental health and access to related services and supports (Hawks, 2023). The number of children ages 3 and older with anxiety and/or depression rose from approximately 5.8 to 7.3 million during the pandemic, with mental health challenges increasing more among children of color than White children (Annie E. Casey Foundation, 2022). Racial disparities in ECMH services also grew during the transition to telehealth and decrease in urban-based mental health treatment (Williams et al., 2023). Improving equitable access to treatment among families of color is critical to promoting ECMH, including working with families to increase their financial stability and overcome barriers to treatment, such as historical and structural racism and related distrust in public services, stigma, lack of child care and transportation, and limited time off from work (Williams et al., 2008). In addition, mental health providers and programs can promote family engagement in treatment by offering services in places that children already spend time (e.g., home, early childhood education program, school, primary care) and at times they are available (Haine-Schlagel & Walsh, 2015).

An Ecological Approach

There has been increasing consensus among experts in the field of ECMH that an ecological approach is most appropriate for understanding risk and resilience in the lives of young children (Cicchetti & Valentino, 2006). An ecological approach is rooted in the notion that environments influence human development (Bronfenbrenner & Morris, 2006). From this perspective, the child is embedded in multiple contexts in varying proximity to the child, such as the family, early childhood education, schools, communities, and sociopolitical contexts (e.g., federal, state, and local policy, climate change, racism, and other forms of oppression), with risk and protective factors interacting at every level over time. Individual characteristics of children (e.g., biology, age, developmental stage) and parents/caregivers (e.g., mental health, prior exposure to trauma), as well as environmental stressors (e.g., unsafe or resource-poor neighborhoods, inadequate or overcrowded housing) and supports (e.g., safe housing, access to mental health care, high-quality child care), all play an important role in ECMH, but the caregiving environment has long been understood to be the most proximal and consequential for young children's mental health and development (Bronfenbrenner & Morris, 2006; National Scientific Council on the Developing Child, 2004).

A Trauma-Informed Approach

A trauma-informed approach to engaging families in young children's mental health treatment is also central to successful treatment given that nearly half of children in the USA – approximately 34 million – experience at least one potentially traumatic experience in early childhood (Bethell et al., 2017). Young children are exposed to a wide range of traumatic events and conditions, such as child abuse and neglect, intimate partner violence, parental mental illness and substance misuse, separation from or loss of a caregiver, unintentional injuries, discrimination, community violence, and natural disasters. A trauma-informed approach aims to "build on consumer and family engagement, empowerment, and collaboration" (SAMHSA, 2014, p. 14), and thus, engaging families in treatment is a cornerstone of successful care. Ames and Loebach (2023) emphasize that trauma-focused treatment and other ECMHC approaches should be applied systemically, at every level of a program, to reap maximum intervention benefits.

Engaging Families in Identifying and Treating Early Childhood Mental Health Challenges

One key factor in effective mental health services for young children is utilizing a two-generation approach that attends to the child, the parents/caregivers, and the caregiver-child relationship (Lieberman & Van Horn, 2008). All children develop bonds, or attachments, with their parents or other caregivers (Ainsworth & Bell, 1970; Bowlby, 1978). Thus, adults are "essential resources for children in managing emotional arousal, coping, and managing behavior" (National Academies of

Sciences, Engineering, and Medicine [NASEM], 2016). On the other hand, limited family engagement in treatment for young children poses serious problems for families and programs alike, such as the reduction of treatment effectiveness and families dropping out of treatment (Haine-Schlagel et al., 2022).

The consequences of poor family engagement in treatment are significant. Treatment may be less effective, and certain groups of families may receive poor-quality treatment or no treatment at all, including those with severe mental health conditions and living in poverty, and historically marginalized families may not receive adequate treatment. Further, mental health agencies incur considerable costs associated with no-shows and cancelled appointments (Kazdin 1996). Families living in poverty, minoritized families (e.g., families of color, LGTBQ families), and families struggling with severe child or adult mental health conditions tend to have particularly high rates of dropout, which warrants further attention from researchers, policymakers, and practitioners related to optimal methods of engaging families facing such adversity in their lives (Snell-Johns et al., 2004).

Family engagement has been conceptualized in myriad ways, but a contemporary view of family engagement is that it extends beyond parent participation in services or compliance with treatment (Staudt, 2007a, b). Staudt (2007a, b) theorized that both behavioral and attitudinal aspects of engagement are relevant to outcomes, and introduced a five-component, empirically based, theoretical framework for engagement of caregivers in treatment for at-risk children:

1. *Treatment relevance and acceptability*: parents need to feel that treatment is justified and palatable.
2. *Cognitions and beliefs about treatment*: parents must view the provider as caring, authentic; and concerned for their well-being.
3. *Daily stressors*: difficulties of daily life are manageable.
4. *External barriers to treatment*: obstacles to treatment access and retention, such as lack of health insurance, stigma, and other obstacles, must be addressed.
5. *Cognitions and beliefs about treatment*: negative perceptions of help-seeking and mental health treatment interfere with engagement and warrant attention from providers and programs.

Staudt's holistic framework serves as the working definition of family engagement throughout this chapter.

Engaging Families in Treatment

Families are integral to early intervention in general and to services that address the mental health needs of young children in particular (Lieberman et al., 2015). Family members typically have extensive knowledge about their child; the quality of parent-child relationships; family functioning; individual family members' strengths and needs; culture (e.g., values, beliefs, and preferences regarding mental health, and parenting); and the social and physical environments in which they live – all essential information for treatment planning (Bartlett, 2020a, b; SAMHSA, 2014). In addition, parents work collaboratively with mental health providers to provide social, emotional, and concrete supports to the child outside of therapy sessions (Lucksted et al., 2012). Strong family engagement also improves transmission of knowledge to parents and enhances engagement of parents in interventions to improve child functioning (Smith et al., 2020). Perhaps most importantly, young children's mental health is inextricably tied to the well-being of their parents and other primary caregivers, and caregiver-child relationships are the primary mechanism for improving young children's mental health (Lieberman et al., 2015).

Effective strategies for enhancing family engagement included outreach to families; telehealth and digital health (i.e., technology to facilitate communication between providers and families, offer psychoeducation coordination of referrals and follow-up, and deliver clinical services); and integrated care approaches, with the strongest evidence found for outreach to families and integrated care. Including extended family (e.g., grandparents, foster, kinship, and adoptive parents) and other important adults (e.g., a friend who provides child care) as defined by the family in early identification (i.e., screening) and treatment of ECMH challenges can enhance information gathering and mobilize support for the child, which may be especially important for families who rely most on natural supports in their own families and communities (e.g., Falicov, 2007). Understanding, expressing curiosity about, and being responsive to diverse family configurations, characteristics, beliefs, and preferences are especially important strategies for engaging the diversity of families who would benefit from ECMH treatment, particularly when the provider and family are from different cultural backgrounds (Conroy et al., 2021).

Engaging Families in Early Identification

Early identification of symptoms and disorders is a crucial element of promotion, prevention, and treatment of mental health problems that emerge among young children. Accordingly, the central aim of early childhood mental health screening and diagnosis is to prevent further suffering and reduce the chances that children develop more severe disorders later in life by identifying and treating problems early (Bartlett, 2020a, b; Cohen & Andujar, 2021).

Engaging families in the process of screening and diagnosis is essential to effective identification of mental health symptoms and conditions, particularly given that parents are experts on their own children and have the most power to improve their mental health. Thus, screening should take place in the context of a partnership with parents and other caregivers. Not surprisingly, parent report is often used to assess mental health symptoms in young children. And while parental report has sometimes been characterized as less subjective and informative than the "gold standard" of assessing parent-child interactions, parents can supply information on their children that others cannot, and they have been found to be especially attuned to the severity of the child's symptoms and to conditions that are challenging to identify in early childhood, such as depression (McGinnis et al., 2022).

To screen children effectively, the first author and colleagues (Bartlett, 2020a, b) recommend a comprehensive, holistic approach to screening that includes the use of a validated, trauma-informed developmentally appropriate, culturally responsive mental health screening tool; assessment of parent child relationships, parent well-being, family functioning, and social determinants of health; as well as identification of child and family strengths. For additional information on early childhood screening, see Halle and Darling-Churchill (2016) for a review of measures to assess young children's social and emotional measures and Bartlett (2020a, b) for a review of screening and assessment of early trauma and adversity.

Following screening and any additional assessment needed, mental health and developmental disorders during early childhood can be classified by licensed mental health providers using the DC:0–5 Diagnostic Classification of Mental Health and Developmental Disorders of Infancy and Early Childhood Version 2.0 (Zero to Three, 2016). The DC:0–5 drew on empirical research and clinical practice to identify childhood disorders that are not otherwise covered in other diagnostic manuals, such as the Diagnostic and Statistical Manual, Version 5 (DSM-5-TR; American Psychological Association, 2022) or International Classification of Diseases, Tenth Revision, Clinical Modification (ICD-10-CM; WHO, 1999), and also provide codes for medical claims reporting. The DC:0–5 facilitates understanding of the young child's social and emotional development, as well as experience in the context of family, community, and culture. The DSM and ICD focus on disorders in older children and adults and do not address parent-child relationships; the DC:0–5 is a nosology of infant and early childhood disorders that integrates relationships into diagnosis (e.g., rating of the primary caregiving relationship(s) and caregiving environment). The next step following early identification of emotional, behavioral, or relational challenges is to support families in obtaining access to effective treatment.

Evidence-Based Early Childhood Mental Health Treatments

Child-Parent Psychotherapy

Child-parent psychotherapy (CPP; Lieberman et al., 2015) is a therapeutic treatment for children from birth to 5 years who have experienced trauma and/or have developed mental health, attachment, and/or behavioral problems and disorders. Based on attachment, psychodynamic, trauma, social learning, cognitive-behavioral, and developmental theories, all sessions include the child and parent or primary caregiver. The primary aim of CPP is to repair and strengthen the relationship between a child and caregiver to support the child's cognitive, behavioral, and social functioning. Weekly sessions are provided by master's or doctoral-level therapists, who facilitate weekly hour-long sessions with parents/caregivers and their young child for a period of 1 year. Caregiver participation is a required element of CPP, and providers are encouraged to tailor their engagement strategies to each family. Evidence from rigorous research with families from diverse backgrounds has shown that CPP improves child behavior (e.g., decreasing child post-traumatic stress) and reduces parental stress and improves their emotional functioning (e.g., Ghosh Ippen et al., 2011).

Parent-Child Interaction Therapy

Parent-child interaction therapy (PCIT; Querido et al., 2002) is an empirically supported intervention, grounded in attachment theory, social learning theory, behavior modification, and system theory, meant to treat behavior challenges in children. During 14–25 weekly sessions, master's level clinicians observe the parent and child through a one-way mirror and provide guidance through a microphone in the parent's ear. Eyberg and Robinson (1982) proposed that identification of interaction patterns in the family and promotion of positive interactions positively influenced young child, parent, and family functioning. Parents and primary caretakers learn child-directed interactions, and are asked to allow the child to direct the play, and parents describe the play, reflect the child's statements, and use praise appropriate behavior. There is also parent-directed interaction, such as giving clear directions for preferred behaviors (not using questions such as "Would you give me the doll now?") and initiating time-outs for inappropriate behaviors that cannot be ignored. Results of a meta-analysis (23 studies) showed that children were more likely to follow instructions, and parental stress decreased after participating in PCIT; this occurred irrespective of length of sessions and type of child behavior problems (Thomas et al., 2017). PCIT also has been found to reduce children's externalizing behavioral problems (e.g., aggression, hyperactivity), with stronger impacts found among families who completed the full course of treatment compared to those who terminated after the first of two phases (Thomas et al., 2017).

Trauma-Focused Cognitive-Behavioral Therapy

Trauma-focused cognitive-behavioral therapy (TF-CBT; Cohen et al., 2018) is an evidence-based treatment model for children, ages 3–18 years, who have experienced and remember at least one form of trauma. The master's or doctoral-level mental health provider facilitates 12–25 sessions, spending about 30 minutes with the child and 30 minutes with the parent, adding conjoint child-parent sessions later in the treatment process to support children-parent communication. This structure was chosen over family sessions based on the belief that child trauma impacts both parents and children and that each derives benefits from individually processing their trauma responses. One of the central principles of TF-CBT is the importance of engaging parents or other primary caregivers in treatment (Cohen & Mannarino, 2015).

A review of two meta-analyses on ten randomized control trials of TF-CBT by de Arellano et al. (2014) found positive outcomes and, notably, reductions in post-traumatic stress disorder (PTSD).

Triple P

The Triple P Positive Parenting Program, is a multilevel, prevention-focused approach to working with families whose children, ages birth to 16 years, have severe behavioral, emotional, and developmental problems by increasing parental knowledge, skills, and confidence (Sanders, 1999). Triple P implements five levels of care with increasing intensity of services: universal prevention; selective and primary care for parents who wish to address specific problems; standard Triple P for children with severe behavior problems; and enhanced Triple P for children with behavior problems and families exhibiting dysfunction. The Triple P program has been studied extensively and found to be effective over time with a range of problems, ages, and settings, including efficacy in preventing child abuse and neglect (Sanders & Mazzucchelli, 2018; Sanders et al., 2022). Research on the enhanced Triple P's group parenting program for mothers with depression shows the program is related to decreases in maternal depression and decreases in children's social, emotional, and behavioral problems (Sanders et al., 2014).

Promising Early Childhood Mental Health Treatment Models

Attachment, Self-Regulation, and Competency (ARC) Model

The Attachment, Regulation, and Competency (ARC; Kinniburgh et al., 2005) Framework is a flexible, component-based intervention for children and youth ages 3–21 who experience complex trauma, as well as their caregiving systems (any and all adults who are primary caregivers for the child). The ARC Framework is an individual practitioner and organization-wide approach with a clinical model designed to treat the child based on the premise that secure attachments are critical for positive development (Kinniburgh et al., 2005). The caregiver learns to respond to consistent routines and establish a secure attachment, and the child learns to recognize, express, and moderate their emotions (Kinniburgh et al., 2005). The therapist and caregiver assist the child in processing traumatic experiences in a developmentally appropriate fashion. The therapist uses child-centered play to help the child work through traumatic experiences. Children who complete ARC treatment have shown reductions in PTSD symptoms and behavior problems in longitudinal studies (e.g., Bartlett et al., 2016).

Circle of Security

The Circle of Security Program is a program for parents of children ages 4 months through 6 years based on attachment theory and three decades of clinical practice (Hoffman et al., 2006). Circle of Security is a relationship-based early intervention program designed to enhance attachment security between parents and children. Parents or other caregivers explore their own attachment issues and also work to establish a secure attachment relationship with their young child. Parents meet in groups, watching videos with a trained facilitator to guide them through psychological issues that can cause them to make negative attributions about attachment behaviors of their child when their child is interacting with them (https://guidebook.eif.org.uk/programme/circle-of-security-parenting). There is a wealth of research and practice evidence, including a randomized clinical trial in Head Start, supporting this intervention (Cassidy et al., 2017; Huber et al., 2019).

Effective Black Parenting Program

The Effective Black Parenting Program (EBPP) is a parenting skill-building program specifically designed for parents of African American children, ages birth to 18 years. It has been identified as a promising intervention in child welfare (Title IV-E Prevention Services Clearinghouse, 2022). Parents select goals for their children from a menu of interventions designed for Black American parents, termed a "Pyramid of Success." Parents learn through discussion of videos showing different scenarios relevant to parenting young children. There typically are about 14 group sessions for groups of 15–30 parents, and trained instructors are from the same cultural group (https://www.hwcmn.org/EffectiveBlackParenting). Studies indicate that this intervention improves secure and positive attachments with young children, use of praise by parents, as well as reduces parental rejection of children and use punishment (hitting and spanking) (Leathers et al., 2011).

Other Services and Supports to Promote Early Childhood Mental Health

Infant and Early Childhood Mental Health Consultation

Infant and early childhood mental health consultation (IECMHC) is a service in which mental health providers partner with early childhood programs (e.g., early childhood education, Head Start, home visiting) to build their capacity to promote healthy social and emotional development among young children before they need more intensive intervention for mental health and behavioral problems (Center of Excellence for Infant and Early Childhood Mental Health Consultation, n.d.).

IECMHC is a preventative approach in which early childhood service providers gain the skills and knowledge they need to promote young children's social and emotional well-being through consultation with a mental health professional. Typically, the mental health consultant works with staff to problem-solve about children's challenging behaviors; observes child behavior and provider-child interactions; offers relevant training for staff and parents; collaborates with families; and supports the referral of children and their families to other services in the community, as needed (Cohen & Kaufmann, 2005). Consultants strive to be nonjudgmental and reflective and express curiosity about individual, family, and broader environmental influences on the psychological well-being of children and adults (Division for Early Childhood of the Council for Exceptional Children, 2017). IECMHC is associated with fewer child emotional and behavioral problems and improved social skills, increased staff self-efficacy, competence in managing children's challenging behaviors, sensitive and less punitive interactions with children, as well as reductions in providers' work-related stress (Silver et al., 2023). At the program level, IECMHC is associated with reductions in staff turnover and improved quality of care in early childhood education settings (Perry et al., 2010; Silver et al., 2023).

Home Visiting

Home visiting is a service strategy that connects young children (birth to age 5) and expectant and parenting adults with a service provider to promote maternal and child health; children's health development and school readiness; family economic self-sufficiency; and positive parent-child relationships, including preventing child abuse and neglect (Kleinman et al., 2023). The federal Maternal, Infant, and Early Childhood Home Visiting (MIECHV) Program is the main source of funding for home visiting in the USA. The Health Resources and Services Administration (HRSA, 2023b) oversees MIECHV and currently awards $400,000 million or more annually to 56 states, territories, and nonprofit organizations. The Administration for Children and Families' Office of Early Childhood Development leads Tribal MIECHV and has provided $140 million to 36 tribal entities to date to implement high-quality, culturally grounded programs in American Indian and Alaska Native (AIAN) communities (ACF, n.d.). Both MIECHV programs require the development and coordination of comprehensive early childhood systems of care, including mental health (ACF, n.d.; HRSA, 2023a). MIECHV is not a mental health program (nor is home visiting), but most local programs require screening for maternal mental health issues and child health, mental health, and development, and three-quarters of programs screen for maternal substance abuse, intimate partner violence, and problematic parenting behaviors. However, home visitors report challenges engaging mothers with mental health challenges, and in these instances, additional professional development on addressing mental health may be especially important (Duggan et al., 2018). Nevertheless, rigorous evaluation of home visiting programs reveals positive impacts, including preventing child abuse and neglect; improving birth outcomes and children's school readiness; and higher maternal high school graduation rates among racially diverse samples, which are empirically linked to positive mental health outcomes for children (National Conference of State Legislatures, 2022).

Integration of Early Childhood Mental Health into Primary Care

Offering mental health services in the context of primary care has advantages, such as the fact that families often go to pediatricians first to seek advice about concerns related to their children's social and emotional well-being; pediatricians follow families over time, and pediatric care is less stigmatized than mental health care (Hodgkinson et al., 2017). The field of pediatrics has increasingly turned attention to its role in supporting children's social and emotional health and through the promotion of safe, stable, and nurturing relationships (SSNRs) that can buffer children from adversity and support resilience in development (Garner & Yogman, 2021).

A family-centered pediatric medical home (FCPMH) is a mechanism for addressing young children's relational and mental health needs (Garner & Yogman, 2021). FCPMHs provide comprehensive, high-quality primary care, with a focus on partnering with families, mental health providers, early childhood professionals, community organizations, educational systems, and other key community resources within a single system of care (American Academy of Pediatrics, 2021). FCPMH is "a family-centered partnership within a community-based system that provides uninterrupted care with appropriate payment to support and sustain optimal health outcomes" (American Academy of Pediatrics, 2021).

One example of the FCPMH model is Zero to Three's Healthy Steps, which embeds a child development expert into primary care. Healthy Steps has eight core components: child developmental, socio-emotional, and behavioral screenings; screening for family needs; a child development support line; three consultation sessions with parents on child development and behavior; interdisciplinary team well-child visits; care coordination and system integration; positive parenting guidance and information; and early learning resources (Valado et al., 2019).

A national multi-site evaluation indicated the program had positive outcomes for children, families, and providers, including improved physician and caregiver satisfaction and continuity of care; better compliance with recommended well-child visits and vaccinations; and higher rates of developmental screening. There were also modest reductions in parents' use of severe physical discipline. Children were more likely to remain in the practice, and parents were more satisfied with care than control group counterparts (Valado et al., 2019).

Barriers to Family Engagement in Mental Health Treatment for Young Children

Some barriers to obtaining mental health treatment for young children pertain to the logistics of accessing and attending therapy sessions, such as a lack of health-care coverage, child care, transportation, time off from work, and geographically accessible services (Garvey et al., 2006; Stevens et al., 2006). Another obstacle identified in the literature is a lack of alignment between a program/provider's approach and the family's beliefs, values, and preferences related to mental health, help-seeking, and parenting (Ingoldsby, 2010; Stevens et al., 2006). In addition, there are not nearly enough treatment providers to meet the current need nor who reflect the racial and ethnic backgrounds of those they serve (Buche et al., 2017).

A review of the research on family engagement in children's mental health treatment by Ingolsby (2010) found that providers were most successful engaging families when they communicated in-depth with the family about the treatment process, such as its potential benefits, realistic expectations for the treatment process and outcomes, and practical and psychological barriers to obtaining treatment for their child. When providers do not address such potential mismatches, families are more likely to drop out of treatment (Miller & Prinz, 2003). Successful strategies for engaging families also include tailoring treatment to each family's needs using a range of approaches engaging multiple family members, and integrating family engagement strategies throughout the program.

Systems of Care for Supporting the Mental Health of Young Children and Their Families

Families often interact with multiple services systems, such as mental health and substance use treatment; health care; early childhood education; housing and financial assistance programs; and others. Typically, service systems do not coordinate services for families with young children, who are burdened by different eligibility requirements, geographical locations, service providers, and organizational policies and practices. Conversely, embedding early childhood mental health treatment within comprehensive systems of care that connect families to the wide range of supports and services they need has been hypothesized to reduce barriers to access and improve child and family outcomes (Stroul et al., 2021). Common components of an early childhood system include interdependent policies, programs, services, and infrastructure among child- and family-serving systems, and the linkages among all elements (BUILD, 2023).

Several federal programs have sought to address service silos and provide comprehensive and coordinated systems of care, such as HRSA's Early Childhood Comprehensive Systems (ECCS) program. The program requires grantees to develop integrated maternal and early childhood systems of care (prenatally to age 3) that promote early developmental health and family well-being using a prevention lens and cross-system collaboration (HRSA, 2023b). More relevant to preschool-age children, the Substance Abuse and Mental Health Services Administration (SAMHSA) developed Project LAUNCH (Linking Actions for Unmet Needs in Children's Health) to promote the social and emotional wellness of young children, birth to 8, by building infrastructure, improving coordination across child-serving systems, and increasing families' access to high-quality services

(SAMHSA, 2023). Grantees (states, tribes, and territories) seek to improve individual, family, and community outcomes by bringing together local child-serving organizations to implement five mental health prevention and promotion strategies: (1) screening and assessment in a variety of child-serving settings, (2) enhanced home visiting through increased focus on social and emotional well-being, (3) mental health consultation in early care and education programs, (4) family strengthening and parent skills training, and (5) integration of behavioral health into primary care settings, although the specific strategies change from year to year. This work is guided by a Young Child Wellness Council, a cross-sector advisory group that requires parent engagement. A cross-site evaluation by Goodson et al. (2014) found that LAUNCH providers in each of the program strategies had increased knowledge of children's socio-emotional development and appropriate service options for children with behavioral concerns, and they used mental health consultation more often; parents reported LAUNCH helped improve their parenting and their child's growth and development.

Caring for the Caregivers

Engaging families is an essential component of effective mental health treatment, but the work can be stressful for providers. Burnout among mental health providers is a common and ongoing phenomenon related to working with families who have experienced trauma (NCTSN, Secondary Traumatic Stress Committee, 2011). Through repeated exposure to children and families who have experienced trauma, mental health providers may develop post-traumatic stress symptoms and become overwhelmed by their clients' difficult experiences, leading to negative consequences for both their personal and professional functioning (Weiss-Dagan et al., 2022). The symptoms of secondary traumatic stress (STS), sometimes referred to as compassion fatigue, develop as professionals learn about the trauma of these families and continuously draw on their own empathy toward their clients (Figley, 2002). Providers may develop detached, negative attitudes toward treatment, leading them to turn that dissatisfaction toward themselves as they feel unhappy in their work (Key & Rider, 2018). Alternatively, providers may need to draw on their emotional memory to express the empathy they display to families. Emotional distress from exposure to firsthand experiences of child and family trauma can trigger their own experience of these emotions (e.g., concern, regret, empathy, post-traumatic stress) and lead to over-involvement in their clients' treatment (Morse et al., 2012). STS symptoms also affect the day-to-day mental state of the provider, leading to feelings of anxiety, depression, fear, withdrawal from personal or work activities, and intrusive thoughts and images (Ogińska-Bulik et al., 2021).

Research indicates that there are multiple protective factors that can promote the psychological well-being of mental health providers (Key & Rider, 2018), which programs and staff can employ to mitigate risk for STS. Self-care through social support is one powerful predictor of compassion satisfaction in mental health professionals (Weiss-Dagan et al., 2015). For example, Killian (2008) found that when therapists felt connected to members of their community and could ask for help from their social network when needed, they reported lower levels of compassion fatigue and higher satisfaction with the client work they performed. Further, the Office of Head Start (OHS, 2021) recommends that programs collect and analyze data on staff wellness to better understand what supports are needed (OHS, 2021). Programs can also determine which positions have high turnover rates, and what resources they can allocate to reduce staff burnout and turnover and increase individual wellness. Programs can also implement strategies in the workplace to support self-care at the system level and show the value in providers' health and well-being. For example, utilizing online platforms for mindfulness and resilience workshops, as well as physical spaces purely for relaxation purposes (soft, calming music, dimmed lighting, etc.), can be restorative for providers' emotional needs (National Child Welfare Work Institute, 2021). When programs communicate with employees about their wellness needs, they can create a work environment built on mutual respect, trust, and collaboration, in turn leading to higher self-efficacy and feelings of support from their employer (OHS, 2021).

Clinician attitudes toward their organization are also related to their experience of burnout (Boyas et al., 2010). The more they feel connected to their employer through the provision of support systems and encouragement, the less emotional exhaustion and detachment they feel (Schmidt, 2007). Staff education about self-care practices, burnout, and STS, especially early on in their work with children and families, can prepare them for trauma exposure, equip them with skills to manage emotional exhaustion, and increase their emotional self-awareness (National Child Welfare Workforce Institute, 2021; OHS, 2021; Killian, 2008). Further, designating time for reflective supervision, where staff meet with their supervisors to discuss challenging cases and emotions that arise as they are supporting families, can be effective at improving care quality, staff retention, and family outcomes (West et al., 2022). When clinicians are empowered to address their own emotional and support needs and struggle less with traumatic stress at work, they better engage with the families and children they seek to help (Key & Rider, 2018; Weiss-Dagan et al., 2022).

Limitations of Current Knowledge

A "robust research agenda on cost-effectiveness, strategy coordination, and cultural challenges should be mounted and drawn upon to inform the next generation of strategies to promote the mental, emotional and behavioral health of children and youth" (Yoshikawa et al., 2012, p. 282). While the field of ECMH has expanded considerably in recent years, research is still needed to identify effective strategies for engaging families from different racial, ethnic, and socioeconomic backgrounds, as well as LGBTQ families and other marginalized groups who often encounter daunting barriers to accessing the services their child needs (Hodgkinson et al.,

2017). Because rigorous research is expensive, is time-consuming, and requires specific research expertise, and thus is not feasible for many smaller, community-developed, culturally grounded ECMH treatment model developers, support from federal, state, and local stakeholders is essential to identifying, testing, and scaling culturally grounded ECMH services, as well as identifying the contextual factors that influence its effectiveness (Goodkind et al., 2017; Lifsey et al., 2015). Increasing the evidence for early intervention to promote ECMH among children from low-income and minoritized backgrounds is particularly important given high levels of exposure to social risk factors associated with poor parental and child mental health; elevated rates of ECMH disorders among Black, Hispanic, and AIAN families compared to non-Hispanic White children; and the lack of access to high-quality, culturally grounded evidence-based treatment (Hodgkinson et al., 2017; Rodgers et al., 2022).

Extant studies suggest that motivational interviewing, family systems work, and support for coping with stress throughout treatment are strategies associated with improved engagement of parents and families, but the wide variation in how they are implemented warrants attention from researchers and practitioners to establish fidelity so they can be replicated and scaled successfully (Ingolsby, 2010). Research is also needed to determine the value-added of tools and frameworks designed to improve parent and family engagement across service sectors. For example, Facilitating Attuned Interaction (FAN; Gilkerson, n.d.) is an "add-on" tool that helps practitioners across disciplines to develop stronger, more respectful, and trusting relationships with families based on the understanding that attunement facilitates a sense of connection and being understood, creating openings for change. Studies of FAN have shown promising results for improving provider attunement and responsiveness to family needs, increasing parental agency, and enhancing collaboration between parents and providers to promote positive parenting (Spielberger et al., 2016). Another example is the Parent, Family, and Community Engagement (PFCE) Framework developed by the Office of Head Start's National Center on PFCE (US Department of Health and Human Services, 2018), which has never been tested empirically yet guides Head Start's family engagement efforts.

Finally, study of the ECMH workforce and evaluation of initiatives aimed at increasing the cadre of well-trained mental health providers in the USA who work across the promotion-prevention-treatment continuum will be vital to developing sufficient capacity to support the mental health and well-being of all families who would benefit from ECMH services (Bartlett & Stratford, 2021). Currently, the shortage of mental health providers, rising rates of mental illness, and scarcity of providers in rural and economically stressed areas are undermining families' ability to access treatment, especially families who are coping with poverty, historical trauma, structural racism, and other serious adversities (Bipartisan Policy Center, 2023). Researchers from the Brookings Institution (Glied & Aguilar, 2023) analyzed 2022 HRSA data and found that HRSA had designated 2774 of the 3144 counties in the country as mental health service shortage areas. Relatedly, increasing knowledge is needed to identify effective organizational staff wellness policies and practices for preventing and addressing secondary traumatic stress to increase retention rates among ECMH providers. A small body of literature suggests that infant and early childhood mental health consultation (IECMHC) and use of evidence-based mental health treatments for children, for example, can have protective effects against job-related provider stress, emotional exhaustion, and turnover (Silver et al., 2023).

Future Directions

Together, the increasing numbers of young children, parents, and providers who develop mental health challenges and disorders, along with the vast unmet need for ECMH services, are cause for alarm. The stigma of mental health treatment along with the traditional approach used by many community mental health agencies (e.g., maintaining traditional work hours, long waitlists, requiring multiple intake visits prior to treatment) can be serious deterrents to families, who in turn may not be able to prioritize their child's or family's mental and physical wellness (Goodman et al. 2013).

In a brief co-authored by this chapter's first author, *A National Agenda for Children's Mental Health*, Bartlett and Stratford (2021) discuss the urgent need to address children's worsening mental health in the USA and related inequities. They recommend adopting a multipronged approach, particularly given the deleterious psychological impacts of the COVID-19 pandemic on children, parents, and service providers alike; the shortage of mental health providers; and inequities in the development of ECMH disorders, access to services, service quality, and outcomes achieved for families experiencing poverty, families of color, LGTBQ families, and those living in rural and other resource-poor geographical areas (Hodgkinson et al., 2017; Rathod et al., 2018). Accordingly, Bartlett and Stratford (2021, pp. 6–11) propose five overarching strategies to promote children's mental health:

1. Establish systems for coordinating mental health with other services that support children, youth, and families, including health care, child welfare, the legal system, home visiting, child care, and education.
2. Develop more flexible and equitable federal, tribal, state, and local funding streams that expand access to mental health promotion, prevention, early intervention, and treatment services.
3. Establish a national, cross-disciplinary initiative to increase workforce capacity in children's mental health.
4. Invest in innovative technology to increase access to mental health supports.
5. Increase children's well-being by reducing family poverty.

The National Academies of Science, Medicine, and Engineering (2023) examined the literature on the impact of the COVID-19 pandemic on child and family well-being and identified support for children's mental health as a high priority. Among the recommendations were developing a task force to address the pandemic's impacts and to focus on families who suffered the worst burdens (i.e., Black, Latino, and Native American children and families, and those living in poverty). They also called for strengthening and expanding Medicaid coverage at the federal level "so that all children and families have consistent access to high-quality, continuous, and affordable physical and mental health services" (p. 8), as well as increasing federal investments to improve access to high-quality treatment and preventive services in clinical settings, communities, and schools. To address the role of poverty in mental health, NASEM asserted that additional efforts are needed to ensure parity across states and to mitigate the economic impacts of the pandemic (e.g., through cash transfers to families).

Ultimately, successful identification and treatment of mental health disorders in early childhood relies heavily on the extent to which providers, programs, and service models promote family engagement among diverse groups of young children. Research, practice, and policy on family engagement in ECMH services are still in the early stages, most services continue to exist in silos, and despite mounting evidence that coordinated and comprehensive systems of care are more likely to achieve the intended outcomes of early interventions, families who are already coping with stress of parenting young children with mental health problems are still required to negotiate the complexity of working with multiple service systems, and our most vulnerable families continue to face the most significant barriers to treatment. Expanded efforts are needed now to successfully engage and retain parents, families, and providers in services to promote the mental health and well-being of young children and their families.

References

Ainsworth, M. D. S., & Bell, S. M. (1970). Attachment, exploration, and separation: Illustrated by the behavior of one-year-olds in a strange situation. *Child Development, 41*(1), 49–67.

American Academy of Pediatrics. (2021). *Patient and family-centered medical home.* American Academy of Pediatrics. https://www.aap.org/en/practice-management/care-delivery-approaches/patient-and-family-centered-medical-home/.

American Psychological Association. (2022). *Diagnostic and statistical manual of mental disorders* (5th ed., text rev.). https://doi.org/10.1176/appi.books.9780890425787.

Ames, R. L., & Loebach, J. E. (2023). Applying trauma-informed design principles to therapeutic residential care facilities to reduce retraumatization and promote resiliency among youth in care. *Journal of Child & Adolescent Trauma*, Advance online publication (13 pages). https://doi.org/10.1007/s40653-023-00528-y.

Annie E. Casey Foundation. (2022). *2022 Kids Count data book.* The Annie E. Casey Foundation. https://assets.aecf.org/m/resourcedoc/aecf-2022kidscountdatabook-2022.pdf

Bartlett, J. D. (2020a). Screening for childhood adversity: Contemporary challenges and recommendations. *Adversity & Resilience Science, 1*, 65–79. https://doi.org/10.1007/s42844-020-00004-8

Bartlett, J. D., Barto, B., Griffin, J. L., Fraser, J. G., Hodgdon, H., & Bodian, R. (2016). Trauma-informed care in the Massachusetts Child Trauma Project. *Child Maltreatment, 21*(2), 101–112. https://doi.org/10.1177/1077559515615700

Bartlett, J. D., & Stratford, B. (2021, January 27). *A national agenda for children's mental health.* Child Trends. https://www.childtrends.org/publications/a-national-agenda-for-childrens-mental-health

Bartlett, J. D. (2020b). Screening for childhood adversity: Contemporary challenges and recommendations. *Adversity and Resilience Science, 1*(33), 65–79. https://doi.org/10.1007/s42844-020-00004-8

Bethell, C., Davis, M. B., Gombojav, N., Stumbo, S., & Powers, K. (2017). *A national and across state profile on adverse childhood experiences among children and possibilities to heal and thrive: Issue brief.* Johns Hopkins Bloomberg School of Public Health.

Bipartisan Policy Center. (2023). *Filling in the gaps in the behavioral health workforce.* Bipartisan Policy Center. https://bipartisanpolicy.org/download/?file=/wp-content/uploads/2023/01/BPC_2022_Behavioral-Health-Integration-Report_RV6Final.pdf

Birnie, M. T., & Baram, T. Z. (2022). Principles of emotional brain circuit maturation. *Science, 376*(6597), 1055–1056. https://doi.org/10.1126/science.abn4016

Bowlby, J. (1978). Attachment theory and its therapeutic implications. *Adolescent Psychiatry, 6*, 5–33.

Boyas, J., & Wind, L. H. (2010). Employment-based social capital, job stress, and employee burnout: A public child welfare employee structural model. *Children and Youth Services Review, 32*(3), 380–388. https://doi.org/10.1016/j.childyouth.2009.10.009

Boyce, W. T., Levitt, P., Martinez, F. D., McEwen, B. S., & Shonkoff J. P. (2021). Genes, environments, and time: The biology of adversity and resilience. *Pediatrics, 147*(2), e20201651. https://doi.org/10.1542/peds.2020-1651. PMID: 33495368.

Bronfenbrenner, U., & Morris, P. A. (2006). The bioecological model of human development. In R. M. Lerner & W. Damon (Eds.), *Handbook of child psychology: Theoretical models of human development* (pp. 793–828). Wiley.

BUILD Initiative. (2023). *What is an early childhood system?* BUILD Initiative. https://buildinitiative.org/approach/early-childhood-system/

Buche, J., Beck, A., & Singer, P. M. (2017, February). *Factors impacting the development of a diverse behavioral health workforce.* Behavioral Health Workforce Research Center, School of Public Health, University of Michigan. https://behavioralhealthworkforce.org/wp-content/uploads/2017/05/FA2P1_Workforce-Diversity_Final-Report.pdf

Cassidy, J., Brett, B., Gross, J., Stern, J., Martin, D., Mohr, J., & Woodhouse, S. (2017). Circle of Security–Parenting: A randomized controlled trial in Head Start. *Development and Psychopathology, 29*(2), 651–673. https://doi.org/10.1017/S0954579417000244

Center of Excellence for Infant & Early Childhood Mental Health Consultation. (n.d.). *About IECMHC.* Georgetown University Center for Child and Human Development. https://www.iecmhc.org/about/

Cicchetti, D., & Valentino, K. (2006). An ecological-transactional perspective on child maltreatment: Failure of the average expectable environment and its influence on child development. In D. Cicchetti & D. J. Cohen (Eds.), *Developmental psychopathology: Risk, disorder, and adaptation* (pp. 129–201). Wiley.

Cohen, J. A., & Andujar, P. (2021). *Integrating DC: 0-5 into state policy systems: 5 years of progress.* Zero to Three. https://www.zerotothree.org/resource/journal/integrating-dc0-5-into-state-policy-and-systems-5-years-of-progress/

Cohen, E., & Kaufmann, R. K. (2005). *Early childhood mental health consultation. Center for Mental Health Services, Substance Abuse and Mental Health Services Administration* (Rev. ed.) https://library.um.edu.mo/ebooks/b15692309a.pdf

Cohen, J. A., Deblinger, E., & Mannarino, A. P. (2018). Trauma-focused cognitive behavioral therapy for children and families. *Psychotherapy Research: Journal of the Society for Psychotherapy Research, 28*(1), 47–57. https://doi.org/10.1080/10503307.2016.1208375

Cohen, J. A., & Mannarino, A. P. (2015). Trauma-focused Cognitive Behavior Therapy for traumatized children and families. *Child and Adolescent Psychiatric Clinics of North America, 24*(3), 557–570. https://doi.org/10.1016/j.chc.2015.02.005

Conroy, K., Frech, N., Sanchez, A. L., Hagan, M. B., Bagner, D. M., & Comer, J. S. (2021). Caregiver stress and cultural identity in families of preschoolers with developmental delay and behavioral problems. *Infant Mental Health Journal, 42*(4), 573–585. https://doi.org/10.1002/imhj.21923

de Arellano, M. A., Lyman, D. R., Jobe-Shields, L., George, P., Dougherty, R. H., Daniels, A. S., Ghose, S. S., Huang, L., & Delphin-Rittmon, M. E. (2014). Trauma-focused cognitive-behavioral therapy for children and adolescents: assessing the evidence. *Psychiatric Services, 65*(5), 591–602. https://doi.org/10.1176/appi.ps.201300255

Division for Early Childhood of the Council for Exceptional Children. (2017). *Position statement on challenging behavior and young children.* National Center for Pyramid Model Innovations. https://challengingbehavior.cbcs.usf.edu/docs/DEC_PositionStatement_ChallengingBehavior.pdf

Duggan, A., Portilla, X. A., Filene, J. H., Crowne, S.S., Hill, C. J., Lee, H., & Knox., V. (2018). *Implementation of evidence-based early childhood home visiting: Results from the Mother and Infant Home Visiting Program Evaluation* (OPRE Report 2018-76A). Office of Planning, Research, and Evaluation, Administration for Children and Families, U.S. Department of Health and Human Services. https://www.acf.hhs.gov/sites/default/files/documents/opre/mihope_implementation_report_2018_10_26_508b.pdf

Eyberg, S. M., & Robinson, E. A. (1982). Parent-child interaction training: Effects on family functioning. *Journal of Clinical Child & Adolescent Psychology, 11*(2), 130–137. https://doi.org/10.1080/15374418209533076

Falicov, C. J. (2007). Working with transnational immigrants: Expanding meanings of family, community, and culture. *Family Process, 46*(2), 157–171. https://doi.org/10.1111/j.1545-5300.2007.00201.x

Figley, C. R. (2002). Compassion fatigue: Psychotherapists' chronic lack of self care. *Journal of Clinical Psychology, 58*(11), 1433–1441. https://doi.org/10.1002/jclp.10090

Garner, A., & Yogman, M. (2021). Preventing childhood toxicity stress: partnering with families and communities to promote relational health. *American Academy of Pediatrics, 48*(2). https://doi.org/10.1542/peds.2021-052582

Garvey, C., Julion, W., Fogg, L., Kratovil, A., & Gross, D. (2006). Measuring participation in a prevention trial with parents of young children. *Research in Nursing and Health, 29*(3), 212–222. https://doi.org/10.1002/nur.20127

Ghosh Ippen, C., Harris, W. W., Van Horn, P., & Lieberman, A. F. (2011). Traumatic and stressful events in early childhood: Can treatment help those at highest risk? *Child Abuse & Neglect, 35*(7), 504–513. https://doi.org/10.1016/j.chiabu.2011.03.009

Gilkerson, L. (n.d.). *Facilitating Attuned Interactions (FAN).* Erikson Institute. https://www.erikson.edu/academics/professional-development/district-infancy-programs/facilitating-attuned-interactions/

Glied, S., & Aguilar, K., (2023). *The behavioral health workforce shortage: Can we make better use of the providers we have?* [White paper]. USC-Brookings Schaeffer Initiative for Health Policy https://www.brookings.edu/wp-content/uploads/2023/04/Glied-and-Aguilar-Workforce-Paper-1.pdf.

Goodkind, J. R., Amer, S., Christian, C., Hess, J. M., Bybee, D., Isakson, B. L., Baca, B., Ndayisenga, M., Greene, R. N., & Shantez, C. (2017). Challenges and innovations in a community-based participatory randomized controlled trial. *Health Education & Behavior, 44*(1), 123–130. https://doi.org/10.1177/1090198116639243

Goodman, L. A., Pugach, M., Skolnik, A., & Smith, L. (2013). Poverty and mental health practice: within and beyond the 50-minute hour. *Journal of Clinical Psychology, 69*(2), 182–190. https://doi.org/10.1002/jclp.21957

Goodson, B., Grindal, T., Darrow, C., Gwaltney, M., Walker, D. K., Wyant, B., Price, C., & Abt Associates Inc. (2014). *Outcomes of Project LAUNCH: Cross-site evaluation findings, volume II* (OPRE Report #2014-88). Office of Planning, Research, and Evaluation, Administration for Children and Families. https://www.acf.hhs.gov/sites/default/files/documents/opre/launch_outcomes_report_12_29_14_final_508.pdf

Haine-Schlagel, R., & Walsh, N. E. (2015). A review of parent participation engagement in child and family mental health treatment. *Clinical Child & Family Psychology Review, 18*(2), 133–150. https://doi.org/10.1007/s10567-015-0182-x

Haine-Schlagel, R., Dickson, K. S., Lind, T., Kim, J. J., May, G. C., Walsh, N. E., Lazarevic, V., Crandal, B. R., & Yeh, M. (2022). Caregiver participation engagement in child mental health prevention Pprograms: A systematic review. *Prevention Science, 23*(2), 321–339. https://doi.org/10.1007/s11121-021-01303-x

Halle, T. G., & Darling-Churchill, K. E. (2016). Review of measures of social and emotional development. *Journal of Applied Developmental Psychology, 45*, 8–18. https://doi.org/10.1016/j.appdev.2016.02.003

Hawks, J. L. (2023). Editorial: The impact of the COVID-19 pandemic on racial disparities in pediatric mental health. *Journal of the American Academy of Child and Adolescent Psychiatry, 62*(4), 398–399. https://doi.org/10.1016/j.jaac.2022.12.015

Health Resources & Services Administration. (2023a). *Early Childhood Comprehensive System (ECCS)*. Health Resources and Services Administration. https://mchb.hrsa.gov/programs-impact/early-childhood-systems/early-childhood-comprehensive-systems

Health Resources & Services Administration. (2023b). *Maternal, Infant, and Early Childhood Home Visiting (MIECHV) Program*. Maternal and Child Health Bureau. https://mchb.hrsa.gov/programs-impact/programs/home-visiting/maternal-infant-early-childhood-home-visiting-miechv-program

Hodgkinson, S., Godoy, L., Beers, L. S., & Lewin, A. (2017). Improving mental health access for low-income children and families in the primary care setting. *Pediatrics, 139*(1). https://doi.org/10.1542/peds.2015-1175

Hoffman, K., Marvin, R., Cooper, G., & Powell, B. (2006). Changing toddlers' and preschoolers' attachment classifications: The Circle of Security intervention. *Journal of Consulting & Clinical Psychology, 74*, 1017–1026. https://doi.org/10.1037/0022-006X.74.6.1017

Huber, A., Hawkins, E., & Cooper, G. (2019). Circle of security. In J. Lebow, A. Chambers, & D. Breunlin (Eds.), *Encyclopedia of couple and family therapy* (pp. 413–418). Springer. https://doi.org/10.1007/978-3-319-15877-8_845-1

Ingolsby, E. M. (2010). Review of interventions to improve family engagement and retention in parent and child mental health programs. *Journal of Child and Family Studies, 19*(5), 629–645. https://doi.org/10.1007/s10826-009-9350-2

Jones, N. L., Gilman, S. E., Cheng, T. L., Drury, S. S., Hill, C. V., & Geronimus, A. T. (2019). Life course approaches to the causes of health disparities. *American Journal of Public Health, 109*(S1), S48–S55. https://10.2105/AJPH.2018.304738

Kazdin, A. E. (1996). Dropping out of child psychotherapy: Issues for research and implications for practice. *Clinical Child Psychology & Psychiatry, 1*(1), 133–156. https://journals.sagepub.com/doi/10.1177/1359104596011012

Key, A., & Rider, K. (2018). Secondary traumatic stress among mental health professionals: implications for graduate training programs. *Graduate Student Journal of Psychology, 17*, 68–77. https://doi.org/10.52214/gsjp.v17i.10921

Kieling, C., Baker-Henningham, H., Belfer, M., Conti, G., Ertem, I., Omigbodun, O., Rohde, L. A., Srinath, S., Ulkuer, N., & Rahman, A. (2011). Child and adolescent mental health worldwide: Evidence for action. *Lancet, 378*(9801), 1515–1525. https://doi.org/10.1016/S0140-6736(11)60827-1

Killian, K. D. (2008). Helping till it hurts? A multimethod study of compassion fatigue, burnout, and self-care in clinicians working with trauma survivors. *Traumatology, 14*(2), 32–44. https://doi.org/10.1177/1534765608319083

Kinniburgh, K., Blaustein, M., Spinazzola, J., & van der Kolk, B. (2005). Attachment, self-regulation and competency: A comprehensive intervention framework for children with complex trauma. *Psychiatric Annals, 35*, 424–430. https://doi.org/10.3928/00485713-20050501-08

Kleinman, R., Del Grosso, P., Harding, J. F., Hsu, R., Kalb, M., O'Brien, J., Rosen, E., Ayoub, C., Caither, M., Mondi-Rago, C., Roberts, J., & Rosengarten, M. (2023). *Understanding family engagement in home visiting: literature synthesis* (OPRE Report #2023-004). Mathematica. https://www.acf.hhs.gov/sites/default/files/documents/opre/hv_reach_literature_synthesis_dec2022.pdf

Leathers, S. J., Spielfogel, J. E., McMeel, L. S., & Atkins, M. S. (2011). Use of a parent management training intervention with urban foster parents: A pilot study. *Children & Youth Services Review, 33*(7), 1270–1279. https://doi.org/10.1016/j.childyouth.2011.02.022
Lieberman, A. E., Ghosh Ippen, C., & Van Horn, P. (2015). Don't hit my mommy: A manual for child-parent psychotherapy with children exposed to violence.. Zero to Three.
Lieberman, A. E., & Van Horn, P. (2008). *Psychotherapy with infants and young children: Repairing the effects of stress and trauma on early attachment*. Guilford Press.
Lifsey, S., Cash, A., Anthony, J., Mathis, S., & Silva, S. (2015). Building the evidence base for population-level interventions: Barriers and opportunities. *Health Education & Behavior, 42*(1 Suppl), 133S–140S. https://doi.org/10.1177/1090198114568429
Lucksted, A., Mcfarlane, W., Downing, D., & Dixon, L. (2012). Recent developments in family psychoeducation as an evidence-based practice. *Journal of Marital and Family Therapy, 38*(1), 101–121. https://doi.org/10.1111/j.1752-0606.2011.00256.x
McGinnis, E. W., Copeland, W., Shanahan, L., & Egger, H. L. (2022). Parental perception of mental health needs in young children. *Child & Adolescent Mental Health, 27*(4), 328–334. https://doi.org/10.1111/camh.12515
Miller, G. E., & Prinz, R. J. (2003). Engagement of families in treatment for childhood conduct Problems. *Behavior Therapy, 34*(4), 517–534. https://doi.org/10.1016/S0005-7894(03)80033-3
Morse, G., Salyers, M. P., Rollins, A. L., Monroe-DeVita, M., & Pfahler, C. (2012). Burnout in mental health services: a review of the problem and its remediation. *Administration and Policy in Mental Health and Mental Health Services Research, 39*(5), 341–352. https://doi.org/10.1007/s10488-011-0352-1
National Academies of Sciences, Engineering, and Medicine. (2016). *Parenting matters: Supporting parents of children ages 0-8*. The National Academies Press. https://doi.org/10.17226/21868.
National Academies of Sciences, Engineering, and Medicine. (2023). *Addressing the long-term impact of the COVID-19 pandemic on children and families*. The National Academies Press. https://doi.org/10.17226/26809.
National Child Traumatic Stress Network. (n.d.). *About child trauma*. https://www.nctsn.org/what-is-child-trauma/about-child-trauma
National Child Traumatic Stress Network, Secondary Traumatic Stress Committee. (2011). *Secondary traumatic stress: A fact sheet for child-serving professionals*. National Center for Child Traumatic Stress. https://www.nctsn.org/sites/default/files/resources/fact-sheet/secondary_traumatic_stress_child_serving_professionals.pdf
National Child Welfare Workforce Institute. (2021). *Supporting self-care at the system level*. National Child Welfare Workforce Institute. https://ncwwi-dms.org/resourcemenu/resource-library/organizational-culture-and-climate/1657-key-takeaways-from-building-a-resilient-workforce-to-address-trauma-and-enhance-well-being-connecting-to-cultural-ways/file
National Conference of State Legislatures. (2022). *Home visiting: improving outcomes for children*. National Conference of State Legislatures. https://www.ncsl.org/human-services/home-visiting-improving-outcomes-for-children
National Scientific Council on the Developing Child. (2004). *Young children develop in an environment of relationships* (Working Paper No. 1). Center on the Developing Child. https://developingchild.harvard.edu/resources/wp1/
National Scientific Council on the Developing Child. (2007). The science of early childhood development: Closing the gap between what we know and what we do. https://www.developingchild.harvard.edu
National Scientific Council on the Developing Child. (2023). *Place matters: The environment we create shapes the foundations of healthy development: Working paper no. 16*. https://harvard-center.wpenginepowered.com/wp-content/uploads/2023/03/HCDC_WP16_R2A.pdf
Office of Head Start (OHS). (2021). *Supporting the wellness of all staff in the Head Start workplace*. Administration for Children and Families. https://eclkc.ohs.acf.hhs.gov/policy/im/acf-im-hs-21-05

Ogińska-Bulik, N., Gurowiec, P. J., Michalska, P., & Kędra, E. (2021). Prevalence and predictors of secondary traumatic stress symptoms in health care professionals working with trauma victims: A cross-sectional study. *PLoS One, 16*(2). https://doi.org/10.1371/journal.pone.0247596

Perry, D. F., Allen, M. D., Brennan, E. M., & Bradley, J. R. (2010). The evidence base for mental health consultation in early childhood settings: A research synthesis addressing children's behavioral outcomes. *Early Education & Development, 21*(6), 795–824. https://doi.org/10.1080/10409280903475444

Querido, J. G., Bearss, K., & Eyberg, S. M. (2002). Parent/child interaction therapy. *Comprehensive handbook of psychotherapy: Cognitive-Behavioral Approaches, 2*, 91–113.

Rathod, S., Gega, L., Degnan, A., Pikard, J., Khan, T., Husain, N., Munshi, T., & Naeem, F. (2018). The current status of culturally adapted mental health interventions: a practice-focused review of meta-analyses. *Neuropsychiatric Disease & Treatment, 14*, 165–178. https://doi.org/10.2147/NDT.S138430

Reiss, F. (2013). Socioeconomic inequalities and mental health problems in children and adolescents: A systematic review. *Social Science & Medicine, 90*, 24–31. https://doi.org/10.1016/j.socscimed.2013.04.026

Rodgers, C. R. R., Flores, M. W., Bassey, O., Augenblick, J. M., & Cook, B. L. (2022). Racial/ethnic disparity trends in children's mental health care access and expenditures from 2010-2017: Disparities remain despite sweeping policy reform. *Journal of the American Academy of Child & Adolescent Psychiatry, 61*(7), 915–925. https://doi.org/10.1016/j.jaac.2021.09.420

Substance Abuse & Mental Health Services Administration. (2014). *SAMHSA's concept of trauma and guidance for a trauma-informed approach*. https://store.samhsa.gov/sites/default/files/d7/priv/sma14-4884.pdf

Sanders, M. R. (1999). Triple P-Positive Parenting Program: Towards an empirically validated multilevel parenting and family support strategy for the prevention of behavior and emotional problems in children. *Clinical Child & Family Psychology Review, 2*, 71–90. https://doi.org/10.1023/A:1021843613840

Sanders, M. R., Kirby, J. N., Tellegen, C. L., & Day, J. J. (2014). The Triple P-Positive Parenting Program: A systematic review and meta-analysis of a multi-level system of parenting support. *Clinical Psychology Review, 34*(4), 337–357. https://doi.org/10.1016/j.cpr.2014.04.003

Sanders, M. R., & Mazzucchelli, T. G. (Eds.). (2018). *The power of positive parenting: Transforming the lives of children, parents, and communities using the Triple P System*. Oxford University Press.

Sanders, M. R., Divan, G., Singhal, M., Turner, K. M., Velleman, R., Michelson, D., & Patel, V. (2022). Scaling up parenting interventions is critical for attaining the sustainable development goals. *Child Psychiatry & Human Development, 53*(5), 941–952. https://doi.org/10.1007/s10578-021-01171-0

Schlack, R., Peerenboom, N., Neuperdt, L., Junker, S., & Beyer, A. K. (2021). The effects of mental health problems in childhood and adolescence in young adults: Results of the KiGGS cohort. *Journal of Health Monitoring, 6*(4), 3–19. https://doi.org/10.25646/8863

Schmidt, S. W. (2007). The relationship between satisfaction with workplace training and overall job satisfaction. *Human Resource Development Quarterly, 18*, 481–498. https://doi.org/10.1002/hrdq.1216

Shonkoff, J. P., Boyce, W. T., & McEwen, B. S. (2009). Neuroscience, molecular biology, and the childhood roots of health disparities: Building a new framework for health promotion and disease prevention. *Journal of the American Medical Association, 301*(21), 2252–2259. https://doi.org/10.1001/jama.2009.754

Silver, H. C., Davis Schoch, A. E., Loomis, A. M., Park, C. E., & Zinsser, K. M. (2023). Updating the evidence: A systematic review of a decade of Infant and Early Childhood Mental Health Consultation (IECMHC) research. *Infant Mental Health Journal, 44*(1), 5–26. https://doi.org/10.1002/imhj.22033

Smith, T. E., Sheridan, S. M., Kim, E. M., Park, S., & Beretvas, S. N. (2020). The effects of family-school partnership interventions on academic and social-emotional functioning: A

meta-analysis exploring what works for whom. *Educational Psychology Review, 32*, 511–544. https://doi.org/10.1007/s10648-019-09509-w
Snell-Johns, J., Mendez, J. L., & Smith, B. H. (2004). Evidence-based solutions for overcoming access barriers, decreasing attrition, and promoting chance with underserved families. *Journal of Family Psychology, 18*, 19–35.
Spielberger, J., Burkhardt, T., Winje, C., Gouvea, M., & Barisik, E. (2016). *Evaluation of the fussy baby network advanced training*. Chicago, IL: Chapin Hall at the University of Chicago. https://www.chapinhall.org/research/relationship-based-approach-to-early-home-visiting-impacts-staff-familyperspectives/
Staudt M. (2007a). Helping children access and use services: A review. *Journal of Child & Family Studies, 12*, 49–60.
Staudt, M. (2007b). Treatment engagement with caregivers of at-risk children: Gaps in research and conceptualization. *Journal of Child and Family Studies, 16*, 183–196.
Stevens, J., Kelleher, K. J., Ward-Estes, J., & Hayes, J. (2006). Perceived barriers to treatment and psychotherapy attendance in child community mental health centers. *Community Mental Health Journal, 42*(5), 449–458. https://doi.org/10.1007/s10597-006-9048-5
Stroul, B. A., Blau, G. M., & Larsen, J. (2021). *The evolution of the system of care approach*. The Institute for Innovation and Implementation, School of Social Work, University of Maryland. https://www.cmhnetwork.org/wp-content/uploads/2021/05/The-Evolution-of-the-SOC-Approach-FINAL-5-27-20211.pdf.
Substance Abuse and Mental Health Services Administration. (2023). *FY 2023 linking actions for unmet needs in child health*. U.S. Department of Health & Human Services, https://www.samhsa.gov/grants/grant-announcements/sm-23-004#:~:text=Description,thrive%20in%20school%20and%20beyond
Swanson, J. D., & Wadhwa, P. M. (2008). Developmental origins of child mental health disorders. *Journal of Child Psychology and Psychiatry, & Allied Disciplines, 49*(10), 1009–1019. https://doi.org/10.1111/j.1469-7610.2008.02014.x
Thomas, R., Abell, B., Webb, H. J., Avdagic, E., & Zimmer-Gembeck, M. J. (2017). Parent-child interaction therapy: A meta-analysis. *Pediatrics, 140*(3). https://doi.org/10.1542/peds.2017-0352
Title IV-E Prevention Services Clearinghouse (2022). *Effective Black parenting program*. Title IV-E Prevention Services Clearinghouse. https://preventionservices.acf.hhs.gov/programs/460/show
U.S. Department of Health and Human Services, Administration for Children and Families, Office of Head Start, National Center on Parent, Family, and Community Engagement (2018). *Head start parent, family, and community engagement framework*. https://eclkc.ohs.acf.hhs.gov/sites/default/files/pdf/pfce-framework.pdf
Valado, T., Tracey, J., Goldfinger, J., & Briggs, R. (2019). Healthy Steps: Transforming the promise of pediatric care. *The Future of Children, 29*(1), 99–122. https://www.jstor.org/stable/26639558
Vasileva, M., Graf, R. K., Reinelt, T., Petermann, U., & Petermann, F. (2021). Research review: A meta-analysis of the international prevalence and comorbidity of mental disorders in children between 1 and 7 years. *Journal of Child Psychology & Psychiatry, 62*(4), 372–381. https://doi.org/10.1111/jcpp.13261
von Klitzing, K., Döhnert, M., Kroll, M., & Grube, M. (2015). Mental disorders in early childhood. *Deutsches Arzteblatt international, 112*(21–22), 375–386. https://doi.org/10.3238/arztebl.2015.0375
Weiss-Dagan, S., Ben-Porat, A., & Itzhaky, H. (2022). Secondary traumatic stress and vicarious post-traumatic growth among social workers who have worked with abused children. *Journal of Social Work, 22*(1), 170–187. https://doi.org/10.1177/1468017320981363
West, A., Madariaga, P., & Sparr, M. (2022). *Reflective supervision: What we know and what we need to know to support and strengthen the home visiting workforce (OPRE Report No. 2022–101)*. Office of Planning, Research, and Evaluation; Administration for Children and Families; U.S. Department of Health and Human Services. https://www.acf.hhs.gov/opre/report/reflective-supervision-what-we-know-and-what-we-need-know-support-and-strengthen-home

Williams, D. R., Costa, M. V., Odunlami, A. O., & Mohammed, S. A. (2008). Moving upstream: How interventions that address the social determinants of health can improve health and reduce disparities. *Journal of Public Health Management and Practice, 14*(6), S8–S17. https://doi.org/10.1097/01.PHH.0000338382.36695.42

Williams, J. C., Ball, M., Roscoe, N., Harowitz, J., Hobbs, R. J., Raman, H. N., Seltzer, M. K., Vo, L. C., Cagande, C. C., Alexander-Bloch, A. F., Glahn, D. C., & Morrow, L. (2023). Widening Racial Disparities During COVID-19 Telemedicine transition: A study of child mental health services at two large children's hospitals. *Journal of the American Academy of Child and Adolescent Psychiatry, 62*(4), 447–456. https://doi.org/10.1016/j.jaac.2022.07.848

World Health Organization (WHO). (1999). *International classification of diseases, tenth revision, clinical modification* (10th ed., text rev.). https://www.cdc.gov/nchs/icd/icd-10-cm.htm

World Health Organization (WHO). (2022, June 17). *Mental health.* https://www.who.int/news-room/fact-sheets/detail/mental-health-strengthening-our-response

Yoshikawa, H., Aber, J. L., & Beardslee, W. R. (2012). The effects of poverty on the mental, emotional, and behavioral health of children and youth: Implications for prevention. *American Psychologist, 67*(4), 272–284. https://doi.org/10.1037/a0028015

Zach, A., Meyer, N., Hendrowarsito, L., Kolb, S., Bolte, G., Nennstiel-Ratzel, U., Stilianakis, N. I., Herr, C., & GME Study Group. (2016). Association of sociodemographic and environmental factors with the mental health status among preschool children—Results from a cross-sectional study in Bavaria, Germany. *International Journal of Hygiene and Environmental Health, 219*(4–5), 458–467. https://doi.org/10.1016/j.ijheh.2016.04.012

Zero to Three. (2016). *DC:0–5: Diagnostic classification of mental health and developmental disorders of infancy and early childhood.* Zero to Three.

Zero to Three. (2017). *The basics of infancy and early childhood mental health: A briefing paper.* https://www.zerotothree.org/resource/the-basics-of-infant-and-early-childhood-mental-health-a-briefing-paper/

Zero to Three. (2023). *Infant and early childhood mental health.* https://www.zerotothree.org/issue-areas/infant-and-early-childhood-mental-health/

Chapter 3
Family Engagement in Mental Health Interventions in the Early Elementary School Years

Jeffrey Waid

Background

The early elementary school years are an important period for children's mental health and well-being. Defined as the time between kindergarten and third grade, the early elementary school years help shape the architecture of children's brain development and provide the foundation for mental health later in life (Center on the Developing Child, 2023). During these years children become increasingly aware of the world around them, begin to show interest in the thoughts and feelings of others, and build capacity for seeing things from another's point of view. During this time children also begin to develop friendships, interact with other children and adults, and begin to develop a sense of identity (McClean, 2020). For some children, this period is also marked by the onset of certain mood, behavioral, and developmental disorders. Common mental health conditions which emerge during the elementary school years include depression, anxiety, attention-deficit/hyperactivity disorder, oppositional defiant disorder, conduct disorder, obsessive-compulsive disorder, eating disorder, post-traumatic stress disorder, Tourette syndrome, and autism spectrum disorder (National Institute of Mental Health, 2021). Prevalence estimates from the United States indicate one in six children aged 2–8 years of age are diagnosed with one or more of these mental health conditions (Perou et al., 2013). Global prevalence estimates for mental illness among children ages 5 and above range from 4 to 16.1%, although these estimates exclude some low- and

A Chapter Submitted to Family Engagement in Mental Health Interventions for Young Children

J. Waid (✉)
School of Social Work, College of Education and Human Development, University of Minnesota – Twin Cities, Saint Paul, MN, USA
e-mail: jdwaid@umn.edu

L. Nabors, J. D. Bartlett (eds.), *Family Engagement in Mental Health Interventions for Young Children*, Springer Series on Child and Family Studies,
https://doi.org/10.1007/978-3-031-47917-5_3

middle-income countries where epidemiological data does not exist or is of poor quality (Erskine et al., 2017).

There are a number of risk and protective factors associated with the development of mental illness during the elementary school years. Risk factors vary by mental health condition, but typically include child, family, community, economic, structural, and historical contributors. Gene-environment interaction, cumulative risk exposure, and social determinants of health are particularly helpful frameworks for understanding the multitude of ways children can develop mental illness (Alegría et al., 2018; Assary et al., 2018; Evans et al., 2013). Protective factors on the other hand can buffer risk processes and promote children's mental health and well-being (Wille et al., 2008). Protective factors are family specific and include individual (e.g., temperament, problem-solving), family (parent-child attachment, nurturing, and support), and extrafamilial processes (e.g., community supports and connections) (Fraser et al., 1999). It is also generally agreed that early engagement with mental health services is an important protective factor which may help reduce the severity and trajectory of mental illness and, in some instances, may help prevent the development of some mental health disorders altogether (McGorry & Mei, 2018; Minnis et al., 2022).

There are currently a range of efficacious and effective practices available to treat and resolve symptoms of mental illness during the early elementary school years (Hoagwood et al., 2001; Ribeiro et al., 2023). Unfortunately, engaging with children's mental health services can be difficult for many families. Prevalence estimates from the United States suggest 18–50% of children with a known mental health condition experience unmet mental health-care needs (Graaf et al., 2022; Merikangas et al., 2010). In low- and middle-income countries, the prevalence of untreated childhood mental health conditions is estimated to be much higher (Patel et al., 2013).

Barriers to accessing and engaging with children's mental health care are complex and multidimensional. A recent review of mental health services research identified a set of common factors which impede engagement with children's mental health care, which include family, provider, community, and health-care system contributors (Waid & Kelly, 2020). At the family level, common barriers to mental health service engagement include individual and family attitudes toward mental illness and help seeking, lack of awareness of available treatment options, concerns related to the logistics scheduling and attending appointments (i.e., transportation, day care, time away from work), negative attitudes toward mental health providers, and concerns for the mental health provider's ability to meet their needs. At the provider level, barriers include long waiting lists and delays to first appointments; limited evening and weekend options; inflexible policies for cancellation and rescheduling; lack of linguistically, culturally, and developmental responsive services; and limited specialist availability. At the community level, lack of services within a family's geographic area, cultural stigma toward mental illness and mental health help seeking, and lack of anonymity in the help seeking process limit access to mental health care. Health-care system barriers include mental health-care costs (i.e., inadequate funding, complex insurance authorization, out-of-pocket expenses), lack of coordination across child-serving systems, and qualified workforce shortages. Families may experience multiple barriers to mental health care concurrently, within and across family, provider, community, and health-care system domains (Waid & Kelly, 2020).

Early and well-timed connection to mental health care can improve the mental health and well-being of children during the early elementary school years. Barriers to mental health care are multidimensional and can delay or inhibit access to effective services, which can be detrimental to children's health and development over time. To meaningfully address the mental health needs of children during the elementary school years, it is important for practitioners, providers, and systems of care to be adept at engaging families, identifying and resolving barriers to care, and facilitating connection to needed services.

Approaches to Intervention

A number of promotive factors and strategies exist to support timely connection to children's mental health care. At the family level, mental health awareness, family resources, support for mental health help seeking, and caregiver-initiated referrals can promote access to children's mental health care. At the provider level, flexibility, culturally centered, and child-friendly services can attract families and facilitate connection and engagement during the treatment process. Mental health services must also be accessible and suitable to the communities being served. At the systems level, embedding services within primary health-care and educational settings, and a commitment to sustained community engagement and relationship development can foster trust between communities and care providers and facilitate engagement with children's mental health care (Waid & Kelly, 2020).

Recently, evidence-informed service navigation strategies have also emerged to support child and family engagement with children's mental health care (Waid et al., 2021). These interventions are diverse with respect to their duration, intensity, and method of delivery, but share a common goal of assisting families in navigating the health-care system and facilitating connection to mental health services. Broadly, strategies to support connection to mental health care include practitioner-mediated, technology-mediated, and integrated care approaches (Waid & Kelly, 2020).

Practitioner-Mediated Interventions

Interventions that are delivered by practitioners and service providers represent the majority of approaches currently available to support family engagement with children's mental health services. These programs typically require sustained engagement with the family and the provision of emotional (i.e., empathy and compassion) and instrumental support (i.e., arranging transportation, sharing information, mediating conversations) to resolve barriers and facilitate access to mental health care. Approaches are diverse and can be delivered in person, remotely, or in combination by peers, paraprofessionals, social workers, nurses, and clinicians (Waid et al., 2021). Common elements of effective programs include engagement, assessment, psychoeducation, empowerment and advocacy, fostering self-efficacy, managing expectations, and encouraging family support (Hoagwood, 2005). To keep families engaged during the service navigation process, it is recommended practitioners continually include family members in the treatment planning process, focus on strengthening coping skills, increasing mental health literacy, and destigmatizing mental illness. For clinician led-programs, cognitive-behavioral strategies targeting negative attributions about mental health treatment and engagement are also indicated (Becker et al., 2015; Ingoldsby, 2010; Lindsey et al., 2014; Xu et al., 2018).

Technology-Mediated Interventions

Technology-mediated strategies such as websites and smartphone applications have also been developed to support family engagement with children's mental health care. These strategies typically are self-guided, with drop-down menus and options for the user to custom-tailor their search for services, email and text reminders for upcoming appointments, and direct message communication with the mental health treatment provider. Research on technology-mediated strategies are inconclusive, but common elements of promising programs include accessibility, ease and efficiency of use, and potential for personalization (Hollis et al., 2017). Technology-mediated strategies are particularly helpful for collaboration and coordination of care (e.g., identification of potential services, scheduling appointments, between-session communication, and reminders) and may be particularly valuable when combined with practitioner-mediated provision of emotional and instrumental supports (McGrath et al., 2011; Peters et al., 2018).

Integrated Care Approaches

Integrating mental health care into other child-serving systems, such as primary care and school settings, can promote service engagement and improve clinical and functional outcomes. Integrated care is achieved by co-locating mental health services within other general medical and specialty care settings (Friedberg & Paternastro, 2019; Yonek et al., 2020). Providers and families engage in intentional collaboration to promote the integration of referrals, assessment, treatment, and progress monitoring. Integrated care in pediatric settings has been shown to improve children's behavioral health outcomes, with a more pronounced treatment effect for intervention- versus prevention-oriented mental health services (Asarnow et al., 2015). Similar treatment effects are observed in school-based mental health programs, again with a more pronounced treatment effect for intervention- versus prevention-oriented programs (Sanchez et al., 2018). Larger effects were also noted for mental health services that were integrated into the child's academic instruction, employed contingency management principles, and were delivered multiple times per week (Sanchez et al., 2018).

Engagement Strategies

A range of evidence-informed strategies exist to support family engagement with children's mental health care during the elementary school years. These strategies can be deployed as a combination of strategies or as part of a larger continuum of integrated care. Engaging in these strategies can help facilitate connection to care and promote child and family well-being.

Rapport

For practitioners, the ability to develop and maintain rapport is foundational to working with families and children in need of mental health care. Broadly, rapport refers to a relationship characterized by mutual understanding, connection, and cooperation (Leach, 2005). Rapport is co-constructed and continually renegotiated over the course of the working relationship. High levels of rapport can build trust, which can lead to more authentic interactions and improved child and family outcomes. Lack of rapport on the other hand can lead to mistrust and disagreement and is disruptive to the helping process. Practitioners can build rapport by centralizing the working relationship, establishing a shared sense of purpose, listening carefully, and prioritizing the family's needs and preferences at each step in the helping process. When rapport is disrupted, practitioners should validate family members' experiences and work intentionally to repair the working relationship before continuing with service navigation activities.

Because rapport is co-constructed, practitioners must also balance the personal and professional dimensions of their practice to create and maintain rapport with families. This can be achieved by creating and maintaining appropriate boundaries, building emotional intelligence (i.e., knowledge and awareness of one's own emotions, ability, and motivation to understand the emotions of others), and creating and sustaining reflexive (e.g., insight-oriented) practices. Approaching families from a strengths-based and solution-focused orientation can help practitioners to build rapport and sustain meaningful working relationships with families over time (DeJong & Miller, 1995; Ingram, 2013).

When working with children during the early elementary school years, it is important to integrate developmental and family systems considerations into the rapport-building process. Because of the younger age of the children, caregivers should be included in all aspects of the navigation planning process. Child-friendly and developmentally appropriate language, vocal tone, and body posture are also important. Children should be engaged authentically, with care taken by the practitioner not to exaggerate or lead the child's communication. If the practitioner is working with the child independently of the caregiver at any time, such as in a school setting, it is important to establish ground rules for what can be expected during the encounters, as well as limits to confidentiality and expectations surrounding communication between the practitioner, child, and parents. If meeting with the child in a clinic or office setting, taking time to ensure the built environment is child-friendly (e.g., child-size furniture, art, games, etc.) can strengthen rapport by signaling to the child the space is designed with them in mind (Cameron, 2005; O'Reilly & Dolan, 2016).

Empathy

The ability to convey and display empathy is a critical skill for practitioners who wish to engage families with children who are experiencing difficulties accessing and engaging mental health services. Broadly, empathy refers to the ability to sense, understand, and imagine what others are experiencing. Like rapport, empathy is critical to establishing trust and authenticity in the helping relationship (Moudatsou et al., 2020). Empathy includes cognitive, affective, and behavioral components. Cognitive empathy involves identifying and understanding another's experiences, from their perspective. Affective empathy involves identifying the emotional state of another and to feel the same way as that person (Watson, 2016). In the helping relationship, behavioral empathy is the compassionate actions taken by the professional to assist the client in resolving the presenting challenges (Gladstein, 1983).

To empathically engage children and families, practitioners must be capable of creating shared representations of the families' lived experience. This requires practitioners to pay careful attention to all aspects of verbal and nonverbal communication from an open and nonjudgmental position. Practitioners must also have a strong sense of self-awareness that allows them to disentangle their own emotions and experiences from the emotions and experiences of the child and family, and an ability to flexibly alternate between empathic engagement and self-regulation in the helping process (Gerdes & Segal, 2011).

The empathy-building process has been described by various scholars and practitioners as a practice which unfolds in a series of steps. The first step requires practitioners to explore the family's situation from a position of openness and curiosity. This allows the practitioner to become familiar with family members' thoughts, feelings, and experiences. Then, there is a deliberate step wherein the practitioner imagines what it is like to have these thoughts, feelings, and experiences personally. The practitioner communicates their sense of the experience to the family to connect with them and to receive feedback. Then, the practitioner decentralizes their personal experiences to continue the helping process. This conscious and cyclical process is undertaken by the practitioner over the course of the helping relationship (Gladstein, 1983).

Family-Centered Care

Family-centered care is an approach to care coordination and service delivery that aligns health-care practices with the family's needs, values, and preferences. In a family-centered framework, care providers work collaboratively with families to address their needs using a whole-person approach which integrates physical, mental health, and social care needs. Services are also coordinated and delivered in ways that are collaborative and responsive to the family's goals (Kokorelias et al., 2019).

There are a number of strategies available to assist practitioners in working with families from a family-centered perspective. First, providers must listen to the family's needs and cultivate two-way communication that is found in mutual respect. This involves actively listening to their needs, values, and goals, attending to nonverbal cues, and asking questions to help clarify concerns and understanding of the service navigation process. Practitioners also must provide families with all the information that is necessary to make informed decisions about their children's care plan, and engage in ongoing discussions to clarify questions and gain consensus. Person-centered care has been shown to improve patients' experiences of the health-care system and improve clinical and functional outcomes (Santana et al., 2018). In the context of children's mental health help-seeking and service engagement, person- and family-centered care helps assure risk and protective factors salient to the development of mental illness are considered and that treatment planning is aligned with the families' values, beliefs, and preferences (Waid et al., 2022, 2023).

Flexibility

Families of elementary school-age children often must manage competing responsibilities, which can result in no-shows and cancellations of appointments and disconnection from the help-seeking process. Practitioner flexibility and intentional consideration of the logistical barrier's families experience can help maintain rapport and keep families connected to the help-seeking process. Offering appointments at times that are convenient for the family, including evenings and weekends, helps reduce the burden of help seeking and time it takes away from other family obligations such as work and school. The ability to flexibly pivot the format of service delivery from in-person navigation to telephone or text message can also help maintain open lines of communication around service needs, barriers and facilitators, and progress toward mental health service access and engagement (Waid et al., 2023).

Collaborative Goal Planning

Collaborative planning and clear articulation of the intended goals of service navigation are essential to promoting children's engagement with mental health care. The process of goal planning provides families and practitioners with a shared vision of the future and what things will look and be like when the barriers to care have been resolved. Typically, the goals of service access are articulated by the family and recorded by the practitioner. Goals are intended to be revisited routinely during the course of service navigation and accompanied by systematic and ongoing evaluation of progress (Poulsen et al., 2015). Goals can be written for individuals (e.g., my child will receive an assessment and begin mental health treatment by a specific date), families (e.g., parents will alternate work shifts to ensure reliable transportation of children to and from appointments), and systems (e.g., family and practitioner will coordinate recommendations from the assessment and mental health-care plan with the child's health-care and school-based providers). Goals should describe how things will be when the presenting problems are resolved, and the course of intervention has been successful. Therefore, goals should be written in strengths-based and solution-focused language. To keep goal planning manageable, practitioners should work with clients to identify the most important things they wish to accomplish (e.g., 3–5 goals).

Once the family has identified, clarified, and prioritized their goals, the practitioner should assist the family in breaking down the goals into objectives and tasks. While goals are the broad, long-term outcomes of intervention (e.g., my child will receive culturally appropriate mental health services from a provider we trust), the objectives are medium-term benchmarks or milestones that, when accomplished, help move the family toward goal completion (e.g., I will identify a provider whose therapeutic approach and cultural orientation are the best-fit provider to my family's needs). Tasks are the behavioral activities and sequential steps taken over days and weeks to accomplish plan objectives (e.g., I will create a list of mental health-care providers who share my culture, work with children, accept my insurance, and have favorable online reviews and ratings). Objectives and tasks should be specific, measurable, attainable, relevant to the goal, and time bound. They should describe who will be involved, what will be done, how frequently the activity will occur, and how long the activity will need to take place for the goal to be accomplished (Bailey, 2017; Centers for Disease Control and Prevention, 2022). Routine and ongoing monitoring of service navigation plans can promote effective mental health service navigation by providing families and practitioners with information about working and what needs to change during the navigation process.

Education and Problem-Solving

Working collaboratively with families to identify and resolve problems that come up is an important part of the service navigation process. The first step in the problem-solving process involves helping families clarify the situation and context surrounding the presenting issues. This requires exploration of circumstances surrounding the problem and its relationship to mental health service engagement. Oftentimes, it can be helpful for practitioners to provide education to address misinterpretation and misunderstanding of mental illness and mental health care during this process (Hoagwood et al., 2010; Miklowitz et al., 2020).

Once awareness of the problem and its context has been clarified, the practitioner explores the families' motivations to address and resolve it. If the family is ambivalent, the practitioner should explore the families' understandings and perceptions in greater detail, and work to uncover the intrinsic and extrinsic factors which motivate them to either resolve the problem or continue with things as they are currently. Once family motivations are clarified, potential solutions can be explored and considered. Potential solutions consider the family's perceptions and understanding of the problem, its antecedents, and contributing factors. Parameters are drawn around potential solutions to determine what is feasible and acceptable to the family. Then, the specific steps required to resolve the problem are clarified in an action plan. This includes specifying what needs to occur, who will be involved, what will happen, and how long specific activities will need to occur to achieve problem resolution (Bagassi & Macchi, 2020; Dostál, 2015).

Self-Efficacy

The process of connecting and engaging with children's mental health care can require sustained efforts on the part of families and practitioners. To maintain motivation and improve the potential for families to resolve barriers independently in the future, it can be helpful to work to promote and strengthen caregiver and family self-efficacy. Self-efficacy is an important driver of health behavior and family wellness (Albanese et al., 2019; Strecher et al., 1986) and, when strengthened, may support engagement and sustained commitment to the help-seeking process (Sheeran et al., 2016). To build and maintain motivation and assist families in resolving barriers to care, practitioners should work to identify, promote, and strengthen family members' self-efficacy.

Self-efficacy refers to an individual's belief in their ability to learn and perform at an expected level (Schunk & DiBenedetto, 2021). In the context of mental health service navigation, self-efficacy refers to the family's expectation that they can access the services they need and that accessing needed services will resolve or ameliorate their child's mental health challenges. Self-efficacy is influenced by personal, social/environmental, and behavior factors (Glatz et al., 2023). Personal factors include one's sense of agency and belief they can access care that will be helpful to them; an ability to consider, plan, and problem-solve barriers to care; and an ability to manage frustration and remain committed in the face of persistent barriers. Social and environmental factors include cues and feedback that signal the family is on the right track, like receiving positive encouragement, learning that others in similar situations have successfully resolved similar challenges, or checking an objective or goal off of their service access plan. Behavioral factors refer to the effort and persistence required to achieve the service goals and objectives.

To strengthen self-efficacy, practitioners should work with families to clarify their expectations for change. If there is little expectation the situation will improve, the practitioner should seek to understand what the family attributes to these expectations. This can be accomplished by exploring the families' previous experiences and efforts to change to the problem, clarifying what happened, and identifying what needs to be happen differently for the problem to be resolved. This can be done during the assessment process, when goals are set and broken down into objectives and tasks. Providing education and demonstration of the skills required to accomplish the plan goals and supporting families as they engage in service navigation activities can build competence and confidence, which can lead to higher feelings of self-efficacy. This can increase family motivation and strengthen their capacity to resolve future barriers independently in the future.

Resilience

Lack of access to children's mental health care can cause stress in the family system and contribute to children's mental health challenges. Promoting and strengthening family resilience can help offset these stressors and promote child and family mental health and well-being. Broadly, resilience refers to the ability to adapt, respond, and thrive despite exposure to significant or persistent adversity (Fraser et al., 1999). Resilience is not a trait or characteristic but instead a dynamic and multisystem process which involves a high degree of interaction between protective and promotive factors within and between individuals, family, and community (Ungar et al., 2013). Personal and interpersonal skills, social support, positive peer and parent-child relationships, family problem-solving, parental resilience, and goal orientation are associated with higher levels of resilience and are associated with fewer mental health problems in childhood and adolescence (Mesman et al., 2021). Working to illuminate and strengthen resilience during the navigation process can improve child and family well-being (Waid et al., 2022).

Practitioners can strengthen child, caregiver, and family resilience by educating families about the nature of resilience, teaching coping and stress management, and reframing difficult situations from a strength's perspective (Walsh 2003, 2016). This can help family members call upon internal and external resources to cope with stressors and address presenting challenges. Helping caregivers learn to identify and manage the sources of stress and response to adversity in healthy and appropriate ways can improve caregiver well-being, which better positions them to help their child. To strengthen family resilience, practitioners should establish a strong rapport, display empathy, and role model problem-solving skills. Practitioners can empower families to call upon internal and external resources by teaching coping and self-care strategies, reframing negative attributions, encouraging connection to their community, and facilitating caregiver connection to their own mental health services (Patterson, 1995; Waid et al., 2022).

Critical Issues, Considerations, and Limitations of Current Knowledge

There are a number of structural factors which limit family access to children's mental health care which are difficult to resolve through family- and organization-level interventions. Lack of transportation, qualified workforce shortages, and mental health care costs are common barriers that require policy solutions. Social and socioeconomic conditions such as poverty, food insecurity, and housing instability are common social determinants of health which are associated with underutilization of children's mental health care (Alegría et al., 2015). To address these issues, practitioners should plan to assess the family's social determinants of mental health and assist them in navigating to basic needs, as part of navigating to children's mental health care.

Social and cultural factors also affect the service navigation process. Racism and mistreatment by the health-care system have affected community trust in mental health services. This, along with cultural and language barriers and a lack of culturally qualified providers, can affect efforts to support family engagement with children's mental health care (Paradies et al., 2015; Silva et al., 2016). To address these issues, it is important to provide information to families that is culturally relevant, including materials that are printed in the family's language, and to assist families in connecting to culturally relevant care. Navigation support can also be provided by a member of the cultural community who can act as a cultural broker and liaison to health-care systems.

Conclusion

The care engagement strategies discussed in this chapter are promising with respect to children's mental health-care access and engagement. Practitioners and care organizations can deploy these practices in part or as a combination of strategies to support family access to children's mental health care. Additional research investigating these strategies across settings, contexts, and populations can strengthen the evidence for children's mental health service navigation approaches. In addition, policy solutions to address social determinants of mental health, qualified workforce shortages, mental health-care costs, and barriers to cross-sector collaboration can help to address systemic barriers to care, promote children's mental health-care access, and improve child and family well-being.

References

Albanese, A. M., Russo, G. R., & Geller, P. A. (2019). The role of parental self-efficacy in parent and child well-being: A systematic review of associated outcomes. *Child: Care, Health and Development, 45*, 333–363. https://doi.org/10.1111/cch.12661

Alegría, M., Green, J. G., McLaughlin, K. A., & Loder, S. (2015). *Disparities in child and adolescent mental health and mental health services in the US*. William T. Grant Foundation.

Alegría, M., NeMoyer, A., Falgàs Bagué, I., Wang, Y, & Alvarez, K. (2018). Social determinants of mental health: Where we are and where we need to go. *Current Psychiatry Reports, 20*, 95 (20 pages). https://doi.org/10.1007/s11920-018-0969

Asarnow, J. R., Rozenman, M., Wiblin, J., & Zeltzer, L. (2015). Integrated medical-behavioral care compared with usual primary care for child and adolescent behavioral health: A meta-analysis. *JAMA Pediatrics, 169*, 929–937. https://doi.org/10.1001/jamapediatrics.2015.1141

Assary, E., Vincent, J. P., Keers, R., & Pluess, M. (2018). Gene-environment interaction and psychiatric disorders: Review and future directions. *Seminars in Cell & Developmental Biology, 77*, 133–143. https://doi.org/10.1016/j.semcdb.2017.10.016

Bagassi, M., & Macchi, L. (2020). Creative problem solving as overcoming a misunderstanding. *Frontiers in Education, 5*, 538202. https://doi.org/10.3389/feduc.2020.538202

Bailey, R. R. (2017). Goal setting and action planning for health behavior change. *American Journal of Lifestyle Medicine, 13*, 615–618. https://doi.org/10.1177/1559827617729634

Becker, K., Lee, B., Daleiden, E., Lindsey, M., Brandt, N., & Chorpita, B. (2015). The common elements of engagement in children's mental health services: Which elements for which outcomes? *Journal of Clinical Child & Adolescent Psychology, 44*, 30–43. https://doi.org/10.1080/15374416.2013.814543

Cameron, H. (2005). Asking the tough questions: a guide to ethical practices in interviewing young children. *Early Child Development and Care, 175*, 597–610. https://doi.org/10.1080/03004430500131387

Center on the Developing Child. (2023). *Early childhood mental health*. Harvard University. Retrieved from https://developingchild.harvard.edu/science/deep-dives/mental-health/

Centers for Disease Control and Prevention. (2022). *SMART framework*. Retrieved from https://www.cdc.gov/healthyyouth/yac/smart-framework.htm#print

DeJong, P., & Miller, S. (1995). How to interview for client strengths. *Social Work, 40*, 729–736. https://doi.org/10.1093/sw/40.6.729

Dostál, J. (2015). Theory of problem solving. *Procedia Social and Behavioral Sciences, 174*, 2798–2805. https://doi.org/10.1016/j.sbspro.2015.01.970

Erskine, H. E., Baxter, A. J., Patton, G., Moffitt, T. E., Patel, V., Whiteford, H. A., & Scott, J. G. (2017). The global coverage of prevalence data for mental disorders in children and adolescents. *Epidemiology and Psychiatric Sciences, 26*(4), 395–402. https://doi.org/10.1017/S2045796015001158

Evans, G. W., Li, D., & Whipple, S. S. (2013). Cumulative risk and child development. *Psychological Bulletin, 139*, 1342–1396. https://doi.org/10.1037/a0031808

Fraser, M. W., Galinsky, M. J., & Richman, J. M. (1999). Risk, protection, and resilience: Towards a conceptual framework for social work practice. *Social Work Research, 23*, 131–143. https://doi.org/10.1093/swr/23.3.131

Friedberg, R. D., & Paternostro, J. K. (2019). The value of integrated pediatric behavioral health care. In R. D. Friedberg & J. K. Paternostro (Eds.), *Handbook of cognitive behavioral therapy for pediatric medical conditions* (pp. 11–20). Springer. https://doi.org/10.1007/978-3-030-21683-2_2

Gerdes, K. E., & Segal, E. (2011). Importance of empathy for social work practice: Integrating new science. *Social Work, 56*, 141–148. https://doi.org/10.1093/sw/56.2.141

Gladstein, G. A. (1983). Understanding empathy: Integrating counseling, developmental, and social psychology perspectives. *American Psychological Association, 30*, 467–482. https://doi.org/10.1037/0022-0167.30.4.467

Glatz, T., Lippold, M., Chung, G., & Jensen, T. (2023). A systematic review of parental self-efficacy among parents of school-age children and adolescents. *Adolescent Research Review, 2023*. https://doi.org/10.1007/s40894-023-00216-w

Graaf, G., Hooley, C., Baiden, P., & Keyes, L. (2022). Parent reported barriers to children's mental health services in the United States. *Social Work in Mental Health*. Advance online publication. https://doi.org/10.1080/15332985.2022.2155503.

Hoagwood, K. E. (2005). Family-based services in children's mental health: A research review and synthesis. *Journal of Child Psychology and Psychiatry, 46*, 690–713. https://doi.org/10.1111/j.1469-7610.2005.01451.x

Hoagwood, K., Burns, B. J., Kiser, L., Ringeisen, H., & Schoenwald, S. K. (2001). Evidence-based practice in child and adolescent mental health services. *Psychiatric Services, 9*, 1179–1189. https://doi.org/10.1176/appi.ps.52.9.1179

Hoagwood, K. E., Cavaleri, M. A., Olin, S. S., Burns, B. J., Slaton, E., Gruttadato, D., & Hughes, R. (2010). Family support in children's mental health: a review and synthesis. *Clinical Child and Family Psychology Review, 13*, 1–45. https://doi.org/10.1007/s10567-009-0060-5

Hollis, C., Falconer, C. J., Martin, J. L., Whittington, C., Stockton, S., Glazebrook, C., & Davies, E. B. (2017). Annual research review: Digital health interventions for children and young people with mental health problems - a systematic and meta-review. *Journal of Child Psychology and Psychiatry, and Allied Disciplines, 58*(4), 474–503.

Ingoldsby, E. M. (2010). Review of interventions to improve family engagement and retention in parent and child mental health programs. *Journal of Child and Family Studies, 19*, 629–645. https://doi.org/10.1007/s10826-009-9350-2

Ingram, R. (2013). Locating emotional intelligence at the heart of social work practice. *British Journal of Social Work, 43*, 987–1004. https://doi.org/10.1093/bjsw/bcs029

Kokorelias, K. M., Gignac, M. A. M., Naglie, G., & Cameron, J. I. (2019). Towards a universal model of family centered care: A scoping review. *BMC Health Services Research, 19*, 564. https://doi.org/10.1186/s12913-019-4394-5

Leach, M. J. (2005). Rapport: A key to treatment success. *Complementary Therapies in Clinical Practice, 11*(4), 262–265. https://doi.org/10.1016/j.ctcp.2005.05.005

Lindsey, M. A., Brandt, N. E., Becker, K. D., Lee, B. R., Barth, R. P., Daleiden, E. L., & Chorpita, B. F. (2014). Identifying the common elements of treatment engagement interventions in children's mental health services. *Clinical Child and Family Psychology Review, 17*, 283–298. https://doi.org/10.1007/s10567-013-0163-x

Mesman, E., Vreeker, A., & Hillegers, M. (2021). Resilience and mental health in children and adolescence: An update of the recent literature and future directions. *Current Opinion in Psychiatry, 34*, 586–592. https://doi.org/10.1097/YCO.0000000000000741

Modatsou, M., Stavropoulou, A., Philalithis, A., & Koukouli, S. (2020). The role of empathy in health and social care professionals. *Healthcare, 8*, 26. https://doi.org/10.3390/healthcare8010026

McClean, S. (2020). *Understanding child development: Ages 5–8 years*. National Workforce Center for Child Mental Health. Retrieved from https://emergingminds.com.au/resources/understanding-child-development-ages-5-8-years.

McGorry, P. D., & Mei, C. (2018). Early intervention in youth mental health: Progress and future directions. *BMJ Mental Health, 21*, 182–184. https://doi.org/10.1136/ebmental-2018-300060

McGrath, P. J., Lingley-Pottie, P., Thurston, C., MacLean, C., Cunningham, C., Waschbusch, D. A., Watters, C., Stewart, S., Bagnell, A., Santor, D., & Chaplin, W. (2011). Telephone-based mental health interventions for child disruptive behavior or anxiety disorders: Randomized trials and overall analysis. *Journal of the American Academy of Child & Adolescent Psychiatry, 50*, 1162–1172. https://doi.org/10.1016/j.jaac.2011.07.013

Merikangas, K. R., He, J.-P., Brody, D., Fisher, P. W., Bourdon, K., & Koretz, D. S. (2010). Prevalence and treatment of mental disorders among US children in the 2001–2004 NHANES. *Pediatrics, 125*(1), 75–81. https://doi.org/10.1542/peds.2008-2598

Miklowitz, D. J., Peris, T. S., & Lord, C. (2020). Helping families to understand and cope with psychiatric disorders in childhood-beyond basic facts. *JAMA Psychiatry, 77*(4), 433–434. https://doi.org/10.1001/jamapsychiatry.2019.4812

Minnis, H., Gajwani, R., & Ougrin, D. (2022). Editorial: Early intervention and prevention of severe mental illness: A child and adolescent psychiatry perspective. *Frontiers in Psychiatry, 13*, 963602. https://doi.org/10.3389/fpsyt.2022.963602

National Institute of Mental Health. (2021). *Children and mental health: Is it just a stage?* Retrieved from https://www.nimh.nih.gov/health/publications/children-and-mental-health

O'Reilly, L., & Dolan, P. (2016). The voice of the child in social work assessments: Age-appropriate communication with children. *British Journal of Social Work, 46*, 1191–1207. https://doi.org/10.1093/bjsw/bcv040

Paradies, Y., Ben, J., Denson, N., Elias, A., Priest, N., Pieterse, A., Gupta, A., Kelager, M., & Gee, G. (2015). Racism as a determinant of health: A systematic review and meta-analysis. *PLoS One, 10*, e0138511. https://doi.org/10.1371/journal.pone.0138511

Patel, V., Kieling, C., Maulik, P. K., & Divan, G. (2013). Improving access to care for children with mental disorders: A global perspective. *Archives of Disease in Childhood, 98*, 323–327. https://doi.org/10.1136/archdischild-2012-302079

Patterson, J. M. (1995). Promoting resilience in families experiencing stress. *Family Focused Pediatrics, 42*, 47–63. https://doi.org/10.1016/S0031-3955(16)38907-6

Perou, R., Bitsko, R. H., Blumberg, S. J., Pastor, P., Ghandour, R. M., Gfroerer, J. C., Hedden, S. L., Crosby, A. E., Visser, S. N., Schieve, L. A., Parks, S. E., Hall, J. E., Brody, D., Simile, C. M., Thompson. W. W., Baio, J., Avenevoli, S., Kogan, M. D., & Huang, L. N. (2013). Mental health surveillance among children – United States, 2005—2011. *Morbidity and Mortality Weekly Report, 62* (Suppl; May 16, 2013), 1–35. Retrieved from https://www.cdc.gov/mmwr/preview/mmwrhtml/su6202a1.htm?s_cid=su6202a1_w

Peters, K. M., Sadler, G., Miller, E., & Radovic, A. (2018). An electronic referral and social work protocol to improve access to mental health services. *Pediatrics, 142*, 1–12. https://doi.org/10.1542/peds.2017-2417

Poulsen, A. A., Ziviani, J., & Cuskelly, M. (2015). *Goal setting and motivation in therapy: engaging children and parents*. Jessica Kingsley Publishers.

Ribeiro, W. S., Grande, A. J., Hoffmann, M. S., Ziebold, C., McDaid, D., Fry, A., Peixoto, C., Miranda, C., King, D., Tomasi, C. D., Faustino, C., Leone, S., Moraes, S., Schäfer, A. A., Alves, V., Rosa, M. I., & Evans-Lacko, S. (2023). A systematic review of evidence-based interventions for child and adolescent mental health problems in low- and middle-income countries. *Comprehensive Psychiatry, 121*, 152358. https://doi.org/10.1016/j.comppsych.2022.152358

Sanchez, A. L., Cornacchio, D., Poznanski, B., Golik, A. M., Chou, T., & Comer, J. S. (2018). The effectiveness of school-based mental health services for elementary-aged children: A meta-analysis. *Journal of the American Academy of Child and Adolescent Psychiatry, 57*, 153–165. https://doi.org/10.1016/j.jaac.2017.11.022

Santana, M. J., Manalili, K., Jolley, R. J., Zelinsky, S., Quan, H., & Lu, M. (2018). How to practice person-centred care: A conceptual framework. *Health Expectations: An International Journal of Public Participation in Health Care and Health Policy, 21*, 429–440. https://doi.org/10.1111/hex.12640

Sheeran, P., Maki, A., Montanaro, E., Avishai-Yitshak, A., Bryan, A., Klein, W. M. P., Miles, E., & Rothman, A. J. (2016). The impact of changing attitudes, norms, and self-efficacy on health-related intentions and behavior: A meta-analysis. *Health Psychology, 35*, 1178–1188. https://doi.org/10.1037/hea0000387

Schunk, D. H., & DiBennedetto, M. K. (2021). Self-efficacy and human motivation. *Advances in Motivation Science, 8*, 153–179. https://doi.org/10.1016/bs.adms.2020.10.001

Silva, M., Loureiro, A., & Cardoso, G. (2016). Social determinants of mental health: A review of the evidence. *European Journal of Psychiatry, 30*, 259–2929.

Strecher, V. J., DeVellis, B. M., Becker, M. H., & Rosenstock, I. M. (1986). The role of self-efficacy in achieving health behavior change. *Health Education Quarterly, 13*, 73–91.

Ungar, M., Ghazinour, M., & Richter, J. (2013). Annual research review: What is resilience within the social ecology of human development? *Journal of Child Psychology and Psychiatry, 54*, 348–366. https://doi.org/10.1111/jcpp.12025

Waid, J., Donaldson, R., & Halpin, K. (2021). Mental health service navigation: A scoping review of programmatic features and research evidence. *Social Work in Mental Health, 19*, 60–79. https://doi.org/10.1080/15332985.2020.1870646

Waid, J., & Kelly, M. (2020). Supporting family engagement with child and adolescent mental health services: A scoping review. *Health and Social Care in the Community, 28*, 1333–1342. https://doi.org/10.1111/HSC.12947

Waid, J., Tomfohrde, O., & Kutzler, C. (2022). Promoting health and social equity through family navigation to prevention and early intervention services. *BMC Public Health, 22*, 1972. https://doi.org/10.1186/s12889-022-14320-4

Waid, J., Tomfohrde, O., & Kutlzer, C. (2023). Connecting and engaging with health and social care: Exploring the core components of a telephone and web-mediated family navigation prevention service. *Child & Family Social Work, 28*, 563–571. https://doi.org/10.1111/cfs.12985

Walsh, F. (2003). Family resilience: A framework for clinical practice. *Family Process, 42*(1), 1–18. https://doi.org/10.1111/j.1545-5300.2003.00001.x

Walsh, F. (2016). *Strengthening Family Resilience: Third Ed.* Guilford Press.

Watson, J. C. (2016). The role of empathy in psychotherapy: Theory, research, and practice. In D. J. Cain, K. Keenan, & S. Rubin (Eds.), *Humanistic psychotherapies: Handbook of research and practice* (pp. 115–145). American Psychological Association. https://doi.org/10.1037/14775-005

Wille, N., Bettge, S., Ravens-Sieberer, U., & the BELLA study group. (2008). Risk and protective factors for children's and adolescents' mental health: Results of the BELLA study. *European Child & Adolescent Psychiatry, 17*(Suppl 1), 133–147. https://doi.org/10.1007/s00787-008-1015-y

Xu, Z., Huang, F., Kösters, M., Staiger, T., Becker, T., Thornicroft, G., & Rüsch, N. (2018). Effectiveness of interventions to promote help-seeking for mental health problems: Systematic review and meta-analysis. *Psychological Medicine, 48*, 2658–2667. https://doi.org/10.1017/S0033291718001265

Yonek, J., Lee, C. M., Harrison, A., Mangurian, C., & Tolou-Shams, M. (2020). Key components of effective pediatric integrated mental health care models: A systematic review. *JAMA Pediatrics, 174*(5), 487–498. https://doi.org/10.1001/jamapediatrics.2020.0023

Chapter 4
Family Engagement in Mental Health Interventions for Children with Developmental Disabilities

Kayla M. Malone, Lee Anne Smith, Kelly W. Cosby, and Jonathan M. Campbell

Children and youth with intellectual and/or developmental disabilities (I/DD), including autistic children and youth, experience mental health challenges at elevated rates compared to general populations. In this chapter, we use the term *mental health conditions* to include *formal psychiatric diagnoses*, such as those identified in the Diagnostic and Statistical Manual of Mental Disorders, Fifth Edition, Text Revision (DSM-5-TR; American Psychiatric Association, 2022), as well as other *behavioral difficulties*, such as aggression and self-injury, which may or may not be formally diagnosed. We discuss prevalence of mental health conditions in I/DD populations; identify evidence-informed practices involving parents or caregivers as interventionists; and outline potential barriers experienced by parents and youth who may be underserved due to social or structural factors like racism and financial barriers. We include a case study illustrating an evidence-informed model for authentic caregiver involvement in interventions and conclude with possibilities for future research and practice.

K. M. Malone · K. W. Cosby
Department of Special Education, University of North Carolina-Chapel Hill, Chapel Hill, NC, USA

L. A. Smith
The Watson Institute, Pittsburgh, PA, USA

J. M. Campbell (✉)
Department of Psychology, Western Carolina University, Cullowhee, NC, USA
e-mail: jmcampbell@wcu.edu

L. Nabors, J. D. Bartlett (eds.), *Family Engagement in Mental Health Interventions for Young Children*, Springer Series on Child and Family Studies,
https://doi.org/10.1007/978-3-031-47917-5_4

I/DD and Co-occurring Mental Health Conditions

Mental health conditions and I/DD can frequently co-occur, even in early childhood. Many children and adolescents with I/DD experience difficulties with anxiety and depression, executive functioning, attentional regulation, and externalizing or internalizing behaviors that may be perceived as oppositional, defiant, or challenging. Formal diagnosis of mental health conditions is reported to be as high as 36% for you with I/DD (Emerson & Hatton, 2007). Rosen et al. (2018) found that up to 70% of autistic individuals meet formal diagnostic criteria for a psychiatric disorder, including among autistic children and youth: approximately 40% experience anxiety disorders and nearly 30% develop clinically significant depression.

Many autistic children and youth present with externalizing behaviors or develop disorders, such as oppositional defiant disorder (ODD) and conduct disorder (CD). Lai et al. (2019) report that up to 28% of autistic children and youth meet criteria for attention-deficit hyperactivity disorder (ADHD), and disruptive behavior, impulse-control disorders, and CD occur for roughly 12%. Mental health conditions differ across age, sex, and gender, with younger individuals showing higher rates of ADHD and older individuals showing higher rates of depressive and affective disorders, with a higher prevalence of depressive disorders among females (Lai et al., 2019).

Behavioral difficulties not formally diagnosed as psychiatric or mental health conditions also occur for many children and youth with I/DD. Common examples include self-injury, aggression, and property destruction. A 2020 meta-analysis (Steenfeldt-Kristensen et al., 2020) found that up to 42% of autistic individuals engage in self-injurious behavior. For autistic children and adolescents, aggression may present as a concern for slightly over half (i.e., 53%; Mazurek et al., 2013), and caregivers frequently end up on the receiving end of aggressive behaviors.

Parents of children and youth with I/DD are critical in clinical planning and care and may engage in various ways in intervention, such as providing information on onset, frequency, duration, and intensity of mental health concerns; supporting the efforts of professionals; or intervening directly with their child.

Evidence-Informed Practices

Parent Implemented Interventions

There has been a steady and growing interest in the identification, dissemination, and implementation of evidence-informed practices (EIPs) for autistic children and youth. Arguably the most well-known efforts are those from the Frank Porter Graham Child Development Institute (FPG), which has published several comprehensive reviews of EIPs over the past 15 years. As of this publication, the identified parent implemented interventions (PIIs) as an EIP for targeting mental health for autistic children and youth, with a PII defined as, "Parent delivery of an intervention to their child that promotes their social communication or other skills or decreases their challenging behavior" (Hume et al., 2021, p. 4024). For PII, "Practitioners teach parents in individual or group formats in home or community settings…The parent's role is to use the intervention practice…Once parents are trained, they implement all or part of the intervention(s) with their child" (Steinbrenner et al., 2020, p. 95). Parents may receive training in PIIs through instruction, therapist modeling, coaching, and feedback within clinic, school, or home settings.

PIIs are identified as EIPs for mental health outcomes from toddlerhood (i.e., ages 0–2) through middle school (i.e., 12–14 years; Steinbrenner et al., 2020). A meta-analysis of randomized controlled trials of PIIs documented moderate effects across varied outcomes, such as language, communication, adaptive behavior, and maladaptive behavior (Cheng et al., 2022). Various PII approaches—such as behavioral parent training, functional communication training, and parent-child interaction therapy (PCIT)—have resulted in statistically significant reductions in maladaptive behavior for young autistic children (*M* age = 5.5 years) (PCIT; Cheng et al., 2022). Here, we highlight two examples of manualized PIIs targeting mental health outcomes for autistic children and those with I/DD: Stepping Stones Triple P (SSTP) and PCIT.

Stepping Stones Triple P (SSTP)

SSTP is a modified version of the Triple P parenting protocol for children with I/DD. Triple-P uses a public health intervention model designed for large-scale implementation of general parent guidance. Delivered within a public health framework, Triple-P and SSTP consist of five intervention levels with each step increasing in intensity and focus (Tellegen & Sanders, 2013). Level 1, for example, involves media and communications strategy; Level 2 delivers intervention via brief large-group seminar; Level 5 consists of intensive intervention for individual families (Tellegen & Sanders, 2013). For children with autism and other I/DD (ages range from 2 to 17 years), SSTP yields significant reductions in child's maladaptive behavior as reported by parents, and improvements in children's behavioral adjustment via behavioral observation (Tellegen & Sanders, 2013). An abbreviated four-session version of SSTP resulted in reduced behavior challenges for young autistic children (Tellegen & Sanders, 2014).

Parent-Child Interaction Therapy

Parent-child interaction therapy (PCIT) is a manualized intervention targeting reduction of children's maladaptive behavior through parent training and enhancement of parent-child interactions. PCIT promotes effective parent behavior management skills in response to children's disruptive behavior and increased positive parent-child interaction. The PCIT protocol involves didactic instruction for parents as well as direct observation, feedback, and coaching by the therapist. PCIT was developed for use with young children without I/DD but has been evaluated with autistic children and children with I/DD and found to be effective in reducing maladaptive behavior with both groups (e.g., Vess & Campbell, 2022).

Many PIIs also address parent functioning through EIPs such as increasing parenting self-efficacy, reducing parenting stress, and improving parents' mental health. Some interventions, such as SSTP and PCIT, target improvements in parent-child relationship quality. Tellegen and Sanders (2013) found that SSTP improved parenting self-efficacy, parental adjustment, and parent-child relationship. Similarly, Vess and Campbell (2022) found that PCIT improved relationship quality between caregivers and young autistic children. Although PIIs have an established and growing evidence base to support child and parent outcomes, effective implementation is more likely to occur within the context of family-professional partnerships (Turnbull et al., 2021).

Models of Family-Professional Partnership

Collaboration between families and professionals is a critical element of supporting children with I/DD. Family engagement in collaboration has conceptually evolved over time by shifting from parent counseling to collective empowerment; approaches to interprofessional collaboration can be linked to these models. Professional organizations, like the Council for Exceptional Children (CEC) and the Division of Early Childhood (DEC), support professionals by identifying collaborative practices to engage families in their children's development and to establish successful family-professional partnerships. Even with identification of these practices, collaboration is not easy, and barriers remain.

This section reviews family-professional partnership models, links them to interprofessional collaboration approaches, and discusses elements of building successful family-professional partnerships in early childhood special education. A case study is integrated throughout this section to illustrate the development of strong family-professional partnerships for children with I/DD. Current research in family-professional relationships in early childhood special education replaces the word *engagement* with *partnership* (Turnbull et al., 2021). We use the term *partnership* in this section as a way to recognize power shifts within collaborative groups, and the key role of families throughout the process.

Arjun and Shreya have been married for 5 years and immigrated to the United States from India shortly after their wedding. Arjun works as a computer scientist for a technology company, and Shreya is an accountant at a local bank. They live with their 3-year-old daughter, Aahna, in a small community with other Indian families. They are active in their community and local church. After Aahna turned 2, they noticed some changes in her behavior: frustration in certain physical environments, challenges during social gatherings, and delays in responding to familiar adults. After talking with some of their community members and Aahna's pediatrician, they contacted early intervention services to ask about an evaluation.

Questions to consider:

- ***What values seem to be important to Arjun and Shreya?***
- ***What might be a positive way to approach Arjun and Shreya to facilitate a partnership?***
- ***What might facilitate further community support for Aahna and her family?***

Family-Professional Partnership Models

In early childhood special education, recommended practices encourage professionals to view and value families as active contributors and decision-makers throughout assessment and planning processes and to provide support and resources to families for goals within their home and community (DEC, 2014). Collaboration among professionals and families extends beyond formal meetings to consistent communication where information is exchanged to support child and family success. When reviewing models of family-professional partnerships, however, it is evident the relationship between family and professional is not always collaborative.

In this section, we discuss five family-professional partnership models: (a) parent counseling/psychotherapy, (b) parent involvement, (c) family-centered services, (d) collective empowerment, and (e) the Sunshine Model of Trusting Family-Professional Partnerships (Sunshine Model). Each model is described by family roles and responsibilities, power dynamics within the model, and intended outcomes of the model's collaborative process.

Parent Counseling Model

During the 1950s and 1960s, the prevailing family-professional partnership approach in early childhood special education was the parent counseling model (Turnbull et al., 2000). This unidirectional model is characterized by de-emphasized, or complete lack of, collaboration between professionals and families, as many professionals did not believe children with I/DD could learn and contribute to society (Turnbull et al., 2000). Consequently, children with I/DD were often institutionalized post-diagnosis, and interventions primarily focused on supporting mothers. Support was primarily provided by medical professionals and often referred to as treatment, which establishes a power differential where professionals are seen as the only experts (Haines et al., 2017). The aim of this family-professional model was to help mothers accept the circumstances around their child's differences (Turnbull et al., 2000).

Parent Involvement Model

The parent involvement model emerged in the 1960s and remained popular through the 1970s (Turnbull et al., 2000). Professionals began to recognize that parents (again mostly mothers) can influence their child's development; therefore, they needed to receive training on how to support their child at home (Bishop et al., 1993). Parents were encouraged to be extensions of their child's teacher. Professionals realized the importance of parent involvement in decision-making processes, but opportunities for input were limited based on how well families were able and willing to implement suggested interventions at home (Hornby, 2011). Professionals continued to be viewed as the sole experts who kept power within their control (Haines et al., 2017). With professionals and parents focusing on the same goals and using the same interventions at school and home, the intention of the parent involvement model was to increase achievement on developmental goals and future outcomes (Turnbull et al., 2000).

Family-Centered Services Model

In the 1980s, family-centered service was the primary family-professional partnership model used in early childhood special education (Turnbull et al., 2000). Focus shifted from the child's mother or parents to inclusion of immediate and extended family and community members (Haines et al., 2017). Families are empowered to make choices throughout special education processes for their child and seen as final decision-makers (Winton & DiVenere, 1995). Professionals focus on family strengths and provide guidance, support, and resources in utilizing those strengths to facilitate their child's development (Douglas et al., 2022). Families are encouraged to access and leverage community assets to support their child, and professionals helped to locate resources within communities (Seeley, 1993). The power dynamic in family-centered services models changed from professionals having power *over* families to sharing power *with* families (Haines et al., 2017). Power is exchanged between families and professionals, and the family is identified as the expert in terms of their own child. This model establishes family-professional collaboration in early childhood special education with the intention to meet child and family needs together (Turnbull et al., 2000). Although family is central to this model, their identified needs are child-focused, which can limit collaboration and support for individual family needs (Turnbull et al., 2000).

Collective Empowerment Model

From the 1990s into the twenty-first century, family-professional partnerships in early childhood special education have emphasized collective empowerment (Turnbull et al., 2000). This model focuses on ensuring that all members of collaborative teams, both family and professionals, have access to the necessary resources for successfully achieving their goals (Haines et al., 2017). Families are no longer viewed as the sole team members lacking resources, and there is a recognition that all team members require support. The power dynamic is different from prior models, with emphasis on capacity building generated through collaboration (Haines et al., 2017). The intended outcome of collective empowerment is for all team members to benefit from the collaboration and to progress together in ways that are possible only through the contributions of every team member (Turnbull et al., 2000).

The Sunshine Model of Trusting Family-Professional Partnerships (Sunshine Model)

The Sunshine Model provides a framework for building capacity within a partnership. Trust is at the core of the sun or partnership (Turnbull et al., 2021). The core contains five dimensions of trusting family-professional partnerships: *equity*, *respect*, *communication*, *advocacy*, and *commitment* (Turnbull et al., 2021). These dimensions provide the framework for strengthening trust within the partnership. There are seven opportunities for families and professionals to utilize the five dimensions as they build trust together: academic learning, social-emotional learning, behavior, student assessment, special meetings, student transitions, and school capacity enhancement (Turnbull et al., 2021).

The Sunshine Model follows a family-systems framework for identifying partnership members. Parents, siblings, partners, and extended family are vital to the child's success and the partnership as a whole; the model recognizes that members will shift and change over time according to the child and family's needs (Turnbull & Turnbull, 2022). The power dynamic is comparable to the collective empowerment model. All members of the partnership share decision-making power, and the group co-generates power and builds individual and collective capacity together (Haines et al., 2017). This model does not explicitly focus on early childhood special education but on all children and individuals across their education trajectories (Turnbull & Turnbull, 2022). The Sunshine Model's primary intended outcome is to co-construct trusting partnerships among families and professionals that support the individual child to grow, develop, and achieve educational goals across their lifespan (Turnbull et al., 2021).

Approaches to Interprofessional Collaboration

Many professional collaborations identify as some sort of disciplinary team. There are three main approaches to interprofessional collaboration: multi-, inter-, and transdisciplinary. Interdisciplinary collaboration is often emphasized for professionals working in the early childhood special education field (Mitsch et al., 2023). Teacher preparation program coursework for future educators and professional development for working teachers both provide guidance on interdisciplinary collaboration; recommended practices encourage families and professionals to utilize this approach (Winton & DiVenere, 1995). Next, we describe three interprofessional collaborative approaches and align them with family-professional partnership models.

Multidisciplinary Approach

When early childhood special education teams use a multidisciplinary approach to collaboration, families and professionals work independent of one another (Hernandez, 2013). For a child with I/DD receiving special education services, their goals are categorized into areas of identified need, and professionals are responsible for goals related to their own discipline. For example, a classroom teacher may solely work on academic related goals, or a speech-language pathologist would only work on communication goals. Team meetings are often an opportunity for professionals to share the child's progress from their discipline's perspective, and family needs or desires for their child are supported by the professional who can best address them (Mortier & Aramburo, 2022). There is little to no overlap in the collaboration. The multidisciplinary interprofessional collaboration approach aligns with parent counseling/psychotherapy and parent involvement models where professionals are siloed within their own discipline and often viewed as specialized experts.

Interdisciplinary Approach

The interdisciplinary approach emphasizes coordination and cooperative opportunities where family and professionals actively collaborate on assessments and planning (Hernandez, 2013). Professionals still primarily work within their disciplines, but there is more opportunity to communicate with other team members for support and input throughout assessment and planning processes (Mortier & Aramburo, 2022). Families are actively engaged when an interdisciplinary approach is used in an educational environment, and resources are shared to support the child and family in their home and community (Winton & DiVenere, 1995). For example, in early childhood special education, a child may demonstrate the ability to use a skill in one environment but not in another. The family and professionals work together and design a plan for how the child will generalize the skill in different environments. The interdisciplinary approach aligns with family-centered services as families are integrated into decision-making processes and power is distributed among team members.

Transdisciplinary Approach

The final interprofessional collaboration approach is transdisciplinary; it emphasizes service integration so all team members share responsibility for the child's development and progress (Hernandez, 2013). While team members are from varying fields, the transdisciplinary approach does not separate professionals. The expectation is that all team members develop capacities for supporting the child across all their areas of need (Mortier & Aramburo, 2022). Team meetings have clear and deliberate communication where families and professionals exchange information to support the child's progress (Hernandez, 2013). This approach aligns with collective empowerment and the Sunshine Model; it is designed to generate power through partnership so all collaboration members can benefit and build capacity (Turnbull et al., 2000).

The evaluation process was overwhelming for Arjun, Shreya, and Aahna. After 3 days in administrative offices, they met to discuss evaluation results with a team of five people: a case manager, psychologist, speech-language pathologist, occupational therapist, and social worker. Each practitioner presented their assessment results and documents; then Arjun and Shreya were asked if they had any questions. Feeling uncertain, they quietly said, "No." They were then asked to sign paperwork. Just before leaving, Arjun and Shreya were informed that, in 2 weeks, Aahna would begin attending a self-contained pre-k class at a school 20 minutes from their home and that the teacher would contact them soon with more information.

Questions to consider:

- ***Which (1) family-professional partnership model and (2) interprofessional collaboration approach were implemented for Aahna and her family?***
- ***How might this process look different in other family-professional partnership models?***
- ***How could the team have supported Aahna's family through the evaluation process?***

Building Effective Family-Professional Partnerships

Multiple elements can support families and professionals in building effective partnerships, but a clear blueprint does not exist as all partnerships are based on individual strengths and needs of the collaborators. As discussed in the Sunshine Model, trust is at the core of all successful collaboration (Turnbull et al., 2021). It is important to nurture trust starting at the beginning of a partnership by focusing on the five dimensions described in the Sunshine Model: *equity*, *respect*, *communication*, *advocacy*, and *commitment*. Trust can take time to build, is easily broken, and benefits from consistency throughout the partnership (Turnbull et al., 2021).

Another cornerstone of building effective family-professional partnerships is for all team members to be treated with dignity (Haines et al., 2017). Dignity in partnership is showing each team member they are worthy of honor and respect (Turnbull & Turnbull, 2022). Team members can identify and build upon strengths that each person brings to the partnership; work to ensure that everyone's voice is heard and understood; and provide a space free of judgement for open collaboration. These efforts can support buy-in from families and professionals.

For children with I/DD, it is especially important that families and professionals work together as consistently as possible through each step of the process. All team members, especially families, should be involved in assessment processes, identifying strengths and needs, writing appropriate goals, and deciding how to reach those goals (DEC, 2014). The goal is for families to feel supported by the professionals on the team and given resources to support their child at home and in their community (Douglas et al., 2022). Most important, the child and their family need adequate time to process and understand information (Mortier & Aramburo, 2022). It is unethical for professionals to rush through evaluations or not fully explain documentation generated during special education processes. These processes can be overwhelming for families, so teams need to plan for sufficient time and support for full team engagement in the partnership.

Aahna's new teacher called Arjun and Shreya the day after the evaluation meeting. She introduced herself, asked how they were feeling after the evaluation process, asked a few questions about Aahna, and scheduled a home visit. She explained that the visit would give them an opportunity to review more information together and discuss questions or concerns.

They spent the first hour of the home visit discussing next steps and addressing questions. The teacher accepted Arjun and Shreya's invitation to stay for lunch, so they had time to chat and continue getting to know one another. The teacher observed Arjun and Shreya with their child and she spent some time playing with Aahna in her playroom. After the home visit, Arjun and Shreya still had some apprehension about transportation to and from school, and about some of the services discussed at the evaluation meeting, but they also felt some relief that Aahna would be in good hands with this teacher.

Questions to consider:

- ***What elements of facilitating effective partnerships are demonstrated in this scenario?***
- ***Which family-professional partnership model does the teacher implement in this scenario?***
- ***What are some next partnership-building steps for Aahna's teacher and family?***

In summary, the perspective of family engagement or partnership has changed drastically from viewing professionals as experts over families to building power through partnership to successfully achieve goals and reach outcomes. The models of family partnership connect to interprofessional collaboration approaches, and the Sunshine Model creates a framework that emphasizes the collective empowerment model of partnership and the transdisciplinary approach to collaboration (Turnbull et al., 2021). Equity, respect, communication, advocacy, and commitment are the five dimensions in the Sunshine Model, and treating all team members with dignity builds trust and leads to successful partnerships (Turnbull et al., 2021). Consistency in collaboration and providing time and resources also supports effective partnerships. While challenges and barriers surely exist, establishing family-professional partnerships in early childhood special education lays the foundation for and is essential for success of the child with developmental disabilities and their family.

Critical Issues Related to Intersectionality, Justice, and Disparities in I/DD Mental Health

Social justice and health disparities are central to this discussion as such disparities pose significant challenges that can marginalize individuals, families, and communities, undermining their health and mental well-being. By identifying and directly addressing these critical issues, we can co-create partnerships that are better equipped to tackle healthcare inequalities and promote more equitable health and life outcomes.

Families from all walks of life find that caring for children with I/DD has its fair share of joys, celebrations, challenges, and obstacles—parents report that their children have taught them unconditional love, compassion, and resilience and do not desire their child to be neurotypical (Di Renzo et al., 2020). Families raising I/DD children are also more likely to experience significant disparities such as economic insecurity, social isolation, and limited access to high-quality education, support services, and healthcare (Zuckerman et al., 2018). A study by Srinivasan et al. (2021) surveyed 263 caregivers raising autistic children and youth; the authors reported 63% of participant families had at least one unmet support need, such as behavioral support, communication aids, or therapies. These disparities can often be exacerbated for racial, ethnic, and linguistically diverse families (e.g., English language learners, ASL) and low-income, nonnuclear and families with an I/DD member (Lovelace et al., 2018).

Disparities by Racial, Ethnic, and Linguistic Identity

Structural barriers in the health and education systems, such as implicit bias of providers, contribute to disparities experienced by families of color raising I/DD children (Malone et al., 2022). Families of color report experiencing racial discrimination such as denial of healthcare and educational services and feeling unsupported and patronized by healthcare and educational service providers (Lovelace et al., 2018). These experiences can cause families to be hesitant to engage with service providers, which can further exacerbate the challenges families face (Pearson et al., 2019).

A family's knowledge and familiarity with I/DD and local service availability impacts how they seek care for their child (Pearson et al., 2019; Zuckerman et al., 2018). Pearson et al. (2019) reported that Black parents raising autistic children were less likely to be aware of available support services in their community. Zuckerman et al. (2018) reported that many Black and Latinx families say they do not know anyone else with I/DD; and, for Hispanic parents, depth of knowledge about autism is the most common barrier to an autism diagnosis (Pearson et al., 2023; Zuckerman et al., 2018).

Students with limited English proficiency are disproportionally represented in special education and are more likely to experience adverse outcomes such as decreased academic achievement when compared to English proficient peers (Counts et al., 2018; Morgan et al., 2015). The culmination of these, and other, barriers for marginalized families has resulted in disparate outcomes for I/DD students of color. I/DD students of color are more likely to be identified later, receive fewer services, and are less likely to receive evidence-informed treatments when compared to White I/DD children (Angell et al., 2018). As a result of these disparities, family members may experience an increased likelihood of developing depression, anxiety, and behavioral health concerns (Song et al., 2018).

Disparities by Socioeconomic Status (SES)

Families whose incomes are below the federal poverty threshold (i.e., low-SES), who are also raising children with I/DD, often face a range of challenges in accessing healthcare, education, and social services. These may include financial constraints, lack of transportation, limited access to information of early developmental milestones, and barriers related to cultural or linguistic mismatch (Campbell et al., 2019; Zuckerman et al., 2018). Special education services can be particularly difficult to access and navigate, and families may not be aware of their rights to these services (Braun, 2017). Low-SES families also face disparities in access to mental health services, which can negatively impact their overall well-being and quality of life (Chen et al., 2022). Few mental healthcare providers are trained to work with I/DD individuals or low-SES families, and as a result are more likely to experience missed diagnosis or misdiagnosis (Fadus et al., 2019). There are limited numbers of culturally competent providers who are responsive to the various needs associated with intersectional identities (Butler et al., 2016). Low-SES families often face discrimination and institutional bias that can lead to increased interactions with the legal system and cascading negative social, economic, health, and functional outcomes (Hinton et al., 2018).

Disparities by Family Structure

Single-parent families often experience higher levels of exhaustion, stress, financial insecurity, and decreased social support and services than two-parent households (Lovelace et al., 2018). Fathers, in particular, report struggling with feelings of inadequacy or guilt, believing they may not do enough for their I/DD child (Thackeray & Eatough, 2016). Hillman and Anderson (2019) report that custodial grandparents experience decreased financial security, social support, and support services when caring for their autistic grandchildren. These challenges can be further compounded for caregivers dealing with their own physical or mental health issues.

There is only emerging research understanding Lesbian, Gay, Bisexual, Transgender, Queer, Intersex, Asexual (LGBTQIA+) families' experiences with raising I/DD children (Hillier et al., 2019). O'Shea et al. (2020) reported that disability service providers often do not understand how inaccessible and inappropriate their services may be to LGBTQIA+ people, while LGBTQIA+ services often fail to provide services that are accessible and appropriate to people with disabilities. Consistent with prior research on I/DD adult outcomes, the overall lack of awareness or knowledge surrounding nonheterosexual orientation and nonbinary gender identities can lead to significant isolation and reduced access to services (e.g., Hillier et al., 2019).

Disparities by I/DD Parenting

I/DD is not a reliable predictor of parenting performance. I/DD parents can demonstrate and develop the skills required to meet their children's needs when provided with adequate support (Aunos et al., 2008). However, there is an overrepresentation of I/DD parents in child protection systems internationally, with 50% more than would be expected given their prevalence in the general population (LaLiberte et al.,

2016). Researchers suggest this is due to ableism, socioeconomic disadvantage, and limited social supports rather than I/DD itself (Feldman et al., 2002; Wade et al., 2011).

I/DD caregivers also experience increased challenges to their mental health and access to related health services compared to other parents, resulting in increased adverse child outcomes (Meppelder et al., 2014). Little is known in the academic literature about I/DD Hispanic and Black parents' experiences (Malone et al., 2022). Magaña et al. (2016) reported that Black and Hispanic adults are more likely to experience challenges in accessing healthcare and more likely to have overall diminished physical and mental health compared to their White peers.

Directions for Future Research and Practice

I/DD and Family-Centered Practices in Mental Health Supports

Adoption of EIPs related to family-centered practices (FCPs) is crucial for families raising children with I/DD due to their complex needs. However, the lack of knowledge or understanding of EIPs among service providers poses a significant barrier to EIP implementation (Dempsey & Keen, 2017). To effectively implement these FCPs, service providers must engage in ongoing professional development that is grounded in EIPs and strategies (Dempsey & Keen, 2017). Investment in professional development can ensure that practitioners have the necessary skills and knowledge to implement FCPs effectively. Organizational culture and service provider values can act as barriers. Effective implementation of FCPs can be hindered if service providers lack commitment to family partnership in service provision and decision-making. It is crucial to explore ways to improve organizational culture around FCPs through research. Service providers could benefit from developing specialized skills and knowledge on effective team partnership and implementation of evidence-informed FCPs to support mental health in children with I/DD.

I/DD and Lifespan Approaches to Mental Health Supports

It is essential to adopt a lifespan approach to gain comprehensive understanding of the complex experiences of individuals with I/DD and their families (Kirby et al., 2023). Only a small portion (~2.5%) of autism research funding is currently dedicated to investigating autistic adults' experiences (Harris et al., 2021). Lack of attention to I/DD populations' strengths, needs, and challenges across the lifespan highlights a significant gap in our understanding. To address this gap, there is a need for more longitudinal studies to track I/DD children and their families to better understand their mental health trajectories and experiences over time, and leverage this information to enhance EIPs, supports, and services. A lifespan approach can improve child outcomes and intrafamily relations, promote overall well-being of individuals with I/DD and their families (Kirby et al., 2023), and facilitate development of interventions tailored to specific needs of I/DD individuals across different stages of life.

I/DD and Cultural Reciprocity in Mental Health Supports

Researchers and support providers must prioritize cultural reciprocity in their approach to understanding and serving the complex intersectional needs of I/DD children and families within diverse communities (Malone et al., 2022). Current knowledge on experiences of families raising autistic children is largely based on majority-white samples (Malone et al., 2022). Researchers and practitioners can work toward increasing and demonstrating their own understanding and appreciation of cultural diversity to provide more effective, inclusive support and scholarship. Collaboration is necessary for authentic cultural reciprocity in practice: cross-cultural exchange, active demonstration of mutual respect, understanding, and appreciation for collective diversity. Cultural reciprocity can actively inform all aspects of research and practice: service providers and researchers can actively seek and listen to perspectives, experiences, and needs of I/DD children and families across diverse backgrounds and communities (Kalyanpur & Harry, 1997). By prioritizing cultural reciprocity, collaborative partnerships in research and practice can nurture positive, trusting relationships across diverse cultural backgrounds to ensure that interventions and services are as culturally responsive, respectful, and effective as possible (Kalyanpur & Harry, 1997).

I/DD, Identity Development, and Mental Health

Facilitating positive disability identity development and embracing neurodiversity are essential for promoting the mental well-being of I/DD youth and adults (Botha & Gillespie-Lynch, 2022). While further research is necessary to understand the impact of masking or camouflaging neurodivergent traits on I/DD youth and adults, current evidence suggests that these behaviors can have detrimental effects on the mental health of non-I/DD autistic individuals (Ross et al., 2022). Therefore, it is important to investigate whether similar negative consequences exist for individuals with I/DD and to consider how existing interventions may exacerbate or encourage masking. Furthermore, to promote the full inclusion and participation of people with I/DD in society, it is crucial to acknowledge their strengths and interests, as well as to eliminate ableism and stigma. This requires a shift in focus from solely addressing I/DD persons to also addressing the broader social and cultural factors that contribute to ableism and stigma.

Toward Collective Care, Equity, and Inclusion

Future research, policies, practices, and collaborative partnerships can intentionally move toward better supporting and advocating for children with I/DD and their families to improve mental health outcomes and overall quality of life. Through more holistically caring for I/DD children's mental health, we can better support and partner with I/DD individuals across the lifespan and promote a more equitable and inclusive society for all.

Possible Answers to Case Study Questions

What values seem to be important to Arjun and Shreya?

The scenario indicates Arjun and Shreya value their community. This would be a good question to add to a questionnaire or to ask a family to build trust.

What might be a positive way to approach Arjun and Shreya to facilitate a partnership?

Asking the family about the possibility of joining them during one of their community or church events would show interest and effort in nurturing a trusting partnership.

What might facilitate further community support for Aahna and her family?

Encouraging the family to ask trusted members of their community to join meetings could expand supportive learning environments for Aahna.

Which (1) family-professional partnership model and (2) interprofessional collaboration approach were implemented for Aahna and her family?

(1) Limited parent input in decision-making processes indicates a parent involvement family-professional partnership model. (2) Individualization while discussing evaluations indicates a multidisciplinary interprofessional collaboration approach.

How might this process look different in other family-professional partnership models?

From the Sunshine Models' perspective, families should be actively involved in every step of the process to ensure understanding and to develop the most effective plan. Family should be given options, not instructions, such as when deciding on classroom placement.

How could the team have supported Aahna's family through the evaluation process?

The team could have tried to get to know the family before evaluations and offered to evaluate Aahna at home where she might be comfortable.

What elements of facilitating effective partnerships are demonstrated in this scenario?

The teacher began building rapport as she introduced herself and did not overwhelm the family over the phone. She approached the family with respect and dignity by following their lead during the home visit. The interaction flowed naturally, giving Arjun, Shreya, and Aahna time to feel more comfortable and to begin developing mutual trust.

Which family-professional partnership model does the teacher implement in this scenario?

The scenario indicates the teacher is utilizing Sunshine Model elements.

What are some next partnership-building steps for Aahna's teacher and family?

It is important for the teacher to establish consistent communication with Arjun and Shreya to exchange information about Aahna's progress and to offer ongoing support.

References

American Psychiatric Association. (2022). *Diagnostic and statistical manual of mental disorders* (5th ed. *Text Revision*). American Psychiatric Association Publishing.

Angell, A. M., Empey, A., & Zuckerman, K. E. (2018). A review of diagnosis and service disparities among children with autism from racial and ethnic minority groups in the United States. *International Review of Research in Developmental Disabilities, 55*, 145–180. https://doi.org/10.1016/bs.irrdd.2018.08.003

Aunos, M., Feldman, M., & Goupil, G. (2008). Mothering with intellectual disabilities: Relationship between social support, health and well-being, parenting and child behaviour outcomes. *Journal of Applied Research in Intellectual Disabilities, 21*(4), 320–330. https://doi.org/10.1111/j.1468-3148.2008.00447.x

Bishop, K., Woll, J., & Arango, P. (1993). *Family/Professional collaboration for children with special health needs and their families*. Retrieved 1 Feb 2023, from https://eric.ed.gov/?id=ED381518

Botha, M., & Gillespie-Lynch, K. (2022). Come as you are: Examining autistic identity development and the neurodiversity movement through an intersectional lens. *Human Development, 66*(2), 93–112. https://doi.org/10.1159/000524123

Braun, C. (2017). *An examination of low-income minority parents' and guardians' experiences with the special education process using a strengths-based perspective* [PhD Dissertation]. Northern Illinois University. Retrieved 1 Feb 2023, from https://www.proquest.com/docview/2013203329

Butler, M., McCreedy, E., Schwer, N., Burgess, D., Call, K., Przedworski, J., Rosser, S., Larson, S., Allen, M., Fu, S., & Kane, R. L. (2016). *Improving cultural competence to reduce health disparities*. Agency for Healthcare Research and Quality (US).

Campbell, J. M., Greenberg, D., Gallagher, P. A., Stoneman, Z., & Simmons, C. (2019). Knowledge of autism for parents of low income with low literacy: Description and relationship to child development knowledge. *Advances in Neurodevelopmental Disorders, 3*(1), 8–16. https://doi.org/10.1007/s41252-018-0079-z

Chen, C. C., Cheng, S. L., Xu, Y., Spence, C., Zhang, F., & Adams, N. B. (2022). Child developmental and special education service receipt: The intersection of health and poverty. *Disability and Health Journal, 15*(3), 101269. https://doi.org/10.1016/j.dhjo.2022.101269

Cheng, W. M., Smith, T. B., Butler, M., Taylor, T. M., & Clayton, D. (2022). Effects of parent-implemented interventions on outcomes of children with autism: A meta-analysis. *Journal of Autism and Developmental Disorders*, 1–17. https://doi.org/10.1007/s10803-022-05688-8

Counts, J., Katsiyannis, A., & Whitford, D. K. (2018). Culturally and linguistically diverse learners in special education: English learners. *NASSP Bulletin, 102*(1), 5–21.

Dempsey, I., & Keen, D. (2017). Desirable outcomes associated with family-centered practices for young children with a disability. In H. Sukkar, C. J. Dunst, & J. Kirkby (Eds.), *Early childhood intervention: Working with families of young children with special needs* (pp. 59–71). Routledge/Taylor & Francis Group. Retrieved 1 Feb 2023, from https://www.taylorfrancis.com/chapters/edit/10.4324/9781315688442-12/

Di Renzo, M., Guerriero, V., Zavattini, G. C., Petrillo, M., Racinaro, L., & Bianchi di Castelbianco, F. (2020). Parental attunement, insightfulness, and acceptance of child diagnosis in parents of children with autism: Clinical implications. *Frontiers in Psychology, 11*, 1849. https://doi.org/10.3389/fpsyg.2020.01849

Division for Early Childhood. (2014). *DEC recommended practices in early intervention/early childhood special education.* https://www.dec-sped.org/dec-recommended-practices

Douglas, S. N., Meadan, H., Biggs, E. E., Bagawan, A., & Terol, A. K. (2022). Building family capacity: Supporting multiple family members to implement aided language modeling. *Journal of Autism and Developmental Disorders*, 1–13. https://doi.org/10.1007/s10803-022-05492-4

Emerson, E., & Hatton, C. (2007). Mental health of children and adolescents with intellectual disabilities in Britain. *British Journal of Psychiatry, 191*, 493–499. https://doi.org/10.1192/bjp.bp.107.038729

Fadus, M. C., Ginsburg, K. R., Sobowale, K., Halliday-Boykins, C. A., Bryant, B. E., Gray, K. M., & Squeglia, L. M. (2019). Unconscious bias and the diagnosis of Disruptive Behavior Disorders and ADHD in African American and Hispanic youth. *Academic Psychiatry, 44*(1), 95–102. https://doi.org/10.1007/s40596-019-01127-6

Feldman, M. A., Varghese, J., Ramsay, J., & Rajska, D. (2002). Relationships between social support, stress and mother-child interactions in mothers with intellectual disabilities. *Journal of Applied Research in Intellectual Disabilities, 15*(4), 314–323. https://doi.org/10.1046/j.1468-3148.2002.00132.x

Haines, S. J., Francis, G. L., Mueller, T. G., Chiu, C.-Y., Burke, M. M., Kyzar, K., Shepherd, K. G., Holdren, N., Aldersey, H. M., & Turnbull, A. P. (2017). Reconceptualizing family-professional partnership for inclusive schools: A call to action. *Inc, 5*(4), 234–247. https://doi.org/10.1352/2326-6988-5.4.234

Harris, L. J., Gilmore, D. W., Longo, A., & Hand, B. N. (2021). Short report: Patterns of US federal autism research funding during 2017–2019. *Autism, 25*(7), 2135–2139. https://doi.org/10.1177/13623613211003430

Hernandez, S. (2013). Collaboration in special education: Its history, evolution, and critical factors necessary for successful implementation. *US China. Education Review, 3*(6), 480–498. Retrieved 1 Feb 2023, from https://eric.ed.gov/?id=ED544122

Hillier, A., Gallop, N., Mendes, E., Tellez, D., Buckingham, A., Nizami, A., & OToole, D. (2019). LGBTQ + and autism spectrum disorder: Experiences and challenges. *International Journal of Transgender Health, 21*(1), 98–110. https://doi.org/10.1080/15532739.2019.1594484

Hillman, J. L., & Anderson, C. M. (2019). It's a battle and a blessing: The experience and needs of custodial grandparents of children with autism spectrum disorder. *Journal of Autism and Developmental Disorders, 49*(1), 260–269. https://doi.org/10.1007/s10803-018-3761-0

Hinton, E., Henderson, L., & Reed, C. (2018). *An unjust burden: The disparate treatment of Black Americans in the criminal justice system.* Vera Institute of Justice. https://www.vera.org/downloads/publications/for-the-record-unjust-burden-racial-disparities.pdf

Hornby, G. (2011). *Parental involvement in childhood education: Building effective school-family partnerships.* Springer Science + Business Media. https://doi.org/10.1007/978-1-4419-8379-4

Hume, K., Steinbrenner, J. R., Odom, S. L., Morin, K. L., Nowell, S. W., Tomaszewski, B., Szendrey, S., McIntyre, N. S., Yucesoy-Ozkan, S., & Savage, M. N. (2021). Evidence-based practices for children, youth, and young adults with autism: Third generation review. *Journal of Autism and Developmental Disorders, 51*, 4013–4032. https://doi.org/10.1007/s10803-020-04844-2

Kalyanpur, M., & Harry, B. (1997). A posture of reciprocity: A practical approach to collaboration between professionals and parents of culturally diverse backgrounds. *Journal of Child and Family Studies, 6*, 487–509. https://doi-org.libproxy.lib.unc.edu/10.1023/A:1025001630436

Kirby, A. V., Morgan, L., & Hilton, C. (2023). Autism and mental health: The role of occupational therapy. *The American Journal of Occupational Therapy, 77*(2). https://doi.org/10.5014/ajot.2023.050303

Lai, M.-C., Kassee, C., Besney, R., Bonato, S., Hull, L., Mandy, W., Szatmari, P., & Ameis, S. H. (2019). Prevalence of co-occurring mental health diagnoses in the autism population: A systematic review and meta-analysis. *Lancet, 6*(10), 819–829. https://doi.org/10.1016/S2215-0366(19)30289-5

LaLiberte, T., Piescher, K., Mickelson, N., & Lee, M. H. (2016). Child protection services and parents with intellectual and developmental disabilities. *Journal of Applied Research in Intellectual Disabilities, 30*(3), 521–532. https://doi.org/10.1111/jar.12323

Lovelace, T. S., Robertson, R. E., & Tamayo, S. (2018). Experiences of African American mothers of sons with autism spectrum disorder: Lessons for improving service delivery. *Education and Training in Autism and Developmental Disabilities, 53*(1), 3–16. https://www.jstor.org/stable/26420423

Magaña, S., Parish, S., Morales, M. A., Li, H., & Fujiura, G. (2016). Racial and ethnic health disparities among people with intellectual and developmental disabilities. *Intellectual and Developmental Disabilities, 54*(3), 161–172. https://doi.org/10.1352/1934-9556-54.3.161

Malone, K. M., Pearson, J. N., Palazzo, K. N., Manns, L. D., Rivera, A. Q., & Mason Martin, D. L. (2022). The scholarly neglect of Black autistic adults in autism research. *Autism in Adulthood, 4*(4), 271–280. https://doi.org/10.1089/aut.2021.0086

Mazurek, M. O., Kanne, S. M., & Wodka, E. L. (2013). Physical aggression in children and adolescents with autism spectrum disorders. *Research in Autism Spectrum Disorders, 7*(3), 455–465. https://doi.org/10.1016/j.rasd.2012.11.004

Meppelder, M., Hodes, M., Kef, S., & Schuengel, C. (2014). Parenting stress and child behaviour problems among parents with intellectual disabilities: The buffering role of resources. *Journal of Intellectual Disability Research, 59*(7), 664–677. https://doi.org/10.1111/jir.12170

Mitsch, M. K., Collins, B., Friesen, A., & Hermoso, J. C. (2023). Social emotional development and early childhood mental health: Special education and social work collaboration. In D. Slanda & L. Pike (Eds.), *Handbook of research on interdisciplinary preparation for equitable special education* (pp. 468–494). IGI Global. https://doi.org/10.4018/978-1-6684-6438-0.ch023

Morgan, P. L., Farkas, G., Hillemeier, M. M., Mattison, R., Maczuga, S., Li, H., & Cook, M. (2015). Minorities are disproportionately underrepresented in special education: Longitudinal evidence across five disability conditions. *Educational Researcher, 44*(5), 278–292.

Mortier, K., & Aramburo, C. (2022). *Collaborative teaming to support quality inclusive education for students with disabilities*. Routledge. https://doi.org/10.4324/9781138609877-REE157-1

O'Shea, A., Latham, J. R., McNair, R., Despott, N., Rose, M., Mountford, R., & Frawley, P. (2020). Experiences of LGBTIQA+ people with disability in healthcare and community services: Towards embracing multiple identities. *International Journal of Environmental Research and Public Health, 17*(21), 8080. https://doi.org/10.3390/ijerph17218080

Pearson, J. N., Akamoglue, Y., Chung, M., & Meadan, H. (2019). Building family-professional partnerships with culturally, linguistically, and economically diverse families of young children. *Multicultural Perspectives, 21*(4), 208–216. https://doi.org/10.1080/15210960.2019.1686381

Pearson, J. N., Malone, K. M., Stewart-Ginsburg, J. H., Manns, L. D., Martin, D. M., & Palazzo, K. M. (2023). "We should all be welcome:" a discourse analysis of religious coping for Black parents raising autistic children. *Journal of Disability & Religion*, 1–25. https://doi.org/10.1080/23312521.2023.2178993

Rosen, T. E., Mazefsky, C. A., Vasa, R. A., & Lerner, M. D. (2018). Co-occurring psychiatric conditions in autism spectrum disorder. *International Review of Psychiatry, 30*, 40–61. https://doi.org/10.1080/09540261.2018.1450229

Ross, A., Grove, R., & McAloon, J. (2022). The relationship between camouflaging and mental health in autistic children and adolescents. *Autism Research, 16*(1), 190–199. https://doi.org/10.1002/aur.2859

Seeley, D. S. (1993). A new paradigm for parent involvement. In N. F. Chavkin (Ed.), *Families and schools in a pluralistic society* (pp. 229–234). State University of New York Press.

Song, J., Mailick, M. R., & Greenberg, J. S. (2018). Health of parents of individuals with developmental disorders or mental health problems: Impacts of stigma. *Social Science & Medicine, 217*, 152–158. https://doi.org/10.1016/j.socscimed.2018.09.044

Srinivasan, S., Ekbladh, A., Freedman, B., & Bhat, A. (2021). Needs assessment in unmet healthcare and family support services: A survey of caregivers of children and youth with autism spectrum disorder in Delaware. *Autism Research, 14*(8), 1736–1758. https://doi.org/10.1002/aur.2514

Steenfeldt-Kristensen, C., Jones, C. A., & Richards, C. (2020). The prevalence of self-injurious behaviour in autism: A meta-analytic study. *Journal of Autism and Developmental Disorders, 50*, 3857–3873. https://doi.org/10.1007/s10803-020-04443-1

Steinbrenner, J. R., Hume, K., Odom, S. L., Morin, K. L., Nowell, S. W., Tomaszewski, B., Szendrey, S., McIntyre, N. S., Yucesoy-Ozkan, S., & Savage, M. N. (2020). *Evidence-based practices for children, youth, and young adults with autism*. The University of North Carolina at Chapel Hill, Frank Porter Graham Child Development Institute, National Clearinghouse on Autism Evidence and Practice Review Team. https://ncaep.fpg.unc.edu/sites/ncaep.fpg.unc.edu/files/imce/documents/EBP%20Report%202020.pdf

Tellegen, C. L., & Sanders, M. R. (2013). Stepping Stones Triple-P Positive Parenting Program for children with disability: A systematic review and meta-analysis. *Research in Developmental Disabilities, 34*, 1556–1571. https://doi.org/10.1016/j.ridd.2013.01.022

Tellegen, C. L., & Sanders, M. R. (2014). Brief report: A randomized controlled trial evaluating a brief parenting program with children with autism spectrum disorders. *Journal of Consulting and Clinical Psychology, 82*(6), 1193–1200. https://doi.org/10.1037/a0037246

Thackeray, L. A., & Eatough, V. (2016). 'Shutting the world out': An interpretative phenomenological analysis exploring the paternal experience of parenting a young adult with a developmental disability. *Journal of Applied Research in Intellectual Disabilities, 31*, 179–190. https://doi.org/10.1111/jar.12313

Turnbull, A., & Turnbull, R. (2022). Trusting partnerships and belonging for families of students with disabilities. In J. Jones & K. Gallus (Eds.), *Belonging and resilience in individuals with developmental disabilities: Community and family engagement* (pp. 35–47). Springer. https://doi.org/10.1007/978-3-030-81277-5_3

Turnbull, A. P., Turbiville, V., & Turnbull, H. R. (2000). Evolution of family–professional partnerships: Collective empowerment as the model for the early twenty-first century. In J. P. Shonkoff & S. J. Meisels (Eds.), *Handbook of early childhood intervention* (pp. 630–650). Cambridge University Press. https://doi.org/10.1017/CBO9780511529320.029

Turnbull, A. P., Turnbull, R. H., Francis, G. L., Burke, M., Kyzar, K., Haines, S. J., Gershwin, T., Shepherd, K. G., Holdren, N., & Singer, G. H. S. (2021). *Families and professionals: Trusting partnerships in general and special education* (8th ed.). Pearson.

Vess, S. F., & Campbell, J. M. (2022). Parent-child interaction therapy (PCIT) with families of children with autism spectrum disorder. *Autism and Developmental Language Impairments, 7*, 1–16. https://doi.org/10.1177/23969415221140707

Wade, C., Llewellyn, G., & Matthews, J. (2011). Modeling contextual influences on parents with intellectual disability and their children. *American Journal on Intellectual and Developmental Disabilities, 116*(6), 419–437. https://doi.org/10.1352/1944-7558-116.6.419

Winton, P. J., & DiVenere, N. (1995). Family-professional partnerships in early intervention personnel preparation: Guidelines and strategies. *Topics in Early Childhood Special Education, 15*(3), 296–313. https://doi.org/10.1177/027112149501500304

Zuckerman, K. E., Chavez, A. E., Regalado Murillo, C., Lindly, O. J., & Reeder, J. A. (2018). Disparities in familiarity with developmental disabilities among low-income parents. *Academic Pediatrics, 18*(8), 944–951. https://doi.org/10.1016/j.acap.2018.06.011

Chapter 5
Family Engagement in Mental Health Interventions for Children with Chronic Illnesses

Laura Nabors, Tabitha Naa Akuyea Addy, and Sachi Shukla

This chapter reviews approaches for parent and family engagement, specifically focusing on parents of children with chronic illnesses, ages birth through 8 years of age. These conditions may include problems related to premature birth (e.g., low birthweight), asthma, developmental disabilities, type I diabetes, cystic fibrosis, heart problems, overweight/obesity, malnutrition, and mental illnesses (Torpy et al., 2010). Chronic illness is a medical condition often lasting a year or longer that limits child activity and daily functioning, requires special medical care or healthcare services, and impacts child development (Consolini, 2022; Kepreotes et al., 2010; van der Lee et al., 2007; Wijlaars et al., 2016). Between 10% and 30% of children suffer from chronic illnesses or health conditions (Consolini, 2022). Common illnesses that carry significant risk for morbidity and mortality for young children (ages 1 through 4 years) include neurological problems, heart conditions, cancer, and respiratory conditions (Wijlaars et al., 2016).

Herzer et al. (2010) reported that, irrespective of the type of chronic illness, about one quarter of families had difficulty functioning as they normally would during a child's chronic illness. These families may feel a lack of engagement in the child's care and are simultaneously coping with disruptions in family functioning (e.g., family separation due to child hospitalization, financial burden related to medical expenses). The behavior of parents and other family members – and functioning of the family unit – has an impact on the child with a chronic illness or medical condition and vice versa. Knafl et al. (2017) proposed that the bidirectional (we prefer the notion of mutual or shared influence among multiple family members) nature of child and family functioning, with the child and parent/family influencing each other, and well-being of the child and family make it critical to study

L. Nabors (✉) · T. N. A. Addy · S. Shukla
University of Cincinnati, Cincinnati, OH, USA
e-mail: naborsla@ucmail.uc.edu

L. Nabors, J. D. Bartlett (eds.), *Family Engagement in Mental Health Interventions for Young Children*, Springer Series on Child and Family Studies,
https://doi.org/10.1007/978-3-031-47917-5_5

interventions that involve the parents and family when an infant or young child has a chronic illness.

Parent and family engagement is critical when children are young because parents have a more significant caregiving role and young children with chronic illnesses are vulnerable and in need of extra care (Balling & McCubbin, 2001). Young children, ages birth through 8 years of age, benefit from significant parent and family involvement in their care. Young children are mastering developmental milestones from infancy through 8 years. For instance, infants are learning to engage the world with their senses. Toddlers are learning to walk and talk, and preschoolers often are learning their first stages of independence. Kindergarteners are learning more academic skills and independence, and these skills increase in the first years of elementary school. There are a host of other tasks, with parents and primary caregivers bridging young children's physical, cognitive, social, emotional, and educational development (see Berk & Meyers, 2016). Children with chronic illnesses can face disruption of these milestones (e.g., Maurice-Stam et al., 2019). Parents, caregivers, and family benefit from support and information sharing from the healthcare team when a young child faces illness, to help them foster child development and engage them in medical care of the child.

Support of the child and the family unit through improved family engagement is a protective factor associated with resilient family functioning and supporting parents (Knafl et al., 2017). Family engagement, involving family contributions to patient care, is defined along a continuum, "…moving from passive (e.g., physical presence at the bedside and receiving and having needs met) to more active activities (e.g., sharing and receiving information, inclusion in decision-making, and making contributions to the care of the patient)" (McAndrew et al., 2022, p. 297). Studies often have a variety of ages in the sample (Lappalainen et al., 2021; Mitchell et al., 2020), and focusing on engagement for families of young children will improve the knowledge base for this vulnerable group. Rolland (1984) emphasized the collaborative, shared nature of family members' influence on each other as the child copes with illness. Consequently, their interactions are integral to child and family adaptation and resilience when a child has a chronic illness. This chapter highlights factors that support the engagement of parents and other family members based on the notion that parent/family engagement will improve family members' abilities to cope with the child's illness, which, in turn, influences the child's adaptation and development as they cope with a chronic disease (Segers et al., 2019).

Consideration of the Family System and Needs of the Young Child

Family systems theory has emphasized the interconnections among family members, which echoes the mutual or shared relationship between child and family, which may contribute to positive adjustment to illness and coping of both the child and family (Knafl et al., 2017). Healthcare providers need to consider the child, parents, and other family members as intertwined, and provide recommendations that will educate and involve parents or guardians in childcare and partner with them to promote child development and well-being. Understanding and providing recommendations to meet parent needs for support and information about medical procedures also is important, because parent confidence and support will strengthen the child's coping. Walsh (2014) posited the essential nature of family relationships and interactions, which promote resilience among children, engage parents and family in care, and bolster a child's emotional functioning, courage, and hope as they cope with stresses and isolation related to dealing with a chronic illness. Balling and McCubbin (2001), family systems theorists, underscored the role of communication among family members and other systems as critical to child and family adjustment. Facilitating communication between the healthcare system and parents or guardians, extended family members, and the child might enhance engagement of the family in helping administer treatments and in supporting the child as he or she copes with multiple medical appointments, invasive medical procedures, and repeated hospitalizations.

Figure 5.1 presents, in broad-brush strokes, our team's ideas of building blocks for promoting parent and family engagement for families of young children with chronic illness. We believe that education has the potential to improve health literacy and health outcomes, thereby reducing morbidities and mortality for young children. Shared decision-making and communication with the parents, family members, and the child can build the resilience of and provide support to the family. Affording healthcare professionals time to communicate and have team meetings to consider engagement is one way to help them foster engagement skills. Having a hospital climate (and policies) in support of engagement can support the family and the healthcare team as they work to develop an alliance and offer coordinated care for the child. The child, parent, and family can engage with the healthcare team and share information to create wraparound care and a long-term relationship to provide child development creating a medical home for the young child (Homer et al., 2008). Hence, support of the healthcare team, the parents and family unit, and the child and a focus on education, communication, and shared decision-making may promote parent and family engagement. Their inclusion and care can, in turn, encourage child well-being and child and family resilience.

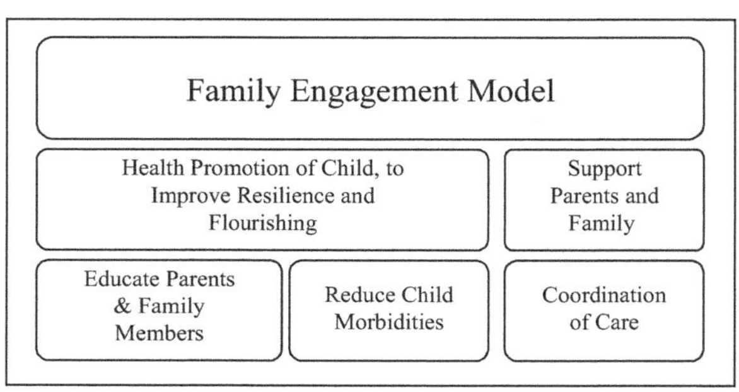

Fig. 5.1 Family engagement model with core ideas: support child, family, and healthcare team. *Note*: We recommend health promotion, education, support, and coordination of care delivered from a strengths-based, culturally sensitive perspective

Engaging Families Through Information Sharing

Healthcare professionals promote parent and family member engagement and health literacy when they discuss information about development and healthcare with the parents, and, as needed, family members (Sanders et al., 2009). For example, if the child is not thriving or their growth is faltering, parents and caregivers may benefit from instruction on feeding practices, as well as instruction on ways to foster adequate sleep (Craig et al., 2015; Tang et al., 2021). Alternately, if the home is food insecure, social workers on staff at the hospital may need to help parents find resources for formula, baby food, or healthy meals for a toddler or preschooler (Tang et al., 2021). They may need to learn new ways to respond to stress, maintain skin-to-skin contact with, and keep their young child safe – ensuring a secure attachment bond between mother and child (Scher et al., 2009; van Der Voort et al., 2014; Widström et al., 2019). Moreover, parents or caregivers may need instructions for operating complex medical equipment or for administering complex treatments at home or for adapting the home for the care of a child with special medical needs (e.g., an infant with respiratory issues) or developmental disabilities (Powell et al., 2019). If the child needs additional therapeutic support, parents may need referrals for care coordination and help locating and accessing specialty services, such as speech, physical, and occupational therapy (Kerber et al., 2007; McManus et al., 2020). Assessment of pain for infants and toddlers should engage parents or caregivers, to understand their perspectives, as part of a multicomponent assessment that also involves behavioral observations (Franck et al., 2000). When involving parents and caregivers in assessing pain, healthcare professionals create opportunities to share information about pain and child distress, such as signs of their child's pain (e.g., grimacing, flinching) as well as ways to assess level of pain, using a facial recognition scale, for example (Franck et al., 2000). It also is important for clinicians to evaluate whether parents need counseling for grief related to their child's condition (e.g., coping with the loss of ideal development for their child; Craig et al., 2015).

Recommendations for Promoting Engagement and Child Functioning

After reviewing the literature on critical care for adults with illnesses (some studies included pregnant women as participants), Mackintosh et al. (2020) proposed recommendations that are appropriate for fostering parent and family engagement when a young child faces a critical illness. Mackintosh et al. (2020) recommended the following approaches, which center on education and coaching so families can secure care for a loved one:

> helping patients and their families to notice changes in a patient's condition and tell healthcare staff about them; (2) empowering patients and families to feel confident about arranging

> for urgent or emergency care; (3) healthcare staff giving patients and families a chance to talk about their concerns, and actively listening to them during an emergency consultation; and (4) training healthcare staff to respond appropriately when patients and their families raise concerns about a patient's condition. (p. 3)

If parents/family members are engaged in care, they may become advocates for a patient, having opportunities to interact with staff, share information, and learn about medical care for their loved one. Healthcare staff need opportunities for training to learn this "listening" and "empowering" mode of care, and the staff may need support as they remain open to giving this type of support to families. Mackintosh et al. (2020) reported that seven of the nine studies they reviewed involved direct instruction to families, while two included staff instruction and support. Engaging families and allowing for shared decision-making take time, expertise, and patience. Ensuring time for team meetings to discuss ideas for family engagement will allow the medical team to plan how to involve parents, and when appropriate young children. Trainings about ways to promote engagement may be another avenue for supporting staff so that they are knowledgeable about ways to engage parents and family members in supporting the medical care and health needs of young children. Mackintosh et al. (2020) stated that more research is needed to determine the effectiveness of interventions, especially what works for whom, in terms of type of illness for the child and family characteristics.

Interventions in Neonatal Intensive Care Units (NICUs) and Critical-Care Units

McAndrew et al. (2022) reviewed interventions to improve family engagement for NICUs and critical-care units for children. Theory and practice of facilitating family learning about medical care, fostering child development, and supporting family voice and engagement in the patient's medical care often guided studies and the development of interventions. For studies conducted in NICUs and hospital-based interventions for young children, a focus on educating parents about care and techniques for helping the child cope (e.g., regulate emotions, understand medical course of treatment) was common. Nurses were typically the chief facilitators of engagement and sharing information about developmentally appropriate healthcare practices to parents/family. The NICU interventions also taught parents how to facilitate sensory and neural development of the infant (McAndrew et al., 2022). Sharing information about or encouraging parents to build infant skills and communicate with staff was positive and could engage and promote the resilience of parents. Behavior-change strategies for parents (e.g., how to care for their child) were presented through role-modeling, and many programs supplied informational pamphlets for parent education. McAndrew et al. (2022) mentioned that interventions decreased parent stress and improved interactions with children and could decrease hospital stays. They cautioned that some of the interventions they reviewed were new, there was variability in outcomes across studies, interventions involved multiple components, specifics on the delivery of interventions were not clear, and the quality of studies was from moderate to low, and thus further research is needed to more fully understand interventions to facilitate engagement.

McAndrew et al. (2022) reported that several of the studies they reviewed examined parental stress as an outcome variable, with mixed results, as sometimes stress levels did not improve over the course of the intervention. Parent emotional functioning and family member/staff satisfaction were other outcomes assessed. Some interventions positively impacted emotional functioning, reducing anxiety and depression for parents by reducing stress. More research will improve understanding of which interventions work better for parents and why this is the case. However, both healthcare staff and family members (namely parents) were satisfied with the interventions, although McAndrew et al. (2022) did recommend that simply assessing satisfaction may not fully capture the impact of interventions to improve engagement. There were not significant changes in physiologic outcomes (e.g., heart rate) for infants, although those families participating in interventions typically had shortened lengths of stay. McAndrew et al. (2022) concluded that results indicated positive outcomes for children and parents; it is important to interpret findings with caution, as several studies were quasi-experimental and only one study was of high quality.

Segers et al. (2019) reviewed parent perceptions of family-centered care interventions and length of stay on pediatric and neonatal and intensive care units. These researchers provided the following definition, "Family centered care emphasizes the importance of a family as a fundamental source of support and it considers involvement of family members in all aspects of the patient's health care" (Segers et al., 2019, p. 63). They found most parents reported satisfaction with interventions. However, they noted satisfaction is difficult to define, making measurement of this variable challenging. Importantly, Segers et al. (2019) reported that some studies they reviewed found reduced hospital stays for children. We recommend continued assessment of hospital stays and health outcomes for the child. Qualitative methods, such as in-depth interviews, may be useful in evaluating the impact of family-centered care on parent and family perceptions of care, emotional functioning, satisfaction, and perceptions of support of the child and family unit.

Approaches to Improve Engagement

Literature reveals approaches that have been successful for improving parent and family engagement. Education is key, either in-person or using informational pamphlets or websites (online support groups) as tools to enhance discussion, to share and talk about medical information with parents or family members (Gurung et al., 2020). Involving parents in sharing what they know and need to know may engage them in the educational process and allow them to ask questions to increase their knowledge about their child's healthcare, allowing them to gain information that will help them in their decision-making regarding their child's medical care. Encouraging communication between the medical team and parents/family also could connect parents and family members and facilitate their engagement as team members (Gurung et al., 2020). Knudsen et al. (2021) recommend that health professionals provide tools for parents (e.g., activities to assist them in caring for their child or building their child's skills/fostering development), to help them care for their child. For example, for premature infants and other infants who have been in the NICU, these tools could include recommendations for child-rearing to optimize child physical, neural, sensory social, and emotional development.

Knafl et al. (2017) conducted a review of 70 family interventions that used a range of approaches to engage the family. Many interventions provided education and involved family members (typically the parent and child) in disease management or presented education about the child's chronic illness (55 of the interventions). Fifteen of the interventions addressed improving family relationships, through a variety of interventions designed to improve family functioning, improve communication, or reduce family conflict. Their findings indicated that engaging the family in disease management improved family engagement as well as child functioning. Knafl et al. (2017) found that other interventions aimed to improve family interaction patterns, and these interventions also could improve both family and child coping. Most interventions were disease-specific (addressing coping with one type of illness, $n = 61$), while seven of the interventions involved assisting families of children with different medical conditions. Interestingly, parents helped to define and determine interventions (e.g., deciding on what problems to address or what skills they wanted to learn) in eight of the interventions. Knafl et al. (2017) noted that to move the field forward, considering the family system or context in design of interventions as well as including parents in the design of interventions would be important. It was surprising that several of the interventions Knafl et al. (2017) reviewed were for parents only or worked with children and parents separately. However, if the influence of the child and parent/family members is mutual or shared, then interventions that address child and parent or family members' needs will be important to improving functioning for the family as a unit.

Roles of Healthcare Providers

Healthcare Team

The team needs to be committed to family engagement and support, and key drivers of engagement may be the behaviors and "stance" of the healthcare team. Misak et al. (2021), authors who have lived experiences coping with critical care of family members, proposed that ideas from critical-care medicine, primarily caring and compassion, are key components for family engagement. Care and compassion can connect the child, parent, and family, especially during "switches" between doctors and medical teams as a child moves in and out of the hospital and goes through different medical experiences. Connecting medical providers (i.e., multiple providers) to each other can promote communication and more "seamless" care, with teams knowing the recommendations of other teams, which can further promote a feeling of connection for the family. Perhaps having a team lead to facilitate communication about multiple health issues could ease communication burdens for parents (Misak et al., 2021). Ensuring that healthcare professionals and teams have opportunities to discuss ways to promote family engagement may optimize chances for promoting family engagement during healthcare appointments and interactions during medical crises.

Pediatricians

Understanding pediatrician's' beliefs about a young child's abilities and social/emotional functioning at different ages (e.g., infancy, toddlerhood, preschool, and early elementary years) will assist research teams and healthcare professionals in designing interventions that consider pediatricians' knowledge about child development (Gabe et al., 2004). It may be that pediatricians need education about social and emotional functioning of young children, so they can help parents understand the importance of improving their connection with their child. They also may need training on communication about sensitive medical issues, such as explaining child discomfort and talking about diagnoses, to improve parent/family engagement (Balling & McCubbin, 2001). Similarly, it may be helpful for pediatricians to think about "readiness" of the parents/family to engage in shared decision-making and take on responsibilities for their child's medical care, and then understand how their readiness might be related to their level of engagement with the doctors and medical team. Medical recommendations and action steps for care that are "user-friendly" and at a level consistent with parent health literacy, cultural and family perspectives and values, knowledge, and readiness to help with care may engage parents and help them understand medical protocols to care for their child (Gurung et al., 2020).

Communication, Decision-Making, and Family-Centered Care

Communication

Establishing effective communication between healthcare professionals, parents, and children may lead to improved health literacy of the child and parents and consequently improved family engagement. On the other hand, poor communication has been associated with lower satisfaction with care, lower levels of adherence to recommendations, and poor health (Porr et al., 2006; Zarcadoolas et al., 2006). Low health literacy can negatively influence patient-provider communication and adherence to recommendations and engagement with the medical team (Bernhardt & Cameron, 2003). A parent with low health literacy may have difficulty communicating the child's problem to the doctor and may not be able to understand questions about the child's health history. If the doctor decides to prescribe medication or a treatment regimen, a parent with low health literacy may not understand how to follow through with recommendations, give medications, and contact the pediatrician if the child's health worsens.

Developing communication programs to share information with patients about the importance of communicating with the doctor about illness, and if they misunderstand treatment recommendations, can foster health literacy (Bernhardt & Cameron, 2003). Health professionals should develop communication programs for parents and family members. When the medical team respects parent expertise and knowledge of their child, they may build a relationship with parents that can foster communication. Communication between the doctor/healthcare professionals, parent, and child is related to mother and child satisfaction with the visit and trust in the doctor, memory of recommendations, self-efficacy for adhering to recommendations, follow-through with recommendations, and recovery to good health for the child (Nutbeam, 2000; Porr et al., 2006). Gurung et al. (2020) also reported that various forms of communication increased family engagement. Results of their review suggested that advisory groups for parents and children, and online communication, such as patient portals (with critical information for healthcare) and online support groups, could engage parents, and other families, in healthcare of child patients.

Family as Decision-Makers

Throughout these changes and the course of the illness, engaging the parents or primary caregiver(s), child, and, as appropriate, the family in decision-making can promote family-centered decision-making and communication, fostering engagement (Segers et al., 2019). Segers et al. (2019) defined family-centered healthcare as care that views family support and engagement as fundamental to healthcare. Additionally, education about options, medical care, and health issues may enhance the child, parent, and family's ability to help "care" for the child and promote better quality of life for the child and further enhance family engagement. Promoting parent knowledge and encouraging their abilities to communicate and make decisions will increase their engagement (Balling & McCubbin, 2001).

Family-Centered Care

One aspect of family-centered care is shared decision-making, where the family and, if possible, the patient share in medical decisions. Critical elements of shared decision-making include common goals for doctors and families (e.g., the patient as well), an absence of a hierarchy in decision-making for the doctor and family to make decisions together, and mutual respect between doctors and parents/children (Coulter, 2002). Describing health issues and effective communication are important to assist parents and children in understanding medical issues (Gabe et al., 2004). This shift can be more challenging in complex, emergent, and serious medical situations. Hence, there must be a readiness on the part of the parents and child to be involved and "take on" decision-making. Health professionals need to have the ability to determine the "readiness" and "willingness" of the parents, family members (if applicable), and child to engage in shared decision-making (Gabe et al., 2004). Parents may want an alliance with health professionals to gain and share knowledge about the care of their child, and it is critical for professionals to work to explain complex health information so that family members can understand medical terms and steps in medical procedures and interventions (Balling & McCubbin, 2001; Nutbeam, 2000).

Health professionals who "partner" with family members can facilitate engagement and shared decision-making (Charles & DeMaio, 1993; Gabe et al., 2004). Misak et al. (2021) discussed shared decision-making in intensive care units (ICUs), where family care and input can be fundamental to care (Segers et al., 2019). Shared decision-making in the ICU is on a continuum, typically occurring with differing levels of family leadership and engagement, and we believe the notion of levels and meeting the parent and family members at the right level is important for engaging families of young children with chronic illnesses. Understanding that the illness, and its waxing and waning course, is a series of traumatic experiences for the family and patient also will help professionals connect with patients and families. Family engagement and education about medical concerns may enhance their ability to engage in conversations about their child's health and well-being, which, in turn, may result in plans that improve quality of life for the child or patient (Misak et al., 2021).

Impact of Trauma

Children and parents facing critical care related to the child's chronic illness may experience medical trauma. Medical trauma is threatening in terms of an injury or a physical or psychological trauma experience and is related to the child's medical condition or experiences related to the child's medical condition (see De Young et al., 2021). Parents, the child, and potentially siblings and other family members (e.g., grandparents) may benefit from participating in therapy with a pediatric psychologist or counselor and receiving guidance from health professionals with expertise in trauma-informed care. In addition to trauma, repeated medical treatments can result in emotional issues for the child. Balling and McCubbin (2001) recommended that health professionals be sensitive to the potential negative impact of repeated hospitalizations on the child, which could result in feelings of depression. Keeping in mind the trauma of multiple emergent care visits and hospitalizations for the child and family will help health professionals provide nurturing and understanding, maximizing family engagement in care and inclusion in the care process for their child, which can be cornerstones of engagement. Misak et al. (2021) recommended a trauma-informed perspective for healthcare providers, which would facilitate "...ensuring safety, establishing trustworthiness, maximizing choice, maximizing collaboration, and prioritizing empowerment" (p. 1397). When health providers can address trauma, ensure a feeling of safety and trust for patients, and develop a stepped model of care (with levels of early intervention to support families to crisis care) that provides the level of care necessary given child medical needs and family values and needs, they may maximize the potential to engage parents and children in care (De Young et al., 2021). Parents of young children with chronic illness may also be facing anxiety and depression, and potential health problems related to stress, related to their child's trauma (Cohn et al., 2020), and healthcare providers should consider their mental health needs when presenting them with information. Moreover, referral may be necessary, if mental health concerns are limiting parent/family member abilities to be engaged in their child's disease management or limiting their abilities to engage in shared decision-making.

Need for More Evidence-Based Approaches

Tailoring approaches to family culture, beliefs, preferences, and needs is an "art" involving care and attention to family "engagement style" and will help healthcare team members to connect with the child, parents, and family members (Misak et al., 2021). To facilitate connection, we recommend an orientation of "putting the family 'first'" and encourage healthcare professionals to recognize that "...the family is the constant in the child's life, whereas the service systems and personnel within those systems fluctuate" (Johnson et al., 1992, p. 3). Thus, there remains a continued need for research on engaging parents and family members to promote child and family functioning. This research also needs to focus on understanding ways to engage families facing health disparities. This type of research will generate interventions that can be disseminated in a variety of settings with children of different ages, who have different chronic illnesses, and with families facing health disparities – which is imperative in promoting social justice.

Critical Issues Related to Social Justice and Health Disparities

Successful parent and family engagement may vary across cultures. We recommend a strengths-based approach to engaging parents and family members. McLendon (2013) mentioned that learning their service provision needs and preferences and considering them as experts on their and their child's lives can provide a starting point for assessment. We recommend asking about and then incorporating family strengths in engagement plans for the family. It also is important to address and try to overcome language and cultural barriers, which may impede understanding of valuable information about the child and family (Isaac et al., 2020; Lambert et al., 2021; Linton et al., 2019). Although their focus was on adults, Lambert et al. (2021) presented points for consideration for working with families from a culture different than that of the provider/health professional. They recommended considering multiple factors, including health perceptions and beliefs, awareness of the course and nature of the illness, awareness of the "acute" nature of the illness, and the parent/family members' and child's ability to express wants and needs. Notably, Lambert et al. (2021) also mentioned that for pamphlets, those parents from different countries may be trying to find words in dictionaries. They may have difficulty understanding terms and information in pamphlets. Consequently, it is important to consider the language in pamphlets and the health literacy levels of parents/family members when presenting them with written information. Talking over written information with families from a different culture while understanding their views about healthcare can assist the healthcare provider in engaging parents and family and improve optimization of the healthcare plan for the child.

Approaches for Engaging Parents and Family Members

We recommend the following steps for guiding professionals in connecting to parents of children with chronic illnesses: (1) learn, discuss, and respect parent/family health beliefs, (2) reflect on parent/family perceptions of the child's illness and the stage of the illness, (3) find out about and address cultural needs of different family members, (4) understand and work through language barriers, and (5) develop an engagement plan that is flexible to meet changing needs of the family. Having "cultural humility" in understanding that all cultural mores and norms are valuable is an essential tool for engagement (Isaac et al., 2020; Linton et al., 2019). In terms of illness stage, it is important to consider the "acuteness" of the medical condition and parent/family emotional reaction to this when communicating, as well as how the parent/family culture might influence reactions of parents and family members. Parent engagement needs differ when a child is extremely ill in the hospital versus when parents attend the clinic for routine care. Hence, the nature of the illness and "stage" is vital to consider for all families, including those facing cultural barriers. Additionally, when providing written material, it may be best to review the material with parents/family members and ensure they understand the material and are interpreting complex medical information and recommendations for care correctly. Healthcare teams at children's hospitals can use interpreters, which can significantly help parents and family with "understanding" medical knowledge.

Considerations for engaging parents include developing strategies to overcome language barriers and offering support to parents, including gaining permission for other family members to come to medical appointments. The engagement plan should be flexible to consider culture and parent health perceptions and knowledge of the illness. Health professionals should be knowledgeable about different diseases and how they impact the child (Isaac et al., 2020; Linton et al., 2019). Knowledge of the illness and its course/severity can help the professional connect to parents and family. For instance, engagement may be different for a child with cancer facing a bone marrow transplant versus a child with asthma. And the phase of illness is important too – engagement approaches may be more critical at diagnosis and the first year after diagnosis compared to later in the course of the illness, when the parent and family have established a secure relationship with the medical team. A "stance" of caring and connection, as well as cultural competence and humility, will help with engagement plans at all phases, and checking in to see how the team's or professional's engagement plan is proceeding can keep engagement as a critical healthcare goal (Linton et al., 2019). Our case study, below, presents the case of a young preschool-age boy facing a bone marrow transplant and discusses connecting the child's mother to a therapist to help her as she navigates the complexities of her child's chronic illness.

Case Study

Denny is a 3-year-old boy with acute lymphoblastic leukemia (ALL). He has battled his cancer for 2 years and received chemotherapy. Currently, he needs a bone marrow transplant. Although brave and involved in his care throughout the rounds of chemotherapy, his mother is hesitant and worried about his bone marrow transplant. She has been avoiding scheduling the hospital stay and talking about her fears and beliefs with Denny's pediatric oncologist. The nurses, with whom she usually easily converses, have noted her hesitancy to speak and her withdrawn nature.

The team decides to consult with the pediatric psychologist to discuss ideas for communicating with Denny's mother to both promote her health literacy, let her know about the procedure, and to find ways to allow her to express her feelings. The pediatric psychologist recommended having a fact-finding meeting between the oncologist and Denny's mother in a more neutral setting than the clinic. They suggest the family room, near the playroom, where Denny and his mother spent time playing during his chemotherapy treatment. The oncologist, nurse, and pediatric psychologist discuss asking Denny's mother her opinion and asking her to direct the session to improve her engagement.

At the meeting, the oncologist offers to answer questions and lets Denny's mother know that she is eager to hear her perspectives. In addition, the oncologist says she hopes she can share any "research knowledge" to help Denny's mother consider medical information related to treatments to help Denny. Denny's mother immediately discusses her worries associated with a potential bone marrow transplant. She is concerned about infection and that the treatment will not be successful. The oncologist listens first and then offers information. She offers Denny's mother the opportunity to "room in" and stay in the hospital room with Denny before and after the procedure. The oncologist adds that she can stay at the nearby Ronald

McDonald House during Denny's hospital stay. The oncologist explains that the Ronald McDonald House is a place for parents of children to stay that is nearby the hospital (Rubin & Franck, 2017). There is a minimal fee or no charge to stay there. Also, Denny's mother will be staying with other parents of children with illnesses, in a supportive environment. Family members, such as Denny's sibling, can stay at the Ronald McDonald House as well. After recovery Denny and his mother could remain at the Ronald McDonald House until he is able to return home. Denny's mother was enthusiastic about staying at the Ronald McDonald house, provided her extended family or another caregiver take care of his older brother and ensure he attends school and some extracurricular activities. Next, the oncologist honestly discussed the pros and cons of the procedure and explains why this type of procedure may be a necessary treatment.

After a few moments, Denny's mother cries. She worries that she and Denny "we can't do through one more thing." The oncologist replies that "I know you have been through so much; I know that so much courage has been needed for you both to keep going through the chemotherapy." Denny's mother mentions that Denny is a "fighter," and his "hope" bolsters her courage. However, she expresses grief over the loss of her son's normal childhood, stating, "He's so young and has been through so much." The doctor recommends a referral to a pediatric psychologist for counseling. The oncologist explains that a pediatric psychologist is a psychologist with experience with children with chronic illness, child development, child therapy, and family therapy, and with working in medical settings, who can help her discuss her concerns (Perricone, 2021). Denny's mother agrees to try an appointment with the pediatric psychologist. Although the oncologist mentioned that the pediatric psychologist can work with Denny to prepare him for his medical procedures, his mother decided that she did not want this option at this time.

During therapy, Denny's mother had opportunities to express her emotions and discuss her need for learning from, "Someone who has been through this." Next, the psychologist referred her to a support group. This group was comprised of parents of children with cancer. After attending three counseling sessions and monthly support group meetings for about 6 months, Denny's mother felt she had increased emotional support and reduced stress. Another meeting with oncology nurses, recommended by another parent in her support group, resulted in her learning useful methods for increasing Denny's calorie intake (e.g., using supplements and a high-protein diet) and helping him get adequate sleep. She was very relieved that she could stay at a local Ronald McDonald House when Denny was in the hospital after his procedure, so she could be close to him. She found a caregiver to stay with Denny's older brother – another referral from a mentor at her support group. His older sibling could also visit and stay with her at the Ronald McDonald House, so that she could remain close to the older child. Denny's mother reported that she could feel her fighting spirit return, so that she could, in turn, foster Denny's resilience.

There are positive steps to facilitate engagement in this case. The medical team took time to discuss this case and think about the perspectives of the mother and child and how to involve them in the healthcare process. The oncologist worked to enhance the mother's health literacy and communicate with her. The doctor allowed her to express feelings and past experiences, which was a positive experience for Denny's mother. The doctor met Denny's mother in the playroom, minimizing the power differential between them. The oncologist was open to hearing Denny's mother and learning about his emotions and empathizing with their perspectives, while trying to improve health literacy, so she had the knowledge she needed to understand the procedure. The oncologist respected Denny's mother's expertise and requests (e.g., rooming in with Denny). Moreover, the doctor did not rush decision-making and encouraged Denny's mother to collaborate with a pediatric psychologist who in turn referred her to other parents with children with cancer. Denny's mother had time to reflect on her feelings, cope with distress over the loss of normalcy for her son, and learn of options for being close to him and caring for her other child, so she could feel more comfortable because she would be there to support Denny during his hospitalization, and that her older child would be supported. His mother did decide to move forward with the bone marrow transplant. During ongoing conversations throughout the process of care, the oncologist, the medical team, and the pediatric psychologist worked to understand family culture and both Denny and his mother's perspectives, and then shared information and engaged them in the decision-making process and recovery care after his bone marrow transplant. This fostered engagement in care, contributing positively to Denny's recovery after the transplant.

Limitations of Current Knowledge

Studies often present multicomponent intervention packages or recommended multicomponent techniques to improve child or family functioning, and this makes it difficult to determine what techniques were related to or drove change processes. Our conclusions after reviewing research for children are consistent with those of a recent Cochrane review for critical care and family engagement with adult patients – high-quality clinical trials will determine how interventions impact family engagement. Although there is information related to the importance of family engagement and the importance of family involvement, more rigorous research will determine the effectiveness of interventions designed to improve family engagement (McAndrew et al., 2022). Gilliss et al. (2019) offered recommendations for improving research on family engagement for adults with chronic illnesses, and their recommendations extend to research for children and their families. Specifically, Gilliss et al. (2019) recommended that researchers need to gain more knowledge about which interventions work for specific diseases, as well as improve knowledge of which types of interventions work for different family members. When considering engagement, it also is important to consider the child's age and developmental stage to understand information about physical, cognitive, social, and emotional development to share with parents and caregivers.

Furthermore, Gilliss et al. (2019) recommended that researchers better explain family and patient change processes that will foster family and child resilience and child development and carefully select outcomes for assessment related to positive change processes. Also, studies have included a broad age range of children in the sample (e.g., Balling & McCubbin, 2001), and therefore enhanced study of parent engagement for young children (e.g., ages birth through 5) may yield information to inform interventions. Studies have often centered on family-level interventions. Policy studies – that investigate hospital and healthcare center policy and practice are needed. The impact of this orientation on family engagement may, in turn, present added information about how systems-level change is related to family engagement when a child has a chronic illness (Gurung et al., 2020).

Future Directions

We propose that, in addition to assessing how engagement impacts mortality and health morbidities, researchers should examine relations among parent and family engagement and quality of life, mental health, and social-emotional functioning for children with chronic illnesses and their family members. Qualitative methods may produce information about the perceptions of parents and the family to guide intervention development. Segers et al. (2019) called for qualitative studies to understand perceptions of care and family needs as well as randomized controlled trials to discover "gaps" in family-centered care and variables that improve family engagement and outcomes for children. Decision-making tools may enhance communication between the medical team and parents (Clarke-Pounder et al., 2015). Specifically, parents may benefit from decision-making tools to inform them about medical developments and information for their children and ideas for promoting healthcare and outcomes for their children (Clarke-Pounder et al., 2015).

McAndrew et al. (2022) recommended that researchers examine data on the safety and efficiency of engaging family (such as parents) in care. Gurung et al. (2020) noted that most studies focused on hospital settings and suggested that researchers turn their lens to understanding family engagement in primary care and community healthcare settings. This would provide information on whether the same or different variables facilitated engagement across settings. Furthermore, enhanced training on parent and family member engagement may improve health professionals' abilities to connect with and engage parents and families in the child's care (Isaac et al., 2020). We had mentioned a need for policy and the study of policy as a direction for the future. Charles and DeMaio (1993) suggested a conceptualization shift to accomplish this, which included having healthcare providers be "accountable" to the communities they serve. Accountability or caring for the family's view and perspective may also ensure that healthcare professionals remain oriented toward family engagement and shared decision-making to enhance health outcomes and quality of life for young children with chronic illnesses.

References

Balling, K., & McCubbin, M. (2001). Hospitalized children with chronic illness: Parental caregiving needs and valuing parental expertise. *Journal of Pediatric Nursing, 16*(2), 110–119. https://doi.org/10.1053/jpdn.2001.23157

Berk, L. E., & Meyers, A. B. (2016). *Infants and children* (8th ed.). Pearson.

Bernhardt, J. M., & Cameron, K. A. (2003). Accessing, understanding, and applying health communication messages: The challenge of health literacy. In T. L. Thompson, A. M. Dorsey, K. I. Miller, & R. Parrott (Eds.), *Handbook of health communication* (pp. 583–605). Lawrence Erlbaum Associates.

Charles, C., & DeMaio, S. (1993). Lay participation in health care decision making: A conceptual framework. *Journal of Health Politics, Policy and Law, 18*(4), 881–904. https://doi.org/10.1215/03616878-18-4-881

Clarke-Pounder, J. P., Boss, R. D., Roter, D. L., Hutton, N., Larson, S., & Donohue, P. K. (2015). Communication intervention in the neonatal intensive care unit: Can it backfire? *Journal of Palliative Medicine, 18*(2), 157–161. https://doi.org/10.1089/jpm.2014.0037

Cohn, L. N., Pechlivanoglou, P., Lee, Y., Mahant, S., Orkin, J., Marson, A., & Cohen, E. (2020). Health outcomes of parents of children with chronic illness: A systematic review and meta-analysis. *Journal of Pediatrics, 218*, 166–177. https://doi.org/10.1016/j.jpeds.2019.10.068

Consolini, D. M. (2022). Children with chronic health conditions. In *Merck manual professional version*. Merck & Co., Inc. https://www.merckmanuals.com/professional/pediatrics/caring-for-sick-children-and-their-families/children-with-chronic-health-conditions

Coulter, A. (2002). *The autonomous patient: Ending paternalism in medical care*. TSO (The Stationery Office). http://hdl.handle.net/10822/951228

Craig, J. W., Glick, C., Phillips, R., Hall, S. L., Smith, J., & Browne, J. (2015). Recommendations for involving the family in developmental care of the NICU baby. *Journal of Perinatology, 35 Suppl 1(Suppl 1), S5–S8*. https://doi.org/10.1038/jp.2015.142

De Young, A. C., Paterson, R. S., Brown, E. A., Egberts, M. R., Le Brocque, R. M., Kenardy, J. A., Landlot, M. A., Marsac, M. L., Alisic, E., & Haag, A. C. (2021). Topical review: Medical trauma during early childhood. *Journal of Pediatric Psychology, 46*(7), 739–746. https://doi.org/10.1093/jpepsy/jsab045

Franck, L. S., Greenberg, C. S., & Stevens, B. (2000). Pain assessment in infants and children. *Pediatric Clinics of North America, 47*(3), 487–512. https://doi.org/10.1016/S0031-3955(05)70222-4

Gabe, J., Olumide, G., & Bury, M. (2004). "It takes three to tango": A framework for understanding patient partnership in paediatric clinics. *Social Science and Medicine, 59*(5), 1070–1079. https://doi.org/10.1016/j.socscimed.2003.09.035

Gilliss, C. L., Pan, W., & Davis, L. L. (2019). Family involvement in adult chronic disease care: Reviewing the systematic reviews. *Journal of Family Nursing, 25*(1), 3–27. https://doi.org/10.1177/1074840718822365

Gurung, G., Richardson, A., Wyeth, E., Edmonds, L., & Derrett, S. (2020). Child/youth, family and public engagement in paediatric services in high-income countries: A systematic scoping review. *Health Expectations, 23*(2), 261–273. https://doi.org/10.1111/hex.13017

Herzer, M., Godiwala, N., Hommel, K. A., Driscoll, K., Mitchell, M., Crosby, L. E., Piazza-Waggoner, C., Zeller, M. H., & Modi, A. C. (2010). Family functioning in the context of pediatric chronic conditions. *Journal of Developmental and Behavioral Pediatrics, 31*(1), 26–34. https://doi.org/10.1097/DBP.0b013e3181c7226b

Homer, C. J., Klatka, K., Romm, D., Kuhlthau, K., Bloom, S., Newacheck, P., Van Cleave, J., & Perrin, J. M. (2008). A review of the evidence for the medical home for children with special health care needs. *Pediatrics, 122*(4), e922–e937. https://doi.org/10.1542/peds.2007-3762

Isaac, E. I., Meisman, A. R., Drucker, K., Violante, S., Behrhorst, K. L., Floyd, A., & Rohan, J. M. (2020). The relationship between health disparities, psychosocial functioning and health outcomes in pediatric hematology-oncology and stem cell transplant populations:

Recommendations for clinical care. *International Journal of Environmental Research and Public Health, 17*(7), Article 2218, 1–14. https://doi.org/10.3390/ijerph17072218
Johnson, B. H., Jeppson, E. S., & Redburn, L. (1992). *Caring for children and families: Guidelines for hospitals* (1st ed.). Association for the Care of Children's Health.
Kepreotes, E., Keatinge, D., & Stone, T. (2010). The experience of parenting children with chronic health conditions: A new reality. *Journal of Nursing and Healthcare of Chronic Illness, 2*, 51–62. https://doi.org/10.1111/j.1752-9824.2010.01047.x
Kerber, K. J., de Graft-Johnson, J. E., Bhutta, Z. A., Okong, P., Starrs, A., & Lawn, J. E. (2007). Continuum of care for maternal, newborn, and child health: From slogan to service delivery. *The Lancet, 370*(9595), 1358–1369. https://doi.org/10.1016/S0140-6736(07)61578-5
Knafl, K. A., Havill, N. L., Leeman, J., Fleming, L., Crandell, J. L., & Sandelowski, M. (2017). The nature of family engagement in interventions for children with chronic conditions. *Western Journal of Nursing Research, 39*(5), 690–723. https://doi.org/10.1177/0193945916664700
Knudsen, K., McGill, G., Waitzman, K. A., Powell, J., Carlson, M., Shaffer, G., & Morris, M. (2021). Collaboration to improve neuroprotection and neuropromotion in the NICU: Team education and family engagement. *Neonatal Network, 40*(4), 212–223. https://doi.org/10.1891/11-T-680
Lambert, S., Loban, E., Li, J., Nghiem, T., Schaffler, J., Maheu, C., Dubois, S., Folch, N., Gélinas-Phaneuf, E., & Laizner, A. M. (2021). Chronic illness management in culturally and linguistically diverse patients: Exploring the needs, access, and understanding of information. *Qualitative Health Research, 31*(13), 2426–2439. https://doi.org/10.1177/10497323211040769
Lappalainen, P., Pakkala, I., Strömmer, J., Sairanen, E., Kaipainen, K., & Lappalainen, R. (2021). Supporting parents of children with chronic conditions: A randomized controlled trial of web-based and self-help ACT interventions. *Internet Interventions, 24, 100382*. https://doi.org/10.1016/j.invent.2021.100382
Linton, J. M., Green, A., the Council on Community Pediatrics, Chilton, L., Duffee, J. H., Dilley, K. J., Gutierrez, J. R., Keane, V. A., Krugman, S. D., McKelvey, C. D., & Nelson, J. L. (2019). Providing care for children in immigrant families. *Pediatrics, 144*(3), e20192077. https://doi.org/10.1542/peds.2019-2077
Mackintosh, N. J., Davis, R. E., Easter, A., Rayment-Jones, H., Sevdalis, N., Wilson, S., Adams, M., & Sandall, J. (2020). Interventions to increase patient and family involvement in escalation of care for acute life-threatening illness in community health and hospital settings. *Cochrane Database of Systematic Reviews, 12*, CD012829. https://doi.org/10.1002/14651858.CD012829.pub2
Maurice-Stam, H., Nijhof, S. L., Monninkhof, A. S., Heymans, H. S. A., & Grootenhuis, M. A. (2019). Review about the impact of growing up with a chronic disease showed delays achieving psychosocial milestones. *Acta Paediatrica, 108*(12), 2157–2169. https://doi.org/10.1111/apa.14918
McAndrew, N. S., Jerofke-Owen, T., Fortney, C. A., Costa, D. K., Hetland, B., Guttormson, J., & Harding, E. (2022). Systematic review of family engagement interventions in neonatal, paediatric, and adult ICUs. *Nursing in Critical Care, 27*(3), 296–325. https://doi.org/10.1111/nicc.12564
McLendon, T. (2013). Family-directed structural assessment: Facilitating strengths-based family assessment and engagement. *Journal of Family Strengths, 13*(1), Article 4. https://digitalcommons.library.tmc.edu/jfs/vol13/iss1/4
McManus, B. M., Richardson, Z., Schenkman, M., Murphy, N. J., Everhart, R. M., Hambidge, S., & Morrato, E. (2020). Child characteristics and early intervention referral and receipt of services: A retrospective cohort study. *BMC Pediatrics, 20*, 1–10. https://doi.org/10.1186/s12887-020-1965-x
Misak, C., Herridge, M., Ely, E. W., Clay, A., & Mikkelsen, M. E. (2021). Patient and family engagement in critical illness. *Critical Care Medicine, 49*(9), 1389–1401. https://doi.org/10.1097/CCM.0000000000005136
Mitchell, A. E., Morawska, A., & Mihelic, M. (2020). A systematic review of parenting interventions for child chronic health conditions. *Journal of Child Health Care, 24*(4), 603–628. https://doi.org/10.1177/1367493519882850

Nutbeam, D. (2000). Health literacy as a public health goal: A challenge for contemporary health education and communication strategies into the 21st century. *Health Promotion International, 15*(3), 259–267. https://doi.org/10.1093/heapro/15.3.259

Perricone, G. (2021). Pediatric psychology. *Pediatric Reports, 13*(1), 135–141. https://doi.org/10.3390/pediatric13010020

Porr, C., Drummond, J., & Richter, S. (2006). Health literacy as an empowerment tool for low-income mothers. *Family & Community Health, 29*, 328–335. https://doi.org/10.1097/00003727-200610000-00011

Powell, R. M., Mitra, M., Smeltzer, S. C., Long-Bellil, L. M., Smith, L. D., Rosenthal, E., & Iezzoni, L. I. (2019). Adaptive parenting strategies used by mothers with physical disabilities caring for infants and toddlers. *Health & Social Care in the Community, 27*(4), 889–898. https://doi.org/10.1111/hsc.12706

Rolland, J. S. (1984). Toward a psychosocial typology of chronic and life-threatening illness. *Family Systems Medicine, 2*(3), 245–262. https://doi.org/10.1037/h0091663

Rubin, N., & Franck, L. (2017). The role of Ronald McDonald House Charities® in keeping families close. *Pediatric Nursing, 43*(4), 202–205.

Sanders, L. M., Shaw, J. S., Guez, G., Baur, C., & Rudd, R. (2009). Health literacy and child health promotion: Implications for research, clinical care, and public policy. *Pediatrics, 124*(Supplement_3), S306–S314. https://doi.org/10.1542/peds.2009-1162G

Scher, M. S., Ludington-Hoe, S., Kaffashi, F., Johnson, M. W., Holditch-Davis, D., & Loparo, K. A. (2009). Neurophysiologic assessment of brain maturation after an 8-week trial of skin-to-skin contact on preterm infants. *Clinical Neurophysiology, 120*(10), 1812–1818. https://doi.org/10.1016/j.clinph.2009.08.004

Segers, E., Ockhuijsen, H., Baarendse, P., van Eerden, I., & van den Hoogen, A. (2019). The impact of family centered care interventions in a neonatal or paediatric intensive care unit on parents' satisfaction and length of stay: A systematic review. *Intensive & Critical Care Nursing, 50*, 63–70. https://doi.org/10.1016/j.iccn.2018.08.008

Tang, M. N., Adolphe, S., Rogers, S. R., & Frank, D. A. (2021). Failure to thrive or growth faltering: Medical, developmental/behavioral, nutritional, and social dimensions. *Pediatrics in Review, 42*(11), 590–603. https://doi.org/10.1542/pir.2020-001883

Torpy, J. M., Campbell, A., & Glass, R. M. (2010). Chronic diseases of children. *Journal of the American Medical Association, 303*(7), 682–682. https://doi.org/10.1001/jama.303.7.682

van der Lee, J. H., Mokkink, L. B., Grootenhuis, M. A., Heymans, H. S., & Offringa, M. (2007). Definitions and measurement of chronic health conditions in childhood: A systematic review. *Journal of the American Medical Association, 297*(24), 2741–2751.

van Der Voort, A., Juffer, F., & Bakermans-Kranenburg, M. J. (2014). Sensitive parenting is the foundation for secure attachment relationships and positive social-emotional development of children. *Journal of Children's Services, 9*(2), 165–176.

Walsh, F. (2014). Family therapy: Systemic approaches to practice. In J. R. Brandell (Ed.), *Essentials of clinical social work* (pp. 160–185). Sage Publications. https://doi.org/10.4135/9781483398266.n7

Widström, A. M., Brimdyr, K., Svensson, K., Cadwell, K., & Nissen, E. (2019). Skin-to-skin contact the first hour after birth, underlying implications, and clinical practice. *Acta Paediatrica (Oslo, Norway: 1992), 108*(7), 1192–1204. https://doi.org/10.1111/apa.14754

Wijlaars, L. P., Gilbert, R., & Hardelid, P. (2016). Chronic conditions in children and young people: Learning from administrative data. *Archives of Disease in Childhood, 101*(10), 881–885. https://doi.org/10.1136/archdischild-2016-310716

Zarcadoolas, C., Pleasant, A. F., & Greer, D. S. (2006). *Advancing health literacy: A framework for understanding and action*. Jossey Bass an Imprint of John Wiley & Sons.

Chapter 6
Trauma-Informed Family Engagement in Mental Health Interventions for Young Children and Their Families

Jessica Dym Bartlett

Although the world is full of suffering, it is also full of the overcoming of it. (Helen Keller)

No child is too young to experience trauma. An extensive and growing body of research has shown that infants and young children are exquisitely attuned to their relationships and environments. They are also more susceptible to the deleterious effects of trauma compared to older children, adolescents, and adults (National Scientific Council on the Developing Child [NSCDC], 2004). While pervasive societal myths suggest infants do not perceive or suffer from trauma exposure, young children can and do develop a wide range of social, emotional, and behavioral challenges and disorders in reaction to serious and prolonged adversity. Conservative estimates suggest that 1 in 6 children between the ages of two and eight have at least one diagnosed mental, behavioral, or developmental disorder (Centers for Disease Control and Prevention [CDC], 2019; Cree et al., 2018).

Trauma that occurs the first years of life is especially detrimental to infants and young children, as early childhood is a sensitive period of development during which children's experiences—both positive and negative—help shape young children's rapidly developing brain, setting the stage for health and development over the life course (Bick & Nelson, 2016). Infants as young as 3 months of age have been observed to exhibit symptoms of post-traumatic stress disorder (PTSD; Cordón et al., 2004). Moreover, a considerable proportion of infants and young children experience more than one form of adversity; over one third experience two or more types of adversity before entering kindergarten (Scheeringa et al., 2011). Overall, young children are disproportionately exposed to trauma. For example, child abuse and neglect occur most often among infants and toddlers. In 2021, children under age two made up 28 percent of all abused and neglected children in the

J. D. Bartlett (✉)
Thriving Together, LLC, West Newton, MA, USA
e-mail: jess@wearethrivingtogether.com

L. Nabors, J. D. Bartlett (eds.), *Family Engagement in Mental Health Interventions for Young Children*, Springer Series on Child and Family Studies,
https://doi.org/10.1007/978-3-031-47917-5_6

USA, and infants under 1 year of age comprised over three quarters of maltreatment-related deaths (U.S. Department of Health & Human Services [USDHHS], 2023).

Fortunately, therapeutic treatment for infant and early childhood trauma has evolved substantially in recent years, and rigorous evaluation has yielded evidence of their effectiveness across diverse groups of families and service settings (for review, see VanDerBeek et al., 2018). The success of treatment, however, is largely predicated on the capacity of infant and early childhood mental health (IECMH) providers and organizations to engage families. As Lieberman and Van Horn (2008) assert, "parents constitute the primary agents of the young child's emotional well-being" (p. 5). Thus, relationships within the family, especially attachment relationships (i.e., with parents and other primary caregivers), play a prominent role in the treatment of IECMH disorders. Engaging families in treatment, however, can be a challenging endeavor. An estimated 80 percent of children in need of mental health services never receive them, and families who begin treatment have a dropout rate of 47 percent (Kataoka et al., 2002; Barrett et al., 2008).

This chapter describes trauma-informed family engagement (TFE) in mental health (i.e., social and emotional development) treatment for infants, young children, and their families. This chapter begins by defining trauma and describing trauma and its effects, noting important distinctions among related concepts and terms (e.g., adversity, adverse childhood experiences [ACEs], early childhood trauma, complex trauma, intergenerational trauma, historical trauma) and describing a trauma-informed approach. A review of evidence-based and promising infant and early childhood mental health trauma treatments follows, accompanied by a discussion of the key components of trauma-informed family engagement in treatment (TFE) with a proposed set of indicators for assessing organizational and provider progress toward TFE. This chapter concludes with a discussion of limitations to current knowledge, such as the dearth of research with historically marginalized groups of families and related implications for future research, policy, and practice.

Early Childhood Trauma

When parent-child bonds are strong, young children feel a sense of safety, love, and predictability that they need to explore and learn from their environments, themselves, and their relationships. Infants and young children are also more likely to recover and return to their typical functioning after experiencing trauma with sensitive and responsive care from the adults in their lives (Lieberman & Van Horn, 2008). Conversely, when parents are unable to buffer children from the damaging effects of trauma, or when they are the source of trauma, chronic overactivation of young children's stress response system, can become toxic (i.e., toxic stress), compromising brain development and increasing their vulnerability to mental and physical health disorders (National Scientific Council on the Developing Child, 2014).

Parents may be unable to protect their children for many reasons, whether due to their own trauma history (e.g., childhood abuse and neglect), the presence of environmental stressors (e.g., poverty, community violence, discrimination), and/or trauma that affects both parent and child (e.g., the loss of a loved one or a serious motor vehicle accident). In other instances, parents are the source of early trauma (e.g., abuse and neglect, parental substance misuse and mental health disorders, intimate partner violence). Such early exposure to multiple adversities over time beginning early in life, often referred to as *complex trauma*, has the most harmful impacts on infants' and young children's brain development, self-concept, and the formation of healthy relationships with peers and adults (National Child Traumatic Stress Network [NCTSNa, b], n.d.).

Trauma has been defined in many ways, but the conceptualization of individual trauma developed by the Substance Abuse and Mental Health Services Administration (SAMHSA, 2014) has been used most widely:

> Individual trauma results from an event, series of events, or set of circumstances that is experienced by an individual as physically or emotionally harmful or life threatening and that has lasting adverse effects on the individual's functioning and mental, physical, social, emotional, or spiritual well-being. (p. 7)

There are several aspects of this definition that are important to note regarding the identification and treatment of early childhood trauma. First, determinations about whether or not trauma has occurred depend on the young child's subjective experience. Second, there is no distinction between the threat of harm and actual harm—both can cause trauma. Third, early childhood trauma can be a physical experience, emotional experience, or a combination of the two, with symptoms typically taking the form of changes in behavior – the primary form of expression for young children. Simply stated, early childhood trauma occurs when infants or young children perceive adverse events or conditions as a threat to their emotional and/or physical well-being (Bartlett et al., 2017; NCTSNb, n.d.). Common types of early adversity associated with early childhood trauma in infants and young children include child abuse and neglect, separation from a caregiver, exposure to intimate partner violence, unintentional injuries, painful medical procedures, and parental anxiety, depression, and substance misuse. Young children have higher rates of exposure to these and other forms of trauma compared to older children and youth (Enlow et al., 2013; USDHHS, 2023).

Impact of Trauma on Infants and Young Children

An extensive body of research across multiple fields of practice, including IECMH (IECMH), early relational health (ERH), maternal-child health (MCH), social-emotional learning (SEL), child development, psychology, social work, and neuroscience, among others, has demonstrated a strong link between early childhood trauma and the development of serious mental health and developmental problems that can persist through adulthood. Common mental health disorders during infancy and early childhood include post-traumatic stress disorder (PTSD), challenging behaviors, difficulties forming healthy relationships, depression, anxiety, attention deficit hyperactivity disorder (ADHD), poor academic achievement and work performance, substance misuse, and physical illness (Woolgar et al., 2022). And yet, almost half of parents believe that infants under 1 year of age are not impacted by adversity and that the quality of care parents provide does not have a long-term impact on infants prior to 6 months of age (Zero to Three, 2016).

The science is clear that infants and young children experience more unfavorable outcomes from trauma than older children and adults, including alterations to brain structure and functioning that compromise the stress response system and reduce children's ability to manage future stress (National Scientific Council on the Developing Child, 2014). Practitioners and researchers have consistently documented that infants and young children are at particularly high risk for developing mental health disorders following trauma. For example, a recent meta-analysis on post-traumatic stress disorder (PTSD) among young children found the prevalence of PTSD among preschoolers exposed to adversity was approximately 21.5 percent (Woolgar et al., 2022). Unfortunately, traumatized young children may remain in a state of hypervigilance and emotional reactivity that can impede the development of foundational skills, such as the ability to form healthy relationships, control one's impulses, and learn (National Scientific Council on the Developing Child, 2014).

Importantly, every child reacts to trauma in their own way, and the nature of a child's trauma reaction is highly dependent on (a) their age and developmental stage, (b) the severity and chronicity of the traumatic event or circumstances, (c) prior trauma exposure, (d) the impact of the trauma on parents and family, if parents are a source of trauma (e.g., child abuse and neglect, mental health problems, substance misuse), and (e) the extent to which parents and other significant people in children's life protect them psychologically and physically. Moreover, not all children are traumatized in the presence of adversity (NCTSNb, n.d.). The distinction between adversity and trauma is important here because conflating these terms implies that adversity inevitably traumatizes children. For example, the "ACE score" developed by Felitti and colleagues (1998) in their seminal study on adverse childhood experiences (ACEs) simply counts the number of adversities, without accounting for whether or not the child was traumatized or the severity of the exposure. Moreover, the ACEs score represents the total number of adversities a child experiences in the home environment but does not account for child functioning or the role of social determinants of health (e.g., discrimination, poverty, natural disasters, school shootings) that disproportionality affect historically marginalized families due to historical and structural racism and discrimination. Clearly stated, these terms should not be used interchangeably (Murphey & Bartlett, 2019). See Table 6.1 for definition of key concepts.

Children also have an innate capacity for resilience in the face of trauma and adversity (Masten, 2001; Luthar et al., 2000). As Masten explains, resilience is "ordinary magic" that "usually arises from the normative functions of human adaptational systems" and "offers a more positive outlook on human development and adaptation" (p. 227). This is evidenced by a large body of literature showing that most children return to their typical levels of functioning after a traumatic experience, as long as they have needed supports, including treatment (SAMHSA, 2014).

Table 6.1 Definition of trauma and related concepts

Term	Definition
Adverse childhood experiences (ACEs)	A subset of childhood adversities occurring in the child's home that were assessed in the ACE study (Felitti et al., 1998) but which are intended for population-level measurement and not for individual screening (Anda et al., 2022, p. 294)
Childhood adversity	Any circumstance or event with the potential to cause trauma and to interfere with a child's physical or mental health and development (SAMHSA, 2014, p. 8)
Complex trauma	Trauma that results from exposure to multiple adversities that begin early in life and typically involve disturbances in the parent-child relationship (NCTSNa, n.d.)
Early childhood trauma	When an infant or young child perceives adverse events or circumstances as a threat to their psychological and/or physical well-being (Bartlett et al., 2017)
Historical trauma	A collective, multigenerational, and cumulative experience of psychological injury in communities and in their descendants (Brave Heart et al., 2012)
Intergenerational trauma	When a child of a parent who has been traumatized develops reactions that are similar to those of the parent (American Psychological Association, n.d.)
Resilience	A dynamic process of positive adaptation in the context of significant risk or adversity, not a personal trait that one does or does not have (Luthar et al., 2000)
Toxic stress	Overactivation of a child's stress response system due to severe and chronic adversity in the absence of support from primary caregivers (National Scientific Council on the Developing Child, 2015)
Trauma	A potential outcome of exposure to adversity in which an individual perceives an event or set of circumstances as extremely frightening, harmful, or threatening—either emotionally, physically, or both (NCTSNc, n.d.)

Adapted from Bartlett and Sacks (2019)

Impact of Early Childhood Trauma on Parents and Families

When infants and young children are traumatized, parents and other primary caregivers are usually their main source of support, and how parents respond to their children can reduce or intensify their post-traumatic reactions. Both ends of caregiving quality continuum—from lack of parental support to overprotection—are associated with the development of PTSD in early childhood (Scheeringa & Zeanah, 2001). Caring for a traumatized child is challenging for most parents and other primary caregivers (e.g., foster and kinship caregivers, other relatives who care for the child, adoptive parents) and can negatively impact caregiving quality. High levels of anxiety among parents coping with children's post-traumatic reactions (e.g., externalizing and internalizing behavior, developmental regression, severe separation anxiety) can reduce a caregiver's sensitivity, attunement, and responsiveness to the child, thereby exacerbating the child's distress (Nugent et al., 2007).

In some instances, when a parent or family is exposed to the same traumatic event (e.g., loss of a close family member, serious car accident, intimate partner violence), emotional reactions among family members can intensify each other's reactions and undermine family support for the child (Scheeringa & Zeanah, 2001). A child's trauma also may trigger strong emotions in a parent with a history of trauma (i.e., intergenerational trauma), leading the parent to prioritize personal needs ahead of attending to the child and recovery process (Lieberman et al., 2015). Given the strong influence of parents' well-being on their young children, engaging at least two generations in treatment for early childhood trauma is a basic tenet of good practice. Further, a family's culture is highly influential in shaping how individual members perceive and react to trauma, and the success of trauma treatment depends on "creating trusting relationships with families rooted in empathy and a responsiveness to their diverse lived experiences and hopes and dreams for their children" (Nicholson et al., 2022, p. 2).

Impact of Early Childhood Trauma on Mental Health Providers

Working with infants, young children, and families exposed to trauma considerably increases the risk of poor mental health among the mental health providers with whom they work. The chronic emotional stress of hearing about someone else's firsthand trauma experiences, often referred to as secondary traumatic stress (STS)/compassion fatigue (CF), can leave mental health providers feeling hopeless, unmotivated, exhausted, hypervigilant, and distressed. Approximately 26 to 50 percent of therapists working with traumatized populations are at high risk for both STS and PTSD (NCTSN, 2011). A combination of psychoeducation, skills training, and reflective supervision are well-proven methods of preventing and addressing STS, but a trauma-informed approach also requires that organizations attend to staff wellness wholistically through organization-wide wellness planning and education to address the effects of trauma on programs and providers (Menschner & Maul, 2016).

Treatment for Traumatized Infants, Young Children, and Their Families

The evidence base for trauma-informed treatment is growing, though the number of evidence-based treatments that are appropriate for infants, toddlers, and preschoolers remains limited – especially for infants. To date, rigorous evaluation (i.e., randomized controlled trials [RCTs] or quasi-experimental designs [QEDs]) reveals only a small number of early childhood trauma treatments that are effective in improving child, parent, and family outcomes, including parenting challenges, child behavior problems, PTSD/post-traumatic stress, depression, and anxiety in young children. Early trauma treatment can also improve children's school readiness, academic achievement, and overall health (Grube & Liming, 2018; VanDerBeek et al., 2018) while producing cost savings. For example, a recent benefit-cost analysis (Oppenheim & Bartlett, 2023) found that Parent-Child Interaction Therapy (PCIT; Funderburk & Eyberg, 2011) has an average return on investment of $15.11 per child and child-parent psychotherapy (CPP; Lieberman et al., 2015) has an average return on investment of $13.82 per child in future savings (Washington State Institute for Public Policy, 2019a, b). While treatment approaches vary widely in their structure and format, most have a number of elements in common, including being relationship based (i.e., attachment based, two generation), trauma informed, culturally responsive, and accounting for the influence of environments on recovery. See Table 6.2 for a description of evidence-based trauma treatments for infants and young children and their approaches to working with families.

Table 6.2 Evidence-based trauma treatments for young children (birth–8 years)

Treatment model	Age range	Approach to working with families
Attachment and Biobehavioral Catch-up (ABC)	Birth to 2 years	ABC is a structured home visiting parenting program (average of 10 sessions) based on attachment theory and stress neurobiology. ABC aims to support parents' ability to nurture and respond sensitively to their infants and toddlers to support their development and strengthen their relationships with their parents
Child First	Prenatal to 5 years	Child First is a two-generation, home-based mental health intervention for young children, prenatal through age five, and their families. It was developed specifically for young children who have experienced trauma and/or have social-emotional, behavioral, developmental, and/or learning problems. Child First's goals are to help children heal from trauma and adversity, improve mental health in both generations, reduce child abuse and neglect, and promote child development
Child-Parent Psychotherapy (CPP)	Birth to 6 years	Dyadic attachment-based therapy that includes the child and parent or primary caregiver in sessions (average of 50 sessions). CPP aims to support and strengthen the relationship between children and their caregivers as the strategy for helping children heal and restore their functioning. Treatment includes attention to social determinants of health that influence the caregiver-child relationship
Parent-Child Interaction Therapy (PCIT)	2–7 years	PCIT uses a structured, step-by-step, live behavioral coaching during sessions with both the parent/caregiver and the child (average of 14–25 sessions). Parents learn skills through PCIT didactic sessions. Using a transmitter and receiver system, parents/caregivers are coached by the therapist as they interact with their child. The therapist typically provides the coaching from behind a one-way mirror with the goal of improving problematic parent/caregiver-child behavior patterns
Trauma-focused-Cognitive Behavioral Therapy (TF-CBT)	3–21 years	TF-CBT is a manualized psychosocial treatment model that combines cognitive-behavioral, attachment, humanistic, empowerment, and family therapy models' brief trauma treatment (12–25 sessions). Sessions are divided between the child and parent/caregiver

There are also several promising trauma treatments and services for infants and young children that have yet to be rigorously evaluated, or their rigorous evaluations do not meet the standards of national clearinghouses (e.g., The Title IV-E Clearinghouse, California Evidence-based Clearinghouse for Child Welfare). The high cost and complexity of conducting randomized controlled trials can be so costly and time intensive that it is not feasible for many treatment developers. It is especially concerning that treatments developed for families from marginalized groups of families often fall into this category. For example, Family Spirit is a promising intervention that aims to break intergenerational cycles of trauma through home visiting with Native American parents and their young children (prenatal to age three), and Effective Black Parenting Program offers culturally specific parenting strategies through group treatment for families at risk for child abuse and neglect. However, neither has undergone an evaluation that supports a designation of the model as "evidence based." Federal, state, and local support are greatly needed to increase the evidence base for programs that offer culturally responsive intervention approaches.

Family Engagement in Early Childhood Trauma Treatment

Family engagement has been defined in many ways, often depending on the service sector of interest. According to the NCTSN (2017):

> Family engagement is the process of identifying, enrolling, and retaining families in treatment services. Because caregivers play a crucial role in the physical and emotional development of their children, it is critical that parents are also involved in their child's mental health treatment. While attendance is important, true engagement is motivating and empowering families to recognize their own needs, strengths, and resources and to take an active role in changing things for the better. (p. 1)

The notion that attendance in treatment sessions is necessary but insufficient has gained widespread agreement among IECMH stakeholders as the definition of family engagement has expanded beyond involvement (e.g., attendance) to include both attitudinal and behavioral components (Staudt, 2007). The underlying assumption of family attitudes that support family engagement is parents' belief that the challenges associated with child trauma treatment will outweigh its costs. True family engagement includes help-seeking, attendance, and meaningful and active participation in treatment as part of a dynamic, ongoing process from the identification of child and family needs to treatment completion (Staudt, 2007). From this viewpoint, family engagement is a process that begins prior to the first treatment session. This is a critical moment for families to begin to form trusting relationships with providers and programs—two thirds of families never attend a first session, even when they report wanting treatment for their child (Ofonedu et al., 2017).

Benefits of Family Engagement in Treatment for Infant and Early Childhood Trauma

Family engagement in clinical treatment for young children has numerous benefits for children, families, service providers, and programs alike. Meta-analyses on family engagement have consistently revealed improvements in child outcomes when parents are well engaged, regardless of the child's particular mental health disorder (Dowell & Ogles, 2010). Children whose parents are more engaged in their treatment tend to have the most positive treatment across multiple outcomes, such as improvements in self-regulation, cooperation and prosocial interactions, self-confidence, attention, motivation to learn, persistence in challenging tasks, school readiness, and academic achievement (for review, see Dowell & Ogles, 2010).

Engaging families in treatment and other services also has advantages for families, providers, and organizations. Parents are better able to cope with challenges, experience a better fit between the family's needs and the treatment received, and have higher quality parent-provider relationships. Further, organizations and providers show increased capacity to provide high-quality services, develop more trusting provider-child relationships, gain more work skills, and have better well-being and staff morale (Child Welfare Information Gateway, 2017).

Barriers to Family Engagement in Infant and Early Childhood Trauma Treatment

Family engagement in children's mental health treatment can be challenging. Half of the 7.7 million children with a mental health disorder that is treatable never receive treatment (Whitney & Peterson, 2019), in large part because obtaining IECMH services often requires families to interact with service systems that are not well coordinated, trauma informed, culturally responsive, or equitable. For example, families of color and LGBTQ families are more likely to experience trauma yet have less access to minimally adequate treatment and receive treatment less often than their White heterosexual counterparts due to language barriers, stigma, lack of health insurance, and shortage of mental health providers (Rodgers et al., 2021).

Barriers to family engagement exist at the individual, program, and societal level. For example, the environments in which parents and children are born and live, or social determinants of health (Healthy People 2030, n.d.), influence individual and relational health, functioning, and quality of life and can pose considerable obstacles to engaging families (Alegría et al., 2018). Families may not be able to afford or obtain transportation, childcare, or time off from work, and the stigma of mental illness and treatment can be a deterrent to treatment engagement for some families. Even parents seeking treatment report high levels of stress and frustration while navigating a fragmented maze of services (Sturm & Sherbourne, 2001).

In addition, mismatches between family and provider expectations about the nature of treatment can impede engagement (Miller & Prinz, 2003).

Certain characteristics of families, parents, and providers also are associated with poor family engagement in children's mental health treatment. For example, parents who view western treatment approaches as poorly aligned with their cultural values, beliefs, and language preferences may be reluctant to seek services or unable to obtain them (Gopalkrishnan, 2018). Family engagement also can be challenging for service providers who feel ill-equipped to work with parents who have mental health and substance use disorders, and organizations are less likely to achieve program and family goals (Ammerman et al., 2010). In addition, both programs and providers can prevent successful engagement due to inflexible scheduling, lack of transportation, telehealth, or home visiting options for families and insufficient staffing of mental health providers trained in evidence-based treatments for infants and young children (Ingolsby, 2010). Such barriers to treatment, particularly for families who lack resources and are marginalized, point to the need for increased professional support and training from organizations (e.g., professional development and coursework on trauma, IECMH, and diversity, equity, and inclusion (DEI); reflective supervision; manageable caseloads; and productivity requirements) to enhance providers' confidence, knowledge, and skills in equitable family engagement (Waid & Kelly, 2020). Accordingly, addressing disparities in trauma exposure, reducing barriers to treatment engagement, and increasing the capacity of the mental health workforce to offer culturally responsive, trauma-informed treatment and supports are all key indicators of trauma-informed family engagement (TFE).

Strategies for Engaging Families in Infant and Early Childhood Trauma Treatment

A synthesis of family engagement definitions across fields of practice identified several successful strategies: child-centered approaches; collaboration with families; joint planning and decision-making; family involvement in services, including children, youth, and extended family; interagency and multisystem collaboration; individualized services; open, honest, and respectful interactions; and family participation at both the system and practice levels. *Family involvement at the system level* refers to engaging families in leadership, policy, and procedures to inform service delivery and ongoing improvement (Child Welfare Information Gateway, 2014, pp. 4–5). In addition, Reardon and colleagues (2017) reviewed the literature on family engagement in children's mental health treatment and found that when parents recognized that their children had a mental health problem, as well as the severity of the problem and its impacts, engagement is stronger.

Collaboration, communication, sustained engagement, and involvement at the systems level are also common strategies for effective family engagement. *Collaboration* is defined as the belief that families are partners in making positive change and that service providers and partners share the responsibility of decision-making to promote positive outcomes for children and families. *Communication* refers to the importance of service providers understanding that families have valuable information and that strong communication is needed to identify and implement the most effective approaches to making progress toward family and program goals. *Sustained engagement* emphasizes that family engagement is a process that entails consistent practice that is sustained over time (Child Welfare Information Gateway, 2014, pp. 4–5).

Along with advancements in our understanding of the pervasive and pernicious nature of early trauma, there has been growing consensus among mental health experts about the importance of TIA to behavioral health services (SAMHSA, 2014). In this chapter, we focus on treatment but with the understanding that supports for children are part of a coordinated system of care with staff at every level capable of implementing TIA—otherwise referred to as a "trauma-informed care," or "trauma-responsive care," or "healing-centered care."

Culturally Responsive Strategies for Treating Infant and Early Childhood Trauma

A trauma-informed approach, as defined here, also incorporates strategies for being culturally responsive and addressing inequities in treatment access, quality, and outcomes (SAMHSA, 2014). However, there is a paucity of research on culturally responsive strategies for engaging families from different racial and ethnic backgrounds in trauma treatment, and this dearth of information remains a serious impediment to mental health equity (American Psychological Association, 2017). In addition to the NCTSN definition above, we propose that cultural responsiveness also requires understanding and addressing inequities in trauma exposure and treatment. For example, the empirical literature clearly shows that Black, Hispanic, Native American, and Alaska Native families are disproportionately exposed to trauma and adversity, routinely experience racialized trauma (i.e., the effects of physical and emotional stress due to racism), and are overrepresented in systems that surveil and refer families to mental health services, such as child welfare (Dettlaff & Boyd, 2021; USDHHS, 2023). As a result, marginalized families are at especially high risk for PTSD, depression, and other mental health and behavioral challenges and concomitantly have less access to treatment (NCTSN, 2020).

Few trauma treatments have been developed and evaluated for families from specific racial and ethnic backgrounds, and treatments that have been tested only with White, heterosexual families of European descent continue to receive a designation of "evidence based" by federally funded clearinghouses (e.g., California Evidence-Based Clearinghouse for Child Welfare, Title IV-E Prevention Services Clearinghouse) regardless of whether or not they are effective with family members from a range racial, ethnic, gender identity, and LGBTQ identities and backgrounds. This begs the question: these interventions are evidence-based for whom? A few IECMH trauma treatments have been tailored to particular communities of color, but most remain "promising" practices, as the rigorous evaluation necessary to be designated an evidence-based treatment is expensive and time-consuming and may require professional skills and resources that are not available to many communities of color. Making matters worse, there is a shortage of IECMH providers who reflect the racial and ethnic backgrounds of families in the communities they serve. The American Psychological Association determined that 86 percent of psychologists and nearly 70 percent of social workers were White, yet they only represent 62 percent of the US population (Lin et al., 2018).

Trauma-Informed Family Engagement (TFE)

Operationalization of a trauma-informed approach – often referred to as trauma-informed care – has been inconsistent across organizations and service systems, and research on the impact of systemically integrated trauma-informed approaches. Research on implementing a trauma-informed approach within and across systems of care is still in the early stages (Hanson et al., 2018). Several studies have found improvements in providers' knowledge, practice, and collaboration, as well as positive child and family treatment among families involved in the child welfare system (Bartlett et al., 2018; Lang et al., 2016). However, a comprehensive review of research found a wide range of implementation approaches with mixed results (Melz et al., 2019). Indeed, better consensus on the essential principles, attitudes, and behaviors of a trauma-informed approach is needed to promote alignment of findings and cross-study comparison, in turn facilitating a shared understanding of how to work toward TFE. SAMHSA's (2014) definition of a trauma-informed approach is among the most widely cited:

> A program, organization, or system that is trauma-informed **realizes** the widespread impact of trauma and understands potential pathways for recovery; **recognizes** the signs and symptoms of trauma in clients, families, staff, and others involved with the system; and **responds** by fully integrating knowledge about trauma into policies, procedures, and practices, and seeks to actively resist **re-traumatization**. (p. 9)

SAMHSA also developed six principles of TIA: (1) safety; (2) trustworthiness and transparency; (3) peer support; (4) collaboration and mutuality; (5) empowerment, voice, and choice; and (6) cultural, historical, and gender issues. For additional information, see SAMHSA, 2014).

Indicators of Trauma-Informed Family Engagement (TFE)

Whereas a trauma-informed approach is inclusive of every step of the screening, assessment, referral, and treatment process, TFE focuses on the engagement process, which begins prior to a first session and is an ongoing process until after treatment completion. TFE emphasizes a collaborative stance with families in which power is shared, providers and parents problem-solve together, and both the attitudes and behaviors of treatment providers and their organizations indicate a strong commitment to family engagement (SAMHSA, 2014).

Because the concepts of family engagement and a trauma-informed approach have been defined and operationalized in many ways, it is useful to develop common indicators of progress toward TFE that can be used across service systems, programs, and organizations. The indicators presented (see Table 6.3) are not intended to be an exhaustive list but rather a set of trauma-informed attitudes and behaviors by providers and their organizations that are grounded in evidence on strong family engagement. The indicators are categorized by SAMHSA's (2014, pp. 10–11) principles of a trauma-informed approach: safety; trustworthiness and transparency; peer support, collaboration, and mutuality; empowerment; voice and choice; and cultural, historical, and gender issues, which are applied here to TFE. The attitude and behavioral indicators are presented separately for each principle (i.e., attitude and behavior indicators relate to each principle but do not directly correspond to one another in Table 6.3).

Limitations of Current Knowledge

Inconsistency in definitions and operationalization of family engagement and a trauma-informed approach has led to confusion about how best to implement and measure progress for either construct or TFE. Research is needed to identify and verify the essential elements of effective TIA broadly and TFE specifically across child and family serving organizations and systems, such as testing the validity of SAMHSA's principles and improving knowledge about the impact of TFE on child and family well-being. Empirical attention is needed to understand if the theorized indicators presented in this chapter are indeed an effective way to monitor progress toward intended outcomes. While they are based on the best evidence available to date, there is surely more to learn about the "essential ingredients" of TFE before indicators can be replicated and scaled. In particular, little is known about effective TIA and TFE strategies for treatments tailored to families from particular racial and ethnic groups, fathers, and LGBTQ families. As Rogoff asserted, "There is not likely to be One Best Way." Thus, investments are needed to support rigorous evaluation of targeted early childhood trauma treatments that might be overlooked due to limited resources for establishing evidence of effectiveness. Similar initiatives have taken place in child welfare (e.g., USDHHS' Supporting Evidence Building in Child Welfare).

In addition, there are multiple pathways to healing and recovery, as well as diverse mechanisms of resilience that operate for different groups of families, but research on TFE strategies that address such variation is scant. A number of

Table 6.3 Indicators of trauma-informed family engagement (TFE) in the treatment for infants, young children, and their families

Attitudes	Behaviors
Safety: Throughout the organization, staff and the people they serve, whether children or adults, feel physically and psychologically safe; the physical setting is safe and interpersonal interactions promote a sense of safety. Understanding safety as defined both those served is a high priority	
1. All young children and families have the right to feel emotionally and physically safe when participating in trauma treatment 2. Early childhood trauma is unique, common, and harmful, particularly due to its negative effects on early brain development 3. Safe, stable, and nurturing relationships and environments are the foundation of mental health in infancy and early childhood and a central focus of treatment 4. Organizations must take proactive steps to avoid re-traumatizing infants, young children, and their families 5. Ensuring that each family can meet their basic need is a critical step in supporting the safety of families with young children 6. Organizations are responsible for the safety and well-being of staff, including preventing and addressing secondary traumatic stress	1. Everyone in the organization receives sufficient training and has knowledge of the impact of early childhood trauma, how to recognize it, and how best to engage families in ways that support their emotional and physical safety 2. The organizational environment is designed to help families feel safe and to reduce the risk of re-traumatization; policies, procedures, and practices are in place to protect the safety and well-being of families 3. The organization and providers ensure that providers are trained in evidence-based, developmentally appropriate, culturally responsive screening, assessment, and treatments for families with young children 4. The organization and providers engage families before treatment begins to start building positive provider-family relationships that promote safety, trust, and communication 5. The organization works with staff to develop, implement, and update a staff wellness plan to promote the safety and well-being of staff, who are routinely exposed to firsthand accounts of trauma

(continued)

Table 6.3 (continued)

Attitudes	Behaviors
Trustworthiness and transparency: Organizational operations and decisions are conducted with transparency with the goal of building and maintaining trust with clients and family members, among staff, and others involved in the organization	
7. Everyone in the organization realizes that parents and other caregivers have the most knowledge about their child and the most potential to help the child heal and thus are essential partners in effective trauma treatment 8. Providers recognize that trust is developed over time and that engaging families is an ongoing process in which providers and families develop mutually respectful partnerships 9. Everyone in the organization understands that some families are forced to seek treatment for their child or themselves (e.g., court-ordered treatment) which may contribute to a family's distrust in service systems 10. Everyone in the organization should be transparent, predictable, and trustworthy in their interactions with families, beginning prior to a first session and continuing until treatment completion 11. Parents and other caregivers who appear "resistant" to treatment may be facing barriers that are not initially clear; intensive engagement efforts may be needed to identify and address psychological barriers and other obstacles to treatment engagement without blaming or shaming them	6. Everyone in the organization works with families to increase their understanding of early childhood trauma and its impacts on infants and young children in a nonjudgmental, unbiased way 7. Everyone in the organization solicits input from families about their beliefs, goals, and preferences related to mental health and treatment and integrates them into policies, procedures, and treatment planning 8. Providers work with families to develop open, honest, and mutually respectful interactions and relationships 9. Everyone in the organization is transparent with families about the selected treatment, what it will entail, and expectations about outcomes 10. The organization offers treatment in the family's preferred language and works toward staffing that reflects the characteristics of families in the community 11. Providers routinely follow-up with families who do not attend a first session or dropped out of treatment to better understand and address the root causes

(continued)

Table 6.3 (continued)

Attitudes	Behaviors
Peer support: Peer support and mutual self-help are key vehicles for establishing safety and hope, building trust, enhancing collaboration, and utilizing their stories and lived experience to promote recovery and healing. The term "peers" refers to individuals with lived experiences of trauma, or in the case of children, this may be family members of children who have experienced traumatic events and are key caregivers in their recovery. Peers have also been referred to as "trauma survivors"	
12. Parents who have lived experience with early childhood trauma are an important resource for supporting family healing and resilience 13. An organization that incorporates peer supports into trauma treatment is communicating the value of provider-consumer partnerships and meaningful engagement of people with lived experience 14. Everyone in the organization understands they have a role in promoting meaningful and mutually beneficial engagement of parents with lived experience trauma treatment and services	12. Parents and other caregivers who have lived experience with early childhood trauma and mental health treatment are integrated into family treatment planning and services 13. Parents and other caregivers who have lived experience with early childhood trauma and mental health treatment are incorporated into decision-making at all levels of the organization (i.e., "nothing about us without us) 14. Everyone in the organization actively participates in promoting meaningful and mutually beneficial engagement of parents with lived experience into trauma treatment and services
Collaboration and mutuality: Importance is placed on partnering and the leveling of power differences between staff and clients and among organizational staff from clerical and housekeeping personnel to professional staff to administrators, demonstrating that healing happens in relationships and in the meaningful sharing of power and decision-making. The organization recognizes that everyone has a role to play in a trauma-informed approach	
15. Effective treatment requires a partnership between family and provider in which power, information, problem-solving, and decision-making are shared 16. Healing occurs in the context of attuned and responsive relationships between parents/caregivers and providers and between parents/caregivers and their children 17. Everyone in an organization has a role to play in a trauma-informed approach to engaging families in mental health treatment	15. Providers and other staff who interact with families routinely inquire about each family's views, preferences, and goals related to treatment and incorporates them into their work with the family 16. Providers and parents/caregivers share information, problem-solving, and decision-making responsibilities; families and providers share information and engage in mutual problem-solving 17. The organization offers professional development and reflective supervision on how each staff member can play a role in a trauma-informed approach to treating early childhood trauma

(continued)

Table 6.3 (continued)

Attitudes	Behaviors
Empowerment, voice, and choice: Throughout the organization and among the clients served, individuals' strengths and experiences are recognized and built upon. The organization fosters a belief in the primacy of the people served, in resilience, and in the ability of individuals, organizations, and communities to heal and promote recovery from trauma. The organization understands that the experience of trauma may be a unifying aspect in the lives of those who run the organization, who provide the services, and/or who come to the organization for assistance and support. As such, operations and workforce development and services are organized to foster empowerment for staff and clients alike. Organizations understand the importance of power differentials and ways in which clients, historically, have been diminished in voice and choice and are often recipients of coercive treatment. Clients are supported in shared decision-making, choice, and goal setting to determine the plan of action they need to heal and move forward. They are supported in cultivating self-advocacy skills. Staff are facilitators of recovery rather than controllers of recovery. Staff are empowered to do their work as well as possible by adequate organizational support	
18. All families have strengths that can be leveraged to support their young child's recovery from trauma 19. All families should be supported in making choices and decisions about treatment and in determining treatment goals for their child and family 20. Providers should be facilitators of recovery and healing rather than experts who try to control how parents and families engage in their child's trauma treatment 21. Staff should be empowered through organizational policies, procedures, information, and supports related to effective work with families and professional/personal well-being	18. All staff who interact with families use a strengths-based approach and resist an exclusive focus on deficits and disorders 19. The organization and providers actively promote parents' capacity to make decisions for their child and family and identify avenues for self-determination even when treatment is not by choice (e.g., court ordered) 20. Organizational policies and procedures are in place to support workforce development, family participation in organizational decision-making, and family's self-determination 21. The organization and providers consistently include parents with lived experience in decisions about trauma services and treatment for parents and children ("nothing about us without us")

(continued)

Table 6.3 (continued)

Attitudes	Behaviors
Cultural, historical, and gender issues: The organization actively moves past cultural stereotypes and biases (e.g., based on race, ethnicity, sexual orientation, age, religion, gender responsive services; leverages the healing value of traditional cultural connections; incorporates policies, protocols, and processes that are responsive to the racial, ethnic, and cultural needs of individuals served; and recognizes and addresses historical trauma	
22. Families who have experienced historical trauma, systemic and structural racism, and marginalization disproportionally experience trauma, have more limited access to treatment, and may have well-founded reservations about treatment given past instances of mistreatment 23. All families should have equitable access to high-quality trauma treatment, as well as outcomes comparable to non-marginalized families 24. The organization must take proactive steps to working with communities to improve equity in access, services, and outcomes for early childhood trauma treatment, particularly for marginalized families 25. The organization should support culturally responsive trauma treatment by providing ongoing training for staff on diversity, equity, and inclusion	22. The organization and providers continually seek knowledge about differences in families' beliefs, attitudes, and preferences related to treating early childhood trauma, as well as potential barriers to treatment engagement and how to address them 23. The organization and providers seek to gain knowledge and improve their skills in successful engagement and treatment of families who have been historically marginalized and disproportionately exposed to trauma based on race, ethnicity, religion, LGBTQ status, age, or gender identity 24. Organizations provide ongoing professional development for all staff on families from different cultural backgrounds and diversity, equity, and inclusion in family engagement early childhood trauma treatment

evidence-based interventions, such as ABC, CPP, PCIT, and TF-CBT, have been tested with racially and socioeconomically diverse families and found to have comparably positive outcomes, both using in-person treatment and tele-mental health to support access (e.g., Stewart et al., 2017). However, evaluation support is needed to test promising treatments and related TFE that were developed for particular racial and ethnic groups (e.g., Effective Black Parenting Program, Family Spirit). Further investigation is needed to clarify which TFE strategies work for whom and under what conditions. Finally, research linking specific trauma-informed and TFE strategies to child and family outcomes could help elucidate the most effective approaches to achieving each intended outcome. Measures often conflate strategies and fail to link activities to the desired results (Epstein, 2011).

Directions for the Future

A substantial evidence base demonstrates that family engagement in trauma treatment for young children and their families can be improved, especially when mental health providers are trained in a holistic approach that moves beyond involvement (i.e., attendance) to include the many attitudes and behaviors of providers that lead to successful TFE in treatment (Becker et al., 2018). However, the literature is scant on TFE practices and policies. Family engagement is essential to TIA, but mental health providers do not necessarily use TFE when working with families. Organizations that offer trauma treatment for infants and young children can promote TFE by offering professional development and supervision on early childhood trauma and engaging a diversity of families and by implementing policies and procedures that are consistent with TFE. Systemwide integration of a trauma-informed approach is also vital to sustaining TFE. Effective TFE will also require that organizations and communities work together to increase the number of mental health providers trained in evidence-based and promising targeted treatments and reduce other barriers to equity in treatment access, service quality, and positive child and family outcomes.

In addition, efforts at the federal, state, tribal, and territory level can be made to support the development and testing of TFE measures so that organizations and providers can better assess their related strengths and needs. For example, the federal government has invested in tools to assess family engagement and family-teacher relationships in early care and education (e.g., Family and Provider/Teacher Relationship Quality [FPTRQ], Kim et al., 2015). Comparable efforts for TFE are needed among IECMH stakeholders to develop and evaluate measures of TFE, such as the indicators presented in this chapter.

References

Alegría, M., NeMoyer, A., Falgàs Bagué, I., Wang, Y., & Alvarez, K. (2018). Social determinants of mental health: Where we are and where we need to go. *Current Psychiatry Reports, 20*(11), 95–114. https://doi.org/10.1007/s11920-018-0969-9

American Psychological Association. (n.d.). *APA dictionary of psychology: Intergenerational trauma*. https://dictionary.apa.org/intergenerational-trauma

American Psychological Association, Working Group for Addressing Racial and Ethnic Disparities in Youth Mental Health. (2017). *Addressing the mental health needs of racial and ethnic minority youth: A guide for practitioners*. https://www.apa.org

Ammerman, R. T., Putnam, F. W., Bosse, N. R., Teers, A. R., & Van Ginkel, J. B. (2010). Maternal depression in home visitation: A systematic review. *Aggression and Violent Behavior, 15*(3), 191–200. https://doi.org/10.1016/j.avb.2009.12.002

Anda, R. F., Porter, L. E., & Brown, D. W. (2022). Inside the Adverse Childhood Experience score: Strengths, limitations, and misapplications. *American Journal of Preventive Medicine, 59*(2), 293–295. https://doi.org/10.1016/j.amepre.2020.01.009

Barrett, M. S., Chua, W. J., Crits-Christoph, P., Gibbons, M. B., Casiano, D., & Thompson, D. (2008). Early withdrawal from mental health treatment: Implications for psychotherapy practice. *Psychotherapy, 45*(2), 247–267. https://doi.org/10.1037/0033-3204.45.2.247

Bartlett, J. D., Kotake, C., Fauth, R., Easterbrooks, M. A. (2017). Intergenerational transmission of child abuse and neglect: Do maltreatment type, perpetrator, and substantiation status matter? *Child Abuse and Neglect, 63, 84–94.* https://doi.org/10.1016/j.chiabu.2016.11.021

Bartlett, J. D., Griffin, J. L., Spinazzola, J., Fraser, J. G., Noroña, C. R., Bodian, R., Todd, M., Montagna, C., & Barto, B. (2018). The impact of a statewide trauma-informed care initiative in child welfare on the well-being of children and youth with complex trauma. *Children & Youth Services Review, 84*, 110–117. https://doi.org/10.1016/j.childyouth.2017.11.015

Bartlett. J. D., & Sacks, V. (2019). *Adverse childhood experiences are different than child trauma, and it's critical to understand why*. https://www.childtrends.org

Becker, K. D., Boustani, M., Gellatly, R., & Chorpita, B. F. (2018). Forty years of engagement research in children's mental health services: Multidimensional measurement and practice elements. *Journal of Clinical Child & Adolescent Psychology, 47*(1), 1–23. https://doi.org/10.1080/15374416.2017.1326121

Bick, J., & Nelson, C. A. (2016). Early adverse experiences and the developing brain. *Neuropsychopharmacology, 41*, 177–196. https://doi.org/10.1038/npp.2015.252
Brave Heart, M. Y. H., Elkins, J., Tafoya, G., Bird, D., & Salvador, M. (2012). Wicasa Was'aka: Restoring the traditional strength of American Indian boys and men. *American Journal of Public Health, 102*(Supplement 2), S177–S183. https://doi.org/10.2105/AJPH.2011.30051
Centers for Disease Control and Prevention. (2019, July). *Identifying, preventing, and treating childhood trauma*. https://www.cdc.gov/washington/testimony/2019/t20190711.htm
Child Welfare Information Gateway. (2014). The Family Engagement Inventory (FEI): A brief cross-disciplinary synthesis. U.S. Department of Health and Human Services, Children's Bureau. https://www.childwelfare.gov/
Child Welfare Information Gateway, Administration on Children, Youth, & Families, Administration for Children & Families, U.S. Department of Health & Human Services. (2017). *The Family Engagement Inventory: A brief cross-disciplinary synthesis*. www.childwelfare.gov/pubPDFs/synthesis.pdf#page=2&zoom=100,-213,716
Cordón, I., Pipe, M., Sayfan, L., Melinder, A., & Goodman, G. (2004). Memory for traumatic experiences in early childhood. *Developmental Review, 24*(1), 101–132. https://doi.org/10.1016/j.dr.2003.09.003
Cree, R. A., Bitsko, R. H., Robinson, L. R., Holbrook, J. R., Danielson, M. L., Smith, C., Kaminski, J. W., Kenney, M. K., & Peacock, G. (2018). Health care, family, and community factors associated with mental, behavioral, and developmental disorders and poverty among children aged 2–8 years – United States, 2016. *Morbidity & Mortality Weekly Report, 67*(50), 1377–1383. https://doi.org/10.15585/mmwr.mm6750a1
Dettlaff, A. J., & Boyd, R. (2021). Racial disproportionality and disparities in the child welfare system: Why do they exist, and what can be done to address them? *Annals of the American Academy of Political & Social Science, 692*, 253–274. https://doi.org/10.1177/0002716220980329
Dowell, K. A., & Ogles, B. M. (2010). The effects of parent participation on child psychotherapy outcome: A meta-analytic review. *Journal of Clinical Child & Adolescent Psychology, 39*(2), 151–162. https://doi.org/10.1080/15374410903532585
Enlow, M. B., Blood, E., & Egeland, B. (2013). Sociodemographic risk, developmental competence, and PTSD symptoms in young children exposed to interpersonal trauma in early life. *Journal of Traumatic Stress, 26*(6), 686–694. https://doi.org/10.1002/jts.21866
Epstein, J. L. (2011). *School, family, and community partnerships: Preparing educators and improving schools* (2nd ed.). Westview.
Felitti, V. J., Anda, R. F., & Nordenberg, D. (1998). Relationship of childhood abuse and household dysfunction to many of the leading causes of death in adults: The Adverse Childhood Experiences (ACE) study. *American Journal of Preventive Medicine, 14*(4), 245–258. https://doi.org/10.1016/S0749-3797(98)00017-8
Funderburk, B. W., & Eyberg, S. (2011). Parent–child interaction therapy. In J. C. Norcross, G. R. VandenBos, & D. K. Freedheim (Eds.), *History of psychotherapy: Continuity and change* (pp. 415–420). American Psychological Association.
Gopalkrishnan, N. (2018). Cultural diversity and mental health: Considerations for policy and practice. *Frontiers in Public Health, 19*(6), 179–187. https://doi.org/10.3389/fpubh.2018.00179
Grube, W. A., & Liming, K. W. (2018). Attachment and Biobehavioral Catch-up: A systematic review. *Infant Mental Health Journal, 39*(6), 656–673. https://doi.org/10.1002/imhj.21745
Hanson, R. F., Lang, J. M., Fraser, J. G., Agosti, J. R., Ake, G. S., Donisch, K. M., & Gewirtz, A. H. (2018). Trauma-informed care: Definitions and statewide initiatives. In J. B. Klika & J. R. Conte (Eds.), *The APSAC handbook on child maltreatment* (4th ed., pp. 272–291). Sage.
Healthy People 2030. (n.d.). *Social determinants of health*. U.S. Department of Health & Human Services, Office of Disease Prevention and Health Promotion. https://health.gov/healthypeople/objectives-and-data/social-determinants-health
Ingolsby, E. (2010). Review of interventions to improve family engagement and retention in parent and child mental health programs. *Journal of Child and Family Studies, 19*(5), 629–645. https://doi.org/10.1007/s10826-009-9350-2
Kataoka, S. H., Zhang, L., & Wells, K. B. (2002). Unmet need for mental health care among U.S. children: Variation by ethnicity and insurance status. *American Journal of Psychiatry, 159*(9), 1548–1555. https://doi.org/10.1176/appi.ajp.159.9.1548

Kim, K., Atkinson, V., Brown, E., Ramos, M., Guzman, L., Forry, N., Porter, T., & Nord, C. (2015). *Family and provider/teacher relationship quality measures*. Office of Planning, Research & Evaluation, U.S. Department of Health & Human Services.

Lang, J. M., Campbell, K., Shanley, P., Crusto, C. A., & Connell, C. M. (2016). Building capacity for trauma-informed care in the child welfare system: Initial results of a statewide implementation. *Child Maltreatment, 21*(2), 113–124. https://doi.org/10.1177/1077559516635273

Lieberman, A. F., & Van Horn, P. (2008). *Psychotherapy with infants and young children: Repairing the effects of stress and trauma on early attachment*. Guilford.

Lieberman, A. F., Ghosh Ippen, C., & Horn, V. (2015). *Don't hit my mommy: A manual for Child-Parent Psychotherapy with young children exposed to violence and other trauma* (2nd ed.). Zero to Three.

Lin, L., Stamm, K., & Christidis, P. (2018). *How diverse is the psychology workforce?* American Psychological Association. www.apa.org/monitor/2018/02/datapoint

Luthar, S. S., Cicchetti, D., & Becker, B. (2000). The construct of resilience: A critical evaluation and guidelines for future work. *Child Development, 71*(3), 543–562. https://doi.org/10.1111/1467-8624.00164

Masten, A. S. (2001). Ordinary magic. Resilience processes in development. *American Psychologist, 56*(3), 227–238. https://doi.org/10.1037//0003-066x.56.3.227

Melz, H., Morrison, C., Ingolsby, E., Cairon, K., & Mackrain, M. (2019, June). *Review of trauma-informed initiatives at the systems level: Trauma-informed approaches: Connecting research, policy, and practice to build resilience in children and families*. https://aspe.hhs.gov/

Menschner, C., & Maul, A. (2016). Key ingredients for successful trauma-informed care implementation. Health Care Strategies. https://www.samhsa.gov/sites/default/files/programs_campaigns/childrens_mental_health/atcwhitepaper-040616.pdf

Miller, G. E., & Prinz, R. J. (2003). Engagement of families in treatment for childhood conduct problems. *Behavior Therapy, 34*, 517–534.

Murphey, D., & Bartlett, J. D. (2019). *Childhood adversity screenings are just one part of an effective policy response to childhood trauma*. Child Trends. https://cms.childtrends.org/

National Child Traumatic Stress Network, Secondary Traumatic Stress Committee. (2011). *Secondary traumatic stress: A fact sheet for child-serving professionals*. https://www.nctsn.org/trauma-informed-care/secondary-traumatic-stress

National Child Traumatic Stress Network (NCTSNa). (n.d.). *Complex trauma*. https://www.nctsn.org/what-is-child-trauma/trauma-types/complex-trauma

National Child Traumatic Stress Network (NCTSNb). (n.d.). *Early childhood trauma*. https://www.nctsn.org/resources/early-childhood-trauma

National Child Traumatic Stress Network (NCTSNc). (n.d.). *About child trauma*. https://www.nctsn.org/what-is-child-trauma/about-child-trauma

National Child Traumatic Stress Network. (2017). *Family engagement and involvement in trauma mental health*. https://www.nctsn.org/sites/default/files/resources/fact-sheet/cac_family_engagement_and_involvement_in_trauma_mental_health.pdf

National Child Traumatic Stress Network. (2020). *Cultural responsiveness to racial trauma: Understanding racial trauma, why it matters, and what to do*. https://www.nctsn.org/resources/cultural-responsiveness-to-racial-trauma

National Scientific Council on the Developing Child. (2004). *Young children develop in an environment of relationships. Working paper no. 1*. http://www.developingchild.net

National Scientific Council on the Developing Child. (2014). *Excessive Stress Disrupts the architecture of the developing brain: Working paper no. 3. Updated edition*. http://www.developingchild.harvard.edu

National Scientific Council on the Developing Child. (2015). *Supportive relationships and active skill-building strengthen foundations of resilience*. www.developingchild.harvard.edu

Nicholson, J., Kurtz, J., Rivas, L., Henneman, T., Peterson, E., Bryant, S., & Lin, B. (2022). *Trauma-responsive family engagement in early childhood: Practices for equity and resilience*. Routledge.

Nugent, N. R., Ostrowski, S., Christopher, N. C., & Delahanty, D. L. (2007). Parental posttraumatic stress symptoms as a moderator of child's acute biological response and subsequent posttraumatic stress symptoms in pediatric injury patients. *Journal of Pediatric Psychology, 32*, 309–318. https://doi.org/10.1093/jpepsy/jsl005

Ofonedu, M. E., Belcher, H. M. E., Budhathoki, C., & Gross, D. A. (2017). Understanding barriers to initial treatment engagement among underserved families seeking mental health services. *Journal of Child and Family Studies, 26*(3), 863–876. https://doi.org/10.1007/s10826-016-0603-6

Oppenheim, J., & Bartlett, J. D. (2023). *Cost-effectiveness of infant and early childhood mental health treatment.* Infant & Early Childhood Technical Assistance Center. https://gucchd.georgetown.edu/Docs/iecmh/Cost-Effectiveness%20of%20Infant%20and%20Early%20Childhood%20Mental%20Health%20Treatment.pdf

Reardon, T., Harvey, K., Baranowska, M., O'Brien, D., Smith, L., & Creswell, C. (2017). What do parents perceive are the barriers and facilitators to accessing psychological treatment for mental health problems in children and adolescents? A systematic review of qualitative and quantitative studies. *European Child and Adolescent Psychiatry, 26(6), 623–647.* https://doi.org/10.1007/s00787-016-0930-6

Rodgers, C. R. R., Flores, M. W., Bassey, O., Augenblick, J. M., & Le Cook, B. (2021). Racial/ethnic disparities trends in children's mental health care access and expenditures from 2010-2017: Disparities remain despite sweeping policy reform. *Child & Adolescent Psychiatry, 61*(7), 915–925. https://doi.org/10.1016/j.jaac.2021.09.420

Scheeringa, M. S., & Zeanah, C. (2001). A relational perspective on PTSD in early childhood. *Journal of Traumatic Stress, 14*, 799–815. https://doi.org/10.1023/A:1013002507972

Scheeringa, M. S., Weems, C. F., Cohen, J. A., Amaya-Jackson, L., & Guthrie, D. (2011). Trauma-focused cognitive-behavioral therapy for posttraumatic stress disorder in three-through six year-old children: a randomized clinical trial. *Journal of Child Psychology and Psychiatry, 52(8), 853–860.* https://doi.org/10.1111/j.1469-7610.2010.02354.x

Staudt, M. (2007). Treatment engagement with caregivers of at-risk children: Gaps in research and conceptualization. *Journal of Child and Family Studies, 16(2), 183–196.* https://doi.org/10.1007/s10826-006-9077-2

Stewart, R. W., Orengo-Aguayo, R. E., Gilmore, A. K., & de Arellano, M. (2017). Addressing barriers to care among hispanic youth: Telehealth delivery of Trauma-Focused Cognitive Behavioral Therapy. *Behavior Therapy, 40*(3), 112–118.

Sturm, R., & Sherbourne, C. D. (2001). Are barriers to mental health and substance abuse care still rising? *Journal of Behavioral Health Services & Research, 28(1), 81–88.*

Substance Abuse and Mental Health Services Administration. (2014). *SAMHSA's concept of trauma and guidance for a trauma-informed approach. HHS Publication No. (SMA) 14–4884.* Author. https://store.samhsa.gov/

U.S. Department of Health & Human Services, Administration for Children & Families, Administration on Children, Youth & Families, Children's Bureau. (2023). *Child maltreatment 2021.* https://www.acf.hhs.gov/cb/data-research/child-maltreatment

VanDerBeek, K. L., Sigel, B. A., Pemberton, J. R., & John, S. G. (2018). Treatments for early childhood trauma: Decision considerations for clinicians. *Journal of Child & Adolescent Trauma, 12*(4), 515–528. https://doi.org/10.1007/s40653-018-0244-6

Waid, J., & Kelly, M. (2020). Supporting family engagement with child and adolescent mental health services: A scoping review. *Health & Social Care in the Community, 28*(5), 1333–1342. https://doi.org/10.1111/hsc.12947

Washington State Institute for Public Policy. (2019a). *Parent-Child Interaction Therapy (PCIT) for families in the child welfare system.* www.wsipp.wa.gov/BenefitCost/Program/77

Washington State Institute for Public Policy. (2019b). *Child-Parent Psychotherapy*. https://www.wsipp.wa.gov/BenefitCost/Program/263

Whitney, D. G., & Peterson, M. D. (2019). U.S. national and state-level prevalence of mental health disorders and disparities of mental health care use in children. *JAMA. Pediatrics, 173*(4), 389–391. https://doi.org/10.1001/jamapediatrics.2018.5399

Woolgar, F., Garfield, H., Dalgleish, T., & Meiser-Stedman, R. (2022). Systematic review and meta-analysis: Prevalence of posttraumatic stress disorder in trauma-exposed preschool-aged children. *Journal of the American Academy of Child & Adolescent Psychiatry, 61*(3), 366–377. https://doi.org/10.1016/j.jaac.2021.05.026

Zero to Three. (2016). *Tuning in: Parents of young children speak up about what they think, know and need.* www.zerotothree.org/resource/national-parent-survey-report/

Chapter 7
Developing Fatherhood: A Cultural Perspective on Engaging Men in the Lives of Children

John Hornstein

This chapter is written from both a research and personal perspective, within the frame of fatherhood as a social and personal construction. Fatherhood may be the most meaningful and gratifying element in a man's life. For many, it is a role embedded in family history and investment in the future. It comes with personal and financial responsibility. Fathering children often takes place within a relational system that encompasses an intimate partnership in parenting and meaningful relations with children. Sometimes, it takes place in the absence of a fulfilling relationship with a partner and separation from family. In many instances, paternal responsibility is gratifying in itself; in some, it is overwhelming. Being the breadwinner is a central role for men in many societies. However, in today's world, that role may be as much for mothers as it is for fathers (Parker & Horowitz, 2015). Father's roles vary greatly between societies and have changed throughout history. What is eminently clear is that men can and do play fundamental and meaningful roles in children's lives. And those roles vary greatly between fathers, families, and societies.

Roles and Identity in Fatherhood

For some men, it is a role not gladly taken or from which they are separated. Fathers can be distant, even absent. If absent, they may still value their identity as fathers (Tamis-LeMonda & McFadden, 2010). Some may choose nurturance but not responsibility. Or, conversely, they can give little in the way of emotional support to children or their mothers but provide economic stability. They can provide moral

J. Hornstein (✉)
Child Development Consultant and Faculty at Napa Infant Parent Mental Health Fellowship Program, University of California – Davis, Davis, CA, USA

L. Nabors, J. D. Bartlett (eds.), *Family Engagement in Mental Health Interventions for Young Children*, Springer Series on Child and Family Studies,
https://doi.org/10.1007/978-3-031-47917-5_7

guidance or model destructive behavior. Fathers can experience delight and pride in seeing a child grow and success or despair at a child's failure or perceived failure. Fathers may emulate their own fathers or consciously choose to parent in a new way or struggle with the balance between the two (Guzzo, 2011).

Becoming a father can bring together many of the elements of a man's identity. Indeed, men often report that becoming a father brings them to a more fulfilling sense of themselves as men. The anthropologist Margaret Mead famously said, "Fathers are biological necessities; but social accidents." It follows that fathers take their cues from those around them, their own families, their communities, and their culture. This includes professionals who seek to join families in the process of caring for children. A fundamental tenet of this chapter is that fathers are created and create themselves within a sociocultural context. Their choices in defining their roles are both driven by the society in which they live and by their individual values and circumstances within that culture.

In *Mothers and Others: The Evolutionary Origins of Mutual Understanding*, Sarah Hrdy (2009) examines alloparenting, the processes by which mothers share the care for their children with fathers and others, as an evolved characteristic of human beings. According to this evolutionary perspective, the survival of the species required cooperative breeding. In human beings, this involves not only shared direct care but also shared cultural beliefs and practices. Fathers in many societies, but not all, care for young children, and the traditions in those societies, transmitted by others, inform men on the nature of their involvement with children. Fathers in even more societies provide food and shelter for their families as well as moral guidance and linkages to the world outside the family. For our purposes, in considering how we engage with fathers in our professional capacities, this perspective both acknowledges that we, as professionals, have a natural role in joining a child's system of care and, more importantly, that we must consider the nature of that caregiving system as we attempt to join it. This requires understanding how a father perceives his role within that system.

Conceiving or adopting a child brings into play the forces that have shaped us. Whether mother or father, experience in one's own family, shared community standards, beliefs about children and their care, societal norms and expectations, personal temperament, and previous love and loss all influence how we parent. Understanding how these forces operate may help professionals working with families effectively join the process of becoming a parent. Indeed, in all societies and throughout history, parents, whether mothers or fathers, rely on others to guide them and help care for children. In some societies, it is the father's father who takes a predominant role as a guide to his son. In others, it is other men or even women who provide such modeling or guidance. In one study, interviews with young fathers found that their role models often included their own fathers, and mothers, but also their spouse's families, and most frequently peer parents (Masciadrelli et al., 2006). The input can be explicit with direct guidance on how to be a responsible father, but most often, it is implicitly transmitted through modeling and shared cultural practices. Whatever the cultural mores, however, men require input and support from others in adopting the role of a parent. Yet, they seem less likely than mothers to seek out that support.

While gender roles do vary both between and within societies in relation to parenting, in today's world, the parenting role is increasingly bounded less by gender than by adopting the responsibilities of parenthood. Men who take on the role, that is, fathers who experience satisfaction and commitment to their role as fathers, are more involved in their children's lives (Henley & Pasley, 2005). Research demonstrates that the child benefits from a sensitive caregiver, an interactive partner, a provider of a safe and healthy environment, and a moral guide regardless of the parent's gender (Grossmann & Grossmann, 2020). The difference, for professionals who wish to engage parents, is often in the parent's perception of his role. This may also include other men in children's lives. Indeed, it is. Often, it is men other than the biological father, stepfathers, boyfriends, uncles, grandparents, and even older siblings, who take on these roles.

While the focus of much of the research on fatherhood focuses on how fathers are different than mothers in their relationships with children, the preponderance of empirical study (Lamb, 2010) demonstrates that strong and growth-enhancing relationships with children develop similarly. Sensitivity to infant and children's cues, playful interactions, caregiving routines, attention to developmental achievements, warmth, and many other behaviors related to the support of strong relationships and healthy development are characteristics of parents of either gender (Partridge et al., 2001). At the same time, the differences are both interesting and useful in that they reflect how fathers see themselves, their role as parents, and in some senses set themselves apart from mothers. The differences are also indicative of how others in families or communities see fathers. From a parent engagement perspective, however, it is useful to consider those areas of difference with the mother as entry points for a relationship with the father, as well as the content of a man's formation of his role as a father.

Historically, in many societies, fathers have played the role of provider and guide toward adulthood. In much of the world, fathers are becoming more involved in the care and nurturance than in the past. In the United States, according to a Pew Research Center Study, the number of stay-at-home fathers almost doubled between 1989 and 2016 (Livingston & Parker, 2019). Those who identify their reason for staying at home as caring for home and family increased from 4% to 24%. Since 1965, the amount of time fathers report providing childcare has tripled. At the same time, about three-fourths of adults indicated that men face a lot of pressure to support their family financially, while almost half said men face a lot of pressure to be an involved parent. Sixty-three percent of fathers say they spend too little time with their children, while only 39% reported that they were doing a very good job raising their children (Livingston & Parker, 2019). Hence, despite the increase in father involvement with their children, many men remain less than satisfied with how they perform those roles.

This chapter uses the term "father" with all of its connotations and manifestations. The roles of other men in children's lives – stepfathers, uncles, brothers, grandfathers, uncles, boyfriends – may or may not overlap with what we discuss here. Similarly, the application of the material to same sex partners and single parents needs to consider the particular conditions in which they parent and how they themselves define their roles. Research on single mothers and single fathers shows that their parenting is far more similar than different (Dufur et al., 2010). Good parenting is not defined by gender. The study and discussion of fatherhood have historically been marked by binary thinking that constrains how both fathers themselves, and those seeking to work with them, see men's relationships with children. This needs to be kept in mind when considering what generations of researchers and clinicians tell us.

Fathers, and other men, are ready to play greater roles in their children's lives. In today's world, taking on larger roles is expected of fathers. Historical and cross-cultural forces play a formative role in how men see themselves in relation to the care and upbringing of children. There are countless models and options. This variability can be challenging for any man attempting to establish his identity as a father. At the same time, it provides a tremendous opportunity for health, education, and social service professionals to have a positive impact on fathers, their families, and the broader society. In this chapter, we focus on three facets of fatherhood, relationships with young children, the social and cultural context of fathering, and a man's construction of his identity as a father. First, we examine these perspectives of fatherhood in today's world, and then, we establish a framework for supporting men via each of those perspectives.

Fatherhood in Today's World

There has been a plethora of research on fatherhood in the last 30 years. Lamb's (2010) *The Role of the Father in Child Development* and Fitzgerald et al.'s (2020) *Handbook of Fathers and Child Development: Prenatal to Preschool* provide extensive and comprehensive reviews of the literature. *Fathering: A Journal of Theory, Research, and Practice about Men as Fathers*, established in 2003, is the first peer-reviewed journal to focus exclusively on fatherhood. A library search on the keyword fatherhood yielded 23,512 results. And, more specific to involvement is Cabrera and Tamis-LeMonda's (2013) *Handbook of Father Involvement: Multidisciplinary Perspectives*. The range of study is as varied as fathers themselves often leading to contradictory findings related to topics such as the influence of divorce, masculinity, and other men in children's lives. In this chapter, we focus on those areas of study most relevant to professionals establishing supporting partnerships with fathers: father-child relationships, fathers in the family and community context, and fatherhood identity.

It is universally clear that competent and involved fatherhood is good for young children, for families, for the fathers themselves, and for communities. Research on father's influence on children's development indicates that such involvement has positive effects on cognitive and language development, self-esteem, self-regulation, academic achievement, and adaptation later in life (Lamb, 2010). In relation to later development, one meta-analysis of 24 studies of the developmental outcomes of involved fatherhood indicated that "father engagement reduces the frequency of behavioral problems in boys and psychological problems in young women; it also enhances cognitive development while decreasing criminality and economic disadvantage in low SES families" (Sarkadi et al., 2008, p. 153). These positive effects may be directly related to interactions with their children or indirectly via support of the other parent and the economic well-being of the family (Allen & Daly, 2007). Interviews with fathers indicate that they find pleasure, pride, love, and personal growth from watching their children grow while at the same time sacrificing time, energy, money, and other personal relationships (Palkovitz, 2002).

Similar to Cabrera et al. (2007a, b), this author's approach is not on fathers as "the other parent" in which the lens is on what is known about mothering but on the fathering role in itself. This role is perhaps complimentary to mothering but with its own characteristics and outcomes. Further, as Belsky (1984) maintains in the multiple determinants of parenting model, fathering is influenced by his social context, by his own personal traits, and by patterns of family functioning including relationships with the mother and level of involvement with his children. The participation of fathers in the system of care of a child can take various forms both through proximal interactions with the child and another parent and more distally as a provider and decision-maker. He may care for and play with his children, he can support the child's other parent in making choices in the care of nurturance of his children, and he can help provide a home and other resources essential to child development, which allow his children to thrive.

Fathers' Relationships with Children

Review of both the nature and benefits of fathers' relationships with young children indicates two interrelated strands of these relationships that might be considered when developing father engagement efforts: attachment, the emotional bonds between father and child, and interaction, the way in which men care for, play with, and communicate with their children. Both can serve as portals to joining men in becoming healthy and nurturing fathers.

New fathers are at risk for postpartum depression (Singley & Edwards, 2015) with roughly 10% of new fathers experiencing anxiety and depression. Prenatal preparation as well as professional support during childbirth has enhanced the father's experience at the birth of his child (Franzen et al., 2021). The traditional focus of both research and intervention has been primarily on the mother. However, the new baby can be "introduced" to both parents by focusing on the child's unique behavioral characteristics.

Singley and Edwards (2015) noted the buffering effect of social support and supporting paternal self-efficacy as a means to improve mental health while acknowledging that traditionally men tend not to ask for support. Noting the effect of maternal gatekeeping, they recommend direct caregiving of the infant as soon as possible and that the new father "can benefit from concrete guidance regarding the need to actively engage their partners on an emotional level about any issues they are experiencing" (Singley & Edwards, 2015, p. 313). Exposure to infants and young children triggers caregiving responses. In one study, researchers found such exposure increased production of oxytocin and prolactin, hormones known to be associated with responsive in the brains of fathers with primary caregiving responsibilities (Abraham et al., 2014). Thus, engaging the infant may be related to paternal mental health.

The preponderance of research on attachment is on mothers and their infants and young children. The secure relationship that is established between mothers and their children is seen by attachment theorists as providing the child with a secure base and as the fundamental model for future relationships (Bowlby, 1969; Bretherton & Munholland, 2016). Ainsworth's (Ainsworth, 1979; Ainsworth et al., 1978, 2015) early study of attachment, in the service of confirming Bowlby's (1969) theses, also found that differential mother-directed responses were fairly quickly followed by differential attachment behavior toward a small number of other figures, including father, grandmother, co-wife, and even siblings. Attachment to fathers seemed to be especially common, even in babies who did not see their fathers often. Indeed, "one of the 26 infants in the Baltimore study showed attachment behavior exclusively to the father… and three others were said to prefer the father as attachment figure over the mother" (Bretherton, 2010, p. 10). Variation in the security of the attachment relationship has been shown to be related to variations in parental behavior as well as child characteristics. For example, babies may form insecure relationships when primary attachment figures are insensitive or intrusive (Ainsworth, 1979; Ainsworth et al., 1978, 2015), or as is maintained by Jerome Kagan and his associates (Kagan, 1995), the child is temperamentally highly reactive to stressful or novel stimuli. The primary measures of the security of the attachment relationship are for the child to seek the attachment figure out when stressed and to use that figure as a base for exploration (Bowlby, 1969).

Nurturant fathers establish emotional ties with their children much as mothers do. Fathers show a strong desire to bond with their infants (Atkinson et al., 2021). Historical review of the accumulated research overwhelmingly demonstrates that secure attachments develop between fathers and children (Bretherton, 2010). And, in cases when the mother is absent, fathers are often the primary source of security and attachment figure. Meta-analysis of studies in which both mothers and fathers' attachments with one-year-olds were assessed showed that of the 950 children for whom measures with father and mother were available, 45% were secure with both parents, 17% were insecure with both, and 38% secure with one parent and insecure with the other (DeWolff & Van Ijzendoorn, 1997). That is, a fairly large proportion of infants demonstrated an independent attachment classification with the father. A more recent summary of research on father attachment (Freeman et al., 2010) concluded that father attachment was not "merely what is left over after subtracting mother attachment" (p. 8). When fathers provide infants with care, their brains change. This is represented in the brain-hormonal-behavioral pathways, which are activated in men and women when they care for infants (Abraham et al., 2014).

There are differences between parents in how attachment relationships are formed (Fernandes et al., 2020). In an early study looking at mother-child and father-child attachment, Lamb (1976) found that infants showed similar behavioral connections with mothers and fathers when both were present. However, infants approached fathers with more positive interactions like offering toys. But when a stranger walked into the room, the infants went to the mother. Another often cited study indicated that fathers' play sensitivity is a better predictor of the child's long-term attachment representation than the early infant-father security of attachment (Grossmann et al., 2002). Such differences may have a differential and complimentary effect on children's development. Paquette (2004) refers to this as the "father-child activation relationship." Contrasted with maternal calming and comforting in times of stress, "men seem to have a tendency to excite, surprise, and momentarily destabilize children; they also tend to encourage children to take risks while at the same time ensuring the latter's safety and security, thus permitting children to learn to be braver in unfamiliar situations, as well as to stand up for themselves" (Paquette, 2004; p. 193). He points out, in relation to attachment, that this interaction style is only effective in the context of a strong emotional bond. Both attachment security and nurturant and playful interactions benefit the child.

Complimentary styles of interaction have their benefits. In a study of resident low-income fathers, Cabrera et al. (2007b) found that supportive paternal interactions with infants and toddlers led to both emotional and cognitive gains. Further, their analysis indicated that the supportiveness of fathers in these interactions had a larger effect than that of mothers. Given the challenges of parenting in poverty, it may be that both the provision of emotional security and growth-enhancing interactions are necessary for optimal development. The nature of the interactions is important. Controlling fathering in a laboratory setting was associated with lower executive functioning scores in their children, whereas paternal support of autonomy was linked to higher executive functioning (Meuwissen & Carlson, 2015).

In general, fathers are more vigorous in their physical play with children (Grossmann & Grossmann, 2020). Responsible rough and tumble play has been found to be related to social competence and to a lesser degree with emotional skills and self-regulation (Stgeorge & Freeman, 2017). Feeling secure and exploring the world are complimentary systems, with both being essential to development. Certainly, parents of either gender can provide either or both. However, the research on fathers indicates that, in general, men tend to provide more support for exploration and women for security (e.g., Grossmann & Grossmann, 2020).

Traditional views of fatherhood often involve that of being a moral authority and, as part of that, a disciplinarian. A study of mothers' and fathers' perceptions of the father's role with children found that contemporary fathers often have difficulty reconciling the two (Bretherton et al., 2005). Many fathers, with expectations from mothers and contemporary society, take on more a more caregiving and nurturant role with children while at the same time necessarily holding on to the job of disciplinarian. Often, they revert to the models they themselves grew up with. In a British study of the transition to fatherhood, researchers found that young fathers intentionally wanted to disrupt traditional gender norms; but they retreated to "patriarchal habits" as the demands of parenting increased (Miller, 2011). The challenge of reconciling sensitive caregiving with moral authority and discipline is real. This is true for both men and women. Some, like the therapist O'Connell (2005), maintain that this requires men to utilize both their masculinity and physical power. Others, like Brazelton (1992), emphasize an understanding of children's development, teaching, and parental self-control. Both require men to adopt moral authority and reflect on their own emotions in setting limits on children's behavior.

Consideration of the benefits and costs of differences in interactive style needs to take into account that, in general, fathers do spend less time with children than mothers do, there is broad variability in the type of play that fathers actually engage in with their children, and cultural variation in father's roles with children may determine the extent to which father's play out interactive activities with children. Most particularly for those who wish to support father involvement, consideration needs to be given to whether and how mothers provide access to children.

The Familial and Cultural Context of Fatherhood

From a letter from my mother to my father when my older brother was two months old: "I want to experience the moment when father and son get to know each other. I can about visualize your face. He would certainly look at you wonderingly and raise one eyebrow with suspicion and move the pacifier to the outer corner of his mouth, just like Mister Daddy when he smokes a cigarette in a somewhat crazy way." Taking on the role of a father varies with how a man defines himself. If the parenting role is overtly part of his identity, his involvement with his children is stronger (McBride et al., 2005).

A recent study of first-time fatherhood (Carlson et al., 2022) in an urban midwestern setting describes this transition as a "developmental engine" starting in the prenatal period. Young fathers "...identified their desire to be "good fathers" and this desire shaped their identity development of being a financial provider and caregiver. The three main themes that emerged were as follows: (1) the desire and motivation to become a good father, (2) the complex understanding of the financial aspect of being a father, and (3) learning caregiving skills." (Carlson et al., 2022; p.189).

Relationships with and responsibility for children take place within a variety of family constellations and community settings. The presence of multiple caregivers in a home may mediate the effects of disturbances in a parent-child relationship. For example, a child's challenging temperament may require a father's greater participation in the care of a child if that child particularly tests the other parent. Marital conflict or dissatisfaction, on the other hand, can alienate one parent from the system of care or enhance that of the other (Harman et al., 2022). Overall, marital satisfaction and communication between parents can support good outcomes for children (Lamb & Lewis, 2010).

Mothers have the largest influence on how a father parents a child. In many cases, if not most, she is the gatekeeper. Bretherton et al. (2005) see father involvement in relation to the mother's influence as bidirectional with parental cooperation yielding higher father involvement and higher father involvement with children leading to greater parental harmony. Further, some research demonstrates that mothers' beliefs about the father's role result in him having access to the child (McBride et al., 2005).

Research from a family systems perspective further demonstrates effects beyond those found in dyadic models of relationships – parent-child and parent-parent. The multiple relationships between parents and their children within the context of extended family and community are a dynamic system in which each element influences the other. Responsible parent engagement requires consideration of these influences on men and their relationships with their children, particularly as the field has relied primarily on a Western and historically recent, nuclear family model (McHale, 2007). A father plays his roles – responsive caregiver, supportive co-parent, and breadwinner – as part of and in relationship to the other moving parts of the relational system around the child or children. He influences, and is influenced by, the other elements of the system. His effect on the well-being of his child may be as much indirectly, through his impact on that system, as his direct interactions with the child (Cabrera et al., 2007a, b).

Another area that bears particular focus is that of attitudes toward low-income fathers. The study of these fathers finds that in taking on their paternal roles these fathers are as diverse as all fathers in relation to interacting with their children, adopting responsibility for their children and, indeed, longing to play a meaningful role in their children's lives. Tamis-LeMonda and McFadden (2010) describe and refute the false characterizations of low-income fathers as nonessential, deadbeat, perpetrators of their own childhood histories and dissenters of marriage. They found that children do benefit from the positive influence of such fathers on their development. The majority of children of low-income fathers do see their nonresident biological fathers. Fathers demonstrated high involvement with their children despite poor personal histories with their own fathers when buffered by positive relationships and better economic circumstances in adulthood. Positive relational histories with their own fathers did not predict high involvement with their children in the face of difficult current circumstances. In studying both resident and nonresident fathers, Coley and Hernandez (2006) conclude that policy efforts aimed at enhancing fathers' responsible parenting should focus both on increasing fathers' human and social capital and on supporting positive family processes.

Engaging Fathers: Responsivity and Responsibility

Years ago, I was on the playground at a childcare center in Maine when I noticed a father with a 3-year-old wrapped around his neck dropping her off for the day. I approached him and noted how attached the child was. He expressed his appreciation for my comment and said that the center staff didn't usually communicate with him.

Whether bound to models of fatherhood grounded in traditional beliefs about masculinity, hindered by poverty or familial conflict, defined by large cultural differences in what fatherhood entails, or committed to changed societal beliefs about nurturant male figures, fathers are ready to be engaged in the lives of their children (Yogman & Eppel, 2022). The most effective strategy we have at our disposal in helping men involve themselves in their children's lives is the children themselves. Caregiving, playing, exploring, holding, observing, and often co-parenting – this is the medium in which men become fathers, preferably in a supportive context. Their investment in their children comes, in large part, from being with them. Overcoming barriers to father engagement, by scheduling sessions outside working hours, specifically targeting concerns and needs expressed by fathers, and enhancing trust in the expertise of therapists, is important (Tully et al., 2017). Thus, a second strategy, emphasized throughout the discussion of father engagement, is the importance of a genuine commitment to connecting with fathers on the part of professionals. Authenticity and the capacity to develop trust through respect and humility are essential ingredients of any effective fatherhood initiative.

Evidence-Based Practices

There are several evidence-based programs that are specifically designed for fathers. The National Responsible Fatherhood Clearinghouse (https://www.fatherhood.gov) is a good resource for clinicians and researchers. As part of efforts for the Clearinghouse, Bronte-Tinkew et al. (2007) established criteria for rating programs as "model," promising," and "emerging." Criteria, common to those used in evaluating other family- and child-focused interventions, included items such as adequate sample size, competent research design, and significant outcomes. The following eight, among 34 examined, were rated as "model" evidence-based fatherhood programs:

1. Dads for Life – for recently divorced noncustodial fathers to improve the father-child relationship and reduce mother-father conflict (Cookston et al., 2007)
2. Family Transition Program – for low-income families receiving public assistance to improve parenting during the transition to self-sufficiency (Bloom et al., 2000)
3. Parents' Education About Children's Emotions (PEACE) Program – for parents who were engaged in divorce proceedings to encourage positive interactions between parents (McKenry et al., 1999)
4. Parenting Together – for first-time expectant parents to increase father involvement and mother-father cooperation (Doherty et al., 2006)
5. Preparing for the Drug Free Years – for parents to prevent their children's drug use (Haggerty et al., 1999)

6. Responsible Fatherhood Program for Incarcerated Dads – for incarcerated fathers to provide information about child development and to improve the father-child relationship (Robbers, 2005)
7. Video Self-Modeling Effects of Parenting Education on First-Time Fathers' Skills – for first-time fathers to improve parents' interactions with infants (Magill-Evans et al., 2007)
8. Young Dads – for African American adolescent fathers to help them become more responsible fathers (Mazza, 2002)

Bronte-Tinkew et al. (2007) identified ten characteristics of effective programs. These included selecting staff who are committed to work with fathers, setting clear goals, implementing the curriculum with skill and fidelity, and providing incentive for involvement. Characteristics that have particular relevance for this chapter are having staff who engage in one-on-one relationships with fathers and using methods that focus on fathers as individuals. Further, effective programs address both fathers' identities as responsible caregivers for their children and their actual interactions with their families (Bronte-Tinkew et al., 2007). My own observation, recorded in a video series on parent engagement for Head Start (ECKLC: https://www.youtube.com/watch?v=2QnAIN5q2gc), is that programs with vibrant fatherhood initiatives were those who had an administrator or outspoken staff member who became a champion for father engagement. Often, if not always, that person had a story to tell about their own father.

A Framework for Father Engagement

In engaging a father, the practitioner, whether therapist, educator, or health or social worker, has a number of entry points into the parent-child-family system. As a mental health therapist, she can focus primarily on the father's emotional well-being and readiness to parent. As a family therapist, she can consider and work with the entire family system. As a pediatrician, she can engage the father through the child's health and behavior. And as an educator, she can form a partnership based upon the child's learning and development. From a system's perspective, regardless of the entry point, the entire system is affected by change (Stern, 1995). The following discussion focuses on how each of these elements of the system – the child's behaviors and representations, the parent's behaviors and representations, and the practitioner' behaviors and representations – can help us define and apply various approaches to father engagement.

The schematic in Fig. 7.1, based upon the work of Daniel Stern (1995) a pioneer in the field of parent-child therapy, shows us various elements of the behavioral and representational world of parents and their children, with a focus on the father's contribution to the system of care around a child. Inside the circle are the behaviors of the child, the father, and the professional. Outside the circle are the mental representations of each participant in the system. The arrows indicate that the behaviors

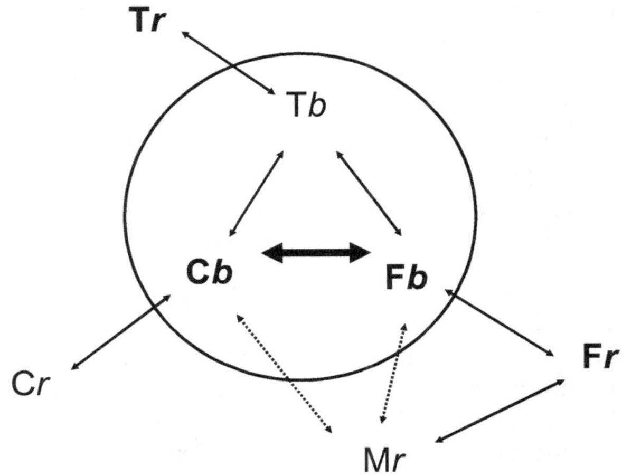

Fig. 7.1 Entry points into the child's system of care showing child (C), father (F) and therapist (T) behaviors (*b*) inside the circle and representations including the mother's (Mr) outside the circle. The arrows indicate relationships between and among the behaviors and representations. Adapted from Stern, 1995

are in response to each other and the various representations of the members of the system. The representations of each participant in this scheme can be affected by those behaviors and vice versa. The mother's representation is added here to indicate that the entire system can be extended beyond an exclusive focus on the father. In this discussion, we focus on three elements (in bold) of this graphic representation of the behavioral and representational system involving a father, a child, and a practitioner. First, and most importantly, the focus is on the behavior of the child (C*b*) as a means of supporting the parent-child relationship as well as of the father's construction of his role as a father. Second, we examine how we can support the construction of paternal identity (F*r*), including the mother's representation (M*r*) of the father's role. And finally, we examine the practitioner's relationship with the father and the parent-child system (T*r*).

The Child's Behaviors and Representations in the Engagement Process

Starting with the child, we can see, for example, behaviors like an infant (C*b*) becoming animated at seeing her father. The father could coo and smile in response (F*b*). The infant's representation (*Cr*) might then become something like, "I enjoy it when this guy shows up." And the father's representation (*Fr*) then becomes something like "She recognizes me. We have a special relationship." We can see thousands, if not tens of thousands of such interactions taking place over time as a father and child form a relationship and the development of each is affected by the other. The child's developmental capacities are influenced by the father's behaviors, which are in turn affected by his representations of himself as a father. A key point here is that the child herself is a route to the father's image of himself as a father.

The entry point into the system then is the behavior of the child (C*b*). Hence, those who effectively engage fathers in this way are astute observers of child behavior. They find words to describe behaviors of the child through which they can affect how the father behaves with the child and perhaps more importantly for the long-term father-child relationship help the father consolidate his image of himself as a contributor to his child's healthy development.

One way to accomplish this, as well as to establish more of a connection between the practitioner and the father, is to use behaviors that the father can identify with. "I notice that he is cautious when trying something new. Were you like that as a child?" It almost does not matter whether he was or was not. What matters is that he considers how he is or is not like his child and that he can tell you what he believes. Another approach is to ask him what he sees in his child's behavior. That makes him the knowledgeable observer. And it provides you, the practitioner, with a picture of what he believes.

The child's representations (C*r*) are reflected in her behavior. "I trust this guy to help me" is expressed in her bringing a toy to him at some point in the interaction. As practitioners, we can simply describe that, or go further, as appropriate, "Did you notice that she brought it to you and not me?" As discussed earlier, the child's representations about herself and her world are influenced by her interactions with her father. Another prompt for a discussion with a father about his own identity as a father might be: "Kids seem to benefit from how fathers play with them differently than how mother's play with them." This could lead to further reflection on how a father has a unique relationship with his child.

Paternal representations in the schematic (Fr) can be influenced and are influenced by the child's behaviors (C*b*) and the practitioner's input into the system (P*b*) as indicated by the arrows between the behaviors. As discussed above, the powerful influence of the child is all important. A father becomes a father when caring for and interacting with a child. His brain changes, he learns from the child, and he is a teacher for the child. Access to the child is essential.

Fathers take on their roles as parents when they are with their children even before they are born. Prenatal visits including the father can "ignite the developmental engine" of fatherhood (Carlson et al., 2015/2016). Healthcare professionals can assess the expectant father's perceptions with questions like, "Tell me what you think you baby will be like?" And perhaps, depending upon the professional role one plays, "How do you think your life will be changed by becoming a father?" This type of inquiry would open the door for a discussion of feelings about impending fatherhood. At the behavioral level, encouraging the father to read to the unborn child with the knowledge that the fetus can hear and begin to recognize her father's voice is one way to encourage the developing relationship.

The COVID pandemic lockdown, as a natural experiment, has shown how the presence of fathers in the home has demonstrated the fundamental tenet that has guided our approach to father involvement; being with children changes men. Results of two nationwide surveys of fathers (Weissbourd et al., 2020) indicated that 64% of fathers felt closer to their children. And more specifically, in the follow-up survey, 51% indicated that they were getting to know their children better, 57%

appreciated their children more, and 43% discovered new shared interests. In looking at the perspective of the children, 53% fathers reported that their children were sharing more of their feelings with them.

Moving to the final person in this schematic, the professional, we can see in the example provided that there are opportunities to support the developing relationship between the father and his child using the child's behavior as a means to enter the system. "I can see that she lights up when she sees you" (T*b*). Part of the therapist's representation, in this case, is the goal of helping the father recognize his unique role with the child. Such representations on the part of the professional are based upon an understanding of her relationship with this father and the goals of her practice.

The Practitioner's Behaviors and Representations in the Engagement Process

As much as the target of a professional's father engagement efforts with fathers may be within the behavioral circle, that is, to help fathers develop their skills in interacting with children, it also works at the representational level, in helping a man construct his identity as a father. Fathers typically know that professionals from various disciplines are working with them in order to benefit children, as a means to an end. Yet, when fathers understand that they are seen as competent and worthwhile individuals, interventions are more likely to be effective and long-standing. The relationship between the practitioner and the father requires authenticity and respect, "...men returned to the programs day after day, in part because the staff members were authentic and ready to engage men, not condemn them" (Roy & Dyson, 2010, p. 147). This capacity – wishing to engage men, particularly those from marginalized communities – runs throughout the literature on effective engagement programs, where spending quality time with the child and participating in activities with the child promote fathers' engagement (Ellis et al., 2014). Further, the characteristics of exciting play, physicality, asserting discipline, providing protection, and providing for all can be seen as elements of a father's role in engaging with young children.

Engaging fathers taken from a broad perspective of men utilizing what their society provides them to take on the various roles of fatherhood is essentially a transmission of cultural knowledge. Specific to the themes developed in this chapter, this includes understanding that being a good father is based not only on what men look like when they are taking on the role but also on what any good caregiver does. Again, the bulk of research on parenthood indicates that both direct caregiving (the processes involved with attachment and interaction with children) and indirect effects (such as breadwinning and provisions for health and education) are not the domain of mothers or fathers but of parents. Even though societies influence how fathers perceive their roles, each man creates his own identity in relation to children.

Joining men in this process of creating their identity in relation to their children is how this author defines engagement. That is, when we as professionals work with a family, we are essentially playing the natural societal function of providing input and support. Of course, the entry point for joining the system of care around a child will vary based upon what role the professional is playing. A preschool educator, for example, might focus on the behaviors of the child while at the same time supporting paternal competence.

What children need is a culturally coherent and safe world to develop in. They require homes, food, and places to play and explore safely. They need relationships, hopefully multiple relationships, which provide nurture, guidance, and support, and indeed playfulness. The presence of a father as a member of this system of care around a child enhances the system by contributing to the material resources that allow children to thrive and by forming relationships with the child and other members of the system that support their health and development. In doing so, the man, the man who chooses to be a father, also grows and thrives. It is not the job of the family engagement professional to decide in what ways the father plays his role. What we can do is enter this system as a guest and support a man as he finds his way into this labyrinth.

A Final Note on Policy

The process of father engagement does not occur in a vacuum. A highly motivated social worker, therapist, or early childhood educator may wish to offer a father's group and yet be told that the resources are not available. Practitioners, program administrators, and researchers are painfully aware of how resources and policies affect whether programs can offer innovative services including father engagement. The inclusion of fathers may lead to adding a new component to a program. Of course, resources are an issue, and we should advocate for those that support parental involvement. But more importantly, engaging fathers is an essential component of working with families that requires an inclusive mindset. Practitioners and programs when working with families should always work with fathers as part of the system of care around a child. The question is how intentionally and effectively they do so.

Program and public policies also define the context in which fathers may or not have access to their children and the support to actually take on parental roles. Antiquated and biased divorce and child custody laws, child welfare practices that literally marginalize fathers and provide incentives for his lack of involvement, and the inhumane incarceration industry all build barriers to father involvement (Cabrera & Tamis-LeMonda, 2013; Lamb, 2010). As a guide to program development and policies affecting paternal involvement, I turn to the Global Fatherhood Charter (Lamb et al., 2019), which was developed by an international group of leaders in the study of fatherhood. The charter stresses that the love of a father is foundational to a child's development and that father engagement takes many forms at different developmental periods (Lamb et al., 2019). Engagement of the father during the first 1000 days of the child's life is important to child development. Familial, societal, and cultural support will foster fathers' engagement. Importantly, engagement and loving care of fathers are pivotal in supporting the health and well-being of the child.

References

Abraham, E., Hendler, T., Shapira-Lichter, I., Kanat-Maymon, Y., Zagoory-Sharon, O., & Feldman, R. (2014). Father's brain is sensitive to childcare experiences. *Proceedings of the National Academy of Sciences, 111*(27), 9792–9797. https://doi.org/10.1073/pnas.1402569111

Ainsworth, M. S. (1979). Infant–mother attachment. *American Psychologist, 34*(10), 932–937. https://doi.org/10.1037/0003-066X.34.10.932

Ainsworth, M. D. S., Blehar, M. C., Waters, E., & Wall, S. (1978). *Strange Situation Procedure (SSP)* [Database record]. APA PsycTests. https://doi.org/10.1037/t28248-000

Ainsworth, M. D. S., Blehar, M. C., Waters, E., & Wall, S. N. (2015). *Patterns of attachment: A psychological study of the strange situation*. Psychology Press.

Allen, S., & Daly, K. (2007). *The effects of father involvement: An updated research summary of the evidence*. Father Involvement Research Alliance, Centre for Families, Work & Well-Being.

Atkinson, L., Silverio, S. A., Bick, D., & Fallon, V. (2021). Relationships between paternal attitudes, paternal involvement, and infant-feeding outcomes: Mixed-methods findings from a global on-line survey of English-speaking fathers. *Maternal & Child Nutrition, 17*(S1), e13147. https://doi.org/10.1111/mcn.13147

Belsky, J. (1984). The determinants of parenting: A process model. *Child Development, 55*(1), 83–96. https://doi.org/10.2307/1129836

Bloom, D., Kemple, J. J., Morris, P., Scrivener, S., Verma, N., Hendra, R., Adams-Ciardullo, D., Seith, D., & Walter, J. (2000). *The Family Transition Program: Final report on Florida's initial time-limited welfare program*. Manpower Demonstration Research Corporation. http://www.mdrc.org/publications/20/overview.html

Bowlby, J. (1969). *Attachment and loss, Vol. 1: Attachment. Attachment and loss*. Basic Books.

Brazelton, T. B. (1992). *Touchpoints. Your child's emotional and behavioral development*. Addison-Wesley Publishing Company.

Bretherton, I. (2010). Fathers in attachment theory and research: A review. *Early Child Development and Care, 180*(1–2), 9–23. https://doi.org/10.1080/03004430903414661

Bretherton, I., & Munholland, K. A. (2016). Internal working models in attachment: A construct revisited. In J. Cassidy & P. R. Shaver (Eds.), *Handbook of attachment theory: Theory, research and application* (3rd ed., pp. 63–88). Guilford Press.

Bretherton, I., Lambert, J. D., & Golby, B. (2005). Involved fathers of preschool children as seen by themselves and their wives: Accounts of attachment, socialization, and companionship. *Attachment & Human Development, 7*(3), 229–251. https://doi.org/10.1080/14616730500138341

Bronte-Tinkew, J., Carrano, J., Allen, T., Bowie, L., Mbwana, K., & Matthews, G. (2007). *Elements of promising practice for fatherhood programs: Evidence-based research findings on programs for fathers*. Report prepared for the U.S. Department of Health and Human Services, Administration for Children and Families, Office of Family Assistance. National Fatherhood Clearinghouse.

Cabrera, N., & Tamis-LeMonda, C. S. (2013). *Handbook of father involvement: Multidisciplinary perspectives* (2nd ed.). Routledge.

Cabrera, N., Fitzgerald, H. E., Bradley, R. H., & Roggman, L. (2007a). Modeling the dynamics of paternal influences on children over the life course. *Applied Development Science, 11*(4), 185–189. https://doi.org/10.1080/10888690701762027

Cabrera, N. J., Shannon, J. D., & Tamis-LeMonda, C. (2007b). Fathers' influence on their children's cognitive and emotional development: From toddlers to pre-K. *Applied Development Science, 11*(4), 208–213.

Carlson, J., Kendall, A., & Edelson, J. L. (2015/2016). Becoming a good father: The developmental engine of first-time fatherhood. *Fathering: A Journal of Theory, Research & Practice about Men as Fathers, 13*(3), 183–202. https://doi.org/10.3149/fth.1303.182

Carlson, D. L., Petts, R. J., & Pepin, J. R. (2022). Changes in US parents' domestic labor during the early days of the COVID-19 pandemic. *Sociological Inquiry, 92*(3), 1217–1244. https://doi.org/10.1111/soin.12459

Coley, R. L., & Hernandez, D. C. (2006). Predictors of paternal involvement for resident and nonresident low-income fathers. *Developmental Psychology, 42*(6), 1041–1056. https://doi.org/10.1037/0012-1649.42.6.1041

Cookston, J. T., Braver, S. L., Griffin, W. A., De Lusé, S. R., & Miles, J. C. (2007). Effects of the dads for life intervention on interparental conflict and coparenting in the two years after divorce. *Family Process, 46*(1), 123–137. https://doi.org/10.1111/j.1545-5300.2006.00196.x

DeWolff, M. S., & Van Ijzendoorn, M. H. (1997). Sensitivity and attachment: A meta-analysis on parental antecedents of infant attachment. *Child Development, 68*(4), 571–591. https://doi.org/10.1111/j.1467-8624.1997.tb04218.x

Doherty, W. J., Erickson, M. F., & LaRossa, R. (2006). An intervention to increase father involvement and skills with infants during the transition to parenthood. *Journal of Family Psychology, 20*(3), 438–447. https://doi.org/10.1037/0893-3200.20.3.438

Dufur, M. J., Howell, N. C., Downey, D. B., Ainsworth, J. W., & Lapray, A. J. (2010). Sex differences in parenting behaviors in single-mother and single-father households. *Journal of Marriage and Family, 72*(5), 1092–1106. https://doi.org/10.1111/j.1741-3737.2010.00752.x

Ellis, S., Khan, Y., Harris, V., McWilliams, R., & Converse, D. (2014). *The impact of fathers on children's well-being 1*. University of Florida/Institute of Food and Agricultural Sciences, Extension Service (FCS3321), Family, Youth, and Community Sciences Department. University of Florida.

Fernandes, C., Monteiro, L., Santos, A. J., Fernandes, M., Antunes, M., Vaughn, B. E., & Veríssimo, M. (2020). Early father–child and mother–child attachment relationships: Contributions to preschoolers' social competence. *Attachment & Human Development, 22*(6), 687–704. https://doi.org/10.1080/14616734.2019.1692045

Fitzgerald, H. E., von Klitzing, K., Cabrera, N., Scarano de Mendonça, J., & Skjøthaug, T. (Eds.). (2020). *Handbook of fathers and child development*. Springer International Publishing.

Franzen, J., Cornet, I., Vendittelli, F., & Guittier, M. J. (2021). First-time fathers' experience of childbirth: A cross-sectional study. *Midwifery, 103*, 103153. https://doi.org/10.1016/j.midw.2021.103153

Freeman, H., Newland, L. A., & Coyl, D. D. (2010). New directions in father attachment. *Early Child Development and Care, 180*(1–2), 18. https://doi.org/10.1080/03004430903414646

Grossmann, K., & Grossmann, K. E. (2020). Essentials when studying child-father attachment: A fundamental view on safe haven and secure base phenomena. *Attachment & Human Development, 22*(1), 9–14. https://doi.org/10.1080/14616734.2019.1589056

Grossmann, K., Grossmann, K. E., Fremmer-Bombik, E., Kindler, H., Scheuerer-Englisch, H., & Zimmermann, A. P. (2002). The uniqueness of the child–father attachment relationship: Fathers' sensitive and challenging play as a pivotal variable in a 16-year longitudinal study. *Social Development, 11*(3), 301–337. https://doi.org/10.1111/1467-9507.00202

Guzzo, K. B. (2011). New father's experiences with their own fathers and attitudes towards fathering. *Fathering, 9*(3), 268–290. https://doi.org/10.3149/fth.0903.268

Haggerty, K., Kosterman, R., Catalano, R. F., & Hawkins, J. D. (1999). Preparing for the drug free years. In *Juvenile Justice Bulletin*. U.S. Department of Justice, Office of Justice Programs, Office of Juvenile Justice and Delinquency Prevention. Juvenile Justice Clearinghouse. https://www.ncjrs.gov/pdffiles1/173408.pdf

Harman, J. J., Warshak, R. A., Lorandos, D., & Florian, M. J. (2022). Developmental psychology and the scientific status of parental alienation. *Developmental Psychology, 58*(10), 1887–1911. https://doi.org/10.1037/dev0001404

Henley, K., & Pasley, K. (2005). Conditions affecting the association between father identity and father involvement. *Fathering: A Journal of Theory, Research, and Practice about Men as Fathers, 3*(1), 59–80. https://doi.org/10.3149/fth.0301.59

Hrdy, S. B. (2009). *Mothers and others: The evolutionary origins of mutual understanding*. Belknap Press, Harvard University Press, Belknap Press. https://www.jstor.org/stable/j.ctt1c84czb

Kagan, J. (1995). On Attachment. *Harvard Review of Psychiatry, 3*(2), 104–106. https://doi.org/10.3109/10673229509017174

Lamb, M. E. (1976). Twelve-month-olds and their parents: Interaction in a laboratory playroom. *Developmental Psychology, 12*(3), 237–244. https://doi.org/10.1037/0012-1649.12.3.237

Lamb, M. (Ed.). (2010). *The role of the father in child development* (5th ed.). New York: Wiley.

Lamb, M. E., & Lewis, C. (2010). The development and significance of father-child relationships in two-parent families. In M. E. Lamb (Ed.), *The role of the father in child development* (pp. 94–153). Wiley.

Lamb, M. E., Cabrera, N. J., Parke, R. D., Hwang, P., Cowan, P. A., Page Cowan, C., Palkovitz, R., & Fisher, D. (2019). Global fatherhood charter. *Child and Family Blog*. https://childandfamilyblog.com/global-fatherhood-charter/

Livingston, G., & Parker, K. (2019). *8 facts about American dads*. Pew Research Center.

Magill-Evans, J., Harrison, M. J., Benzies, K., Gierl, M., & Kimak, C. (2007). Effects of parenting education on first-time father's skills in interactions with their infants. *Fathering, 5*(1), 42–57. https://doi.org/10.3149/fth.0501.42

Masciadrelli, B. P., Pleck, J. H., & Stueve, J. L. (2006). Fathers' role model perceptions: Themes and linkages with involvement. *Men and Masculinities, 9*(1), 23–34. https://doi.org/10.1177/1097184X04270377

Mazza, C. (2002). Young dads: The effects of a parenting program on urban African-American adolescent fathers. *Adolescence, 37*(148), 681–694. https://link.gale.com/apps/doc/A97723206/AONE?u=anon~3577a239&sid=googleScholar&xid=059c7766

McBride, B. A., Brown, G. L., Bost, K. K., Shin, N., Vaughn, B., & Korth, B. (2005). Paternal identity, maternal gatekeeping, and father involvement. *Family Relations, 54*(3), 360–372. https://doi.org/10.1111/j.1741-3729.2005.00323.x

McHale, J. P. (2007). When infants grow up in multiperson relationship systems. *Infant Mental Health Journal, 28*(4), 370–392. https://doi.org/10.1002/imhj.20142

McKenry, P. C., Clark, K. A., & Stone, G. (1999). Evaluation of a parent education program for divorcing parents. *Family Relations*, 129–137. https://doi.org/10.2307/585076

Meuwissen, A. S., & Carlson, S. M. (2015). Fathers matter: The role of father parenting in preschoolers' executive function development. *Journal of Experimental Child Psychology, 140*, 1–15. https://doi.org/10.1016/j.jecp.2015.06.010

Miller, T. (2011). Falling back into gender? Men's narratives and practices around first-time fatherhood. *Sociology, 45*(6), 1094–1109. https://doi.org/10.1177/0038038511419180

O'Connell, M. (2005). *The good father: On men, masculinity, and life in the family*. Scribner.

Palkovitz. R. (2002). *Involved fathering and men's adult development: Provisional balances*. Lawrence Erlbaum Associates.

Paquette, D. (2004). Theorizing the father-child relationship: Mechanisms and developmental outcomes. *Human Development, 47*(4), 193–219. https://doi.org/10.1159/000078723

Parker, K., & Horowitz, J. M. (2015). *Parenting in America: Outlook, worries, aspirations are strongly linked to financial situation*. Pew Research Center. https://www.pewresearch.org/social-trends/2015/12/17/parenting-in-america/

Partridge, S. E., Hornstein, J., & Marsh, M. S. N. (2001). *Strengthening the foundations of emotional health in early childhood: A handbook for practitioners*. Edmund S. Muskie School of Public Service, Institute for Child and Family Policy, University of Southern Maine.

Robbers, M. L. (2005). Focus on family and fatherhood: Lessons from Fairfax County's responsible fatherhood program for incarcerated dads. *Justice Policy Journal, 2*(1), 1–27.

Roy, K. M., & Dyson, O. (2010). Making daddies into fathers: Community-based fatherhood programs and the construction of masculinities for low-income African American men. *American Journal of Community Psychology, 45*, 139–154. https://doi.org/10.1007/s10464-009-9282-4

Sarkadi, A., Kristiansson, R., Oberklaid, F., & Bremberg, S. (2008). Fathers' involvement and children's developmental outcomes: A systematic review of longitudinal studies. *Acta Paediatrica, 97*(2), 153–158. https://doi.org/10.1111/j.1651-2227.2007.00572.x

Singley, D. B., & Edwards, L. M. (2015). Men's perinatal mental health in the transition to fatherhood. *Professional Psychology: Research and Practice, 46*(5), 309–316. https://doi.org/10.1037/pro0000032

Stern, D. N. (1995). *The motherhood constellation. A unified view of parent-infant psychotherapy.* Basic Books.

Stgeorge, J., & Freeman, E. (2017). Measurement of father-child rough and tumble play and its relation to child behavior. *Infant Mental Health Journal, 38*(6), 709–725. https://doi.org/10.1002/imhj.21676

Tamis-LeMonda, C., & McFadden, K. (2010). Fathers from low-income backgrounds: Myths and evidence. In M. E. Lamb (Ed.), *The role of the father in child development* (5th ed., pp. 296–318). Wiley.

Tully, L., Piotrowska, P. J., Collins, D. A. J., Mairet, K. S., Black, N., Kimonis, E. R., Hawes, D. J., Moul, C., Lenroot, R. K., Frick, P. J., Anderson, V., & Dadds, M. R. (2017). Optimising child outcomes from parenting interventions: Fathers' experiences, preferences and barriers to participation. *BMC Public Health, 17*(1), 550–550. https://doi.org/10.1186/s12889-017-4426-1

Weissbourd, R., Batanova, M., McIntyre, J., & Torres, E. (2020, June). *How the pandemic is strengthening fathers' relationships with their children.* Making Caring Common Project. Harvard Graduate School of Education. Retrieved from https://mcc.gse.harvard.edu/

Yogman, M. W., & Eppel, A. M. (2022). The role of fathers in child and family health. In M. Grau, M. I. H. Maestro, & H. R. Bowles (Eds.), *Engaged fatherhood for men, families and gender equality: Healthcare, social policy and work perspectives* (pp. 15–30). Springer.

Chapter 8
Family Engagement in Systems of Care

Genevieve Graaf and Millie Sweeney

Family Engagement and Family Partnership in Children's Behavioral Health Systems of Care

In children's mental health research, child and family engagement has broadly been conceptualized as a multistage process that begins with a child's mental health problem being recognized, the child and family accessing services for the first time, and the continued use of—and active participation in—mental health services as needed (McKay & Bannon, 2004). It is frequently measured through assessment of family enrollment or intent to enroll in services, mental health services attendance, family-reported barriers to care, adherence to treatment requirements, cognitive preparation for engaging in services ("...expectations about roles or outcomes, attitudes toward therapy, or understanding of services by the identified participant in therapy."; Becker et al., 2015, p. 35), and satisfaction with services.

According to Lindsey et al. (2014), these processes and outcomes may be impacted by one or more of four dimensions of family engagement in services. The attitudinal dimension of engagement refers to a family's emotional investment in and commitment to mental healthcare, whereas the behavioral dimension is a family's performance of the activities needed to implement treatment and achieve treatment goals. The facilitative dimension of family engagement includes the logistical and systemic access barriers to services. Finally, the socializing dimensions of engagement address families' experiences of mutual support and the interactions

G. Graaf (✉)
School of Social Work, University of Texas at Arlington, Arlington, TX, USA
e-mail: genevieve.graaf@uta.edu

M. Sweeney
Director, Learning & Workforce Development, Family-Run Executive Director Leadership Association (FREDLA), Turner, ME, USA

L. Nabors, J. D. Bartlett (eds.), *Family Engagement in Mental Health Interventions for Young Children*, Springer Series on Child and Family Studies,
https://doi.org/10.1007/978-3-031-47917-5_8

with providers that honor the challenges families encounter when navigating services and validate their experiences (Lindsey et al., 2014).

Family engagement is defined more broadly by family advocates and in medical or health services research and policy. In these settings, family engagement refers primarily to the collaborative relationship between care providers and their patients and families. This relationship is aimed at promoting and supporting patient and family voice in their healthcare decisions and incorporating their priorities and values into shaping the healthcare system (Coulter, 2011). In this context, engagement can range from family involvement—in which families provide input and participate in service decisions—to full partnership in which families are included as equal members of the treatment team and participate in organizational and policy decision-making (Carman et al., 2013). Suggested measures of this type of family engagement or partnership include monitoring family and patient capacity for engagement and relying on consumers' assessment of their experiences in shared decision-making with healthcare providers and systems (Carman et al., 2013).

The Family-Run Executive Director Leadership Association (FREDLA), a national family-run organization and association of family-run organizations, adapted Carman et al.'s (2013) model for understanding the range of family engagement in child mental healthcare (https://www.fredla.org/wp-content/uploads/2018/09/SEC-1-FREDLA-MODELS-OF-FAMILY-ORGS.pdf). They assert that communicating with families, providing supports for them, and including them in interventions merely qualifies as family involvement. Family engagement is a midrange, program-level commitment to working with families. In FREDLA's model, family-driven care is full family partnership and is the gold standard for family engagement. Their model asserts that family partnership means that families, youth, and children are involved in decision-making in system-level policies, procedures, and priorities at the local, state, and national level (Stroul et al., 2021). For this reason, and to distinguish it conceptually from how family engagement is defined in child mental health research, FREDLA's conceptualization of family engagement will be referred to as "family partnership." Activities involved in family partnership and how they differ from family involvement or family engagement, adapted from FREDLA's model (https://www.fredla.org/wp-content/uploads/2018/09/SEC-1-FREDLA-MODELS-OF-FAMILY-ORGS.pdf; https://www.fredla.org/wp-content/uploads/2016/01/Checklist_of_Family_Roles_in_SOC_Work_PDF.pdf), are illustrated in Fig. 8.1.

FREDLA promotes multiple levels of family partnership in children's mental healthcare (Carman et al., 2013). At the service delivery level, this can include employing parent peers as part of the professional team of supportive providers. Families can provide the following types of services: parent peer support, intake and assessment, respite care, information and referrals, helpline services, system navigation support, support group facilitation, family and child psychoeducation, and community outreach. Families can also provide training to providers and other children and families participating in mental health services, and they can participate as members of continuous quality improvement teams. At the organizational level, families can participate in policy and procedure review and development; help to

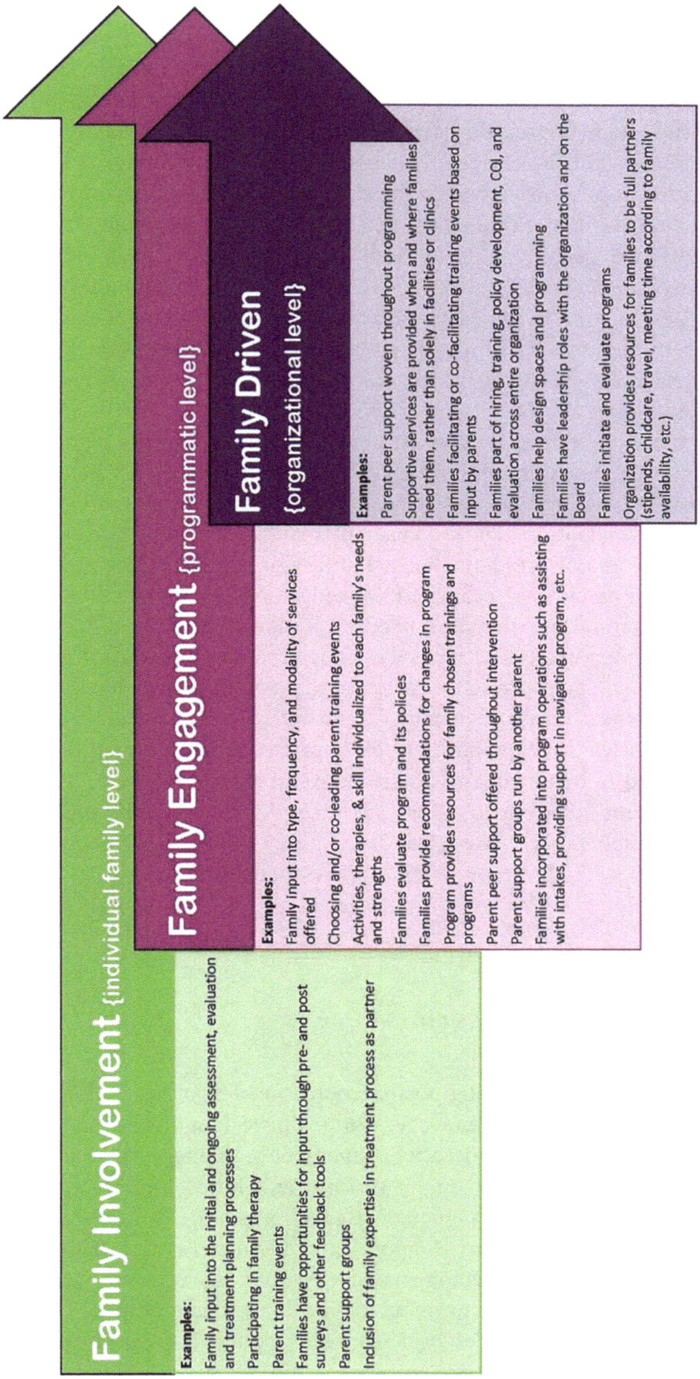

Fig. 8.1 Adaptation of FREDLA's conceptualization of family engagement

design and implement services and supports; assist in recruiting, training, and supporting families in system- or policy-level participation; participate as board and committee members; and coauthor community service or evaluation grants. At the policy and system level, families can help to provide education to policymakers; assist in drafting legislation and system or service guidelines, governance, and oversight processes; establish service standards; and provide training and certification for parent peer support providers. In these roles, families can inform the development, implementation, and evaluation of services; they can help to ensure that services are designed based on family and young children's input, when possible, about what works and best practices for service delivery. Behavioral health policymakers and administrators can establish policy and funding processes that incorporate family representation (with voting authority) at all levels and can help to design and implement policy, regulatory, and contractual requirements around partnering with families.

Because the focus of this book is on mental healthcare for young children, ages birth through eight years, it is important to address the extent to which young children can provide meaningful input in treatment decisions as well as organizational- and policy-level system design. Because very young children, especially children younger than 4 years of age, have limited ability to express their preferences, they must rely on their caregivers' intimate knowledge and communication of their preferences and emotional or behavioral needs (Gutman et al., 2018). For school-aged young children, interventions using psychoeducation, discussion prompts, and decision aids have been demonstrated to successfully assist children in expressing their feelings and perspectives in regard to healthcare (Segers et al., 2022). For these reasons, going forward, when family or child partnership, participation, or engagement is discussed in this chapter, we will be referring to caregivers' expression of their own preferences and needs, their advocacy for their child's preferences and needs based on their expert knowledge of their child, as well as the participation—to the extent that is developmentally appropriate—of school-age children in decision-making.

Predictors of Family Engagement

Given its importance in achieving positive outcomes for young children and families in behavioral healthcare, numerous studies have identified child, family, and environmental factors associated with engagement in mental healthcare. These can impact each stage of the engagement process and reflect points of intervention across dimensions of family engagement (Becker et al., 2018). Engagement studies have generally operationalized behavioral and facilitative dimensions of family engagement by measuring mental health service attendance, family-reported barriers to treatment, and enrollment or intent to enroll in services (Lindsey et al., 2014). These dimensions of engagement are negatively impacted by family, provider, and health system factors. Family difficulty scheduling childcare, competing family obligations, or lack of transportation, combined with provider inflexibility in the timing of appointment availability, deter family engagement. Organizational barriers include complex intake or referral processes and delays; lack of service availability; less experienced or underqualified providers; service tools and environments that are not individualized and developmentally appropriate for young children; a lack of culturally competent providers; and providers failing to center child preferences and family perspectives. A lack of coordination between referring and collaborating service providers can also inhibit service utilization (Waid & Kelly, 2020). In particular, many families with young children report being unaware of where or how to access mental healthcare or lack of cooperation from their healthcare providers in providing relevant information or referrals (Hansen et al., 2021a).

Individual, family, or community attitudes toward mental illness, help seeking, and mental health service providers themselves influence the behavioral, attitudinal, and social dimensions of family engagement (Waid & Kelly, 2020). Inability to recognize symptoms, social stigma, feelings of shame related to mental illness and help seeking, reliance on self or informal support systems, and a lack of knowledge about the resources available and low confidence in the ability of such resources to help are associated with reduced identification of mental health need, service enrollment, attendance and adherence, cognitive preparation, and satisfaction with care (Hansen et al., 2021a; Waid & Kelly, 2020).

Interventions to Increase Family Engagement

Many interventions can address facilitative and attitudinal dimensions of engagement for families with young children by increasing attendance and reducing barriers to access and enrollment. The development of evidence-based interventions specifically for young children, as well as sustainable funding sources to ensure their availability, can be critical to facilitating access to care (Hickey et al., 2023). Digital health technologies that deliver mental health interventions, information sharing, or enable scheduling and coordinated management of care (Hickey et al., 2023; Waid & Kelly, 2020) can increase service use and active participation in therapeutic interventions for these families. Additionally, culturally responsive family outreach activities such as psychoeducation that acknowledges family attitudes about mental healthcare and mental illness, logistical barriers to access, and the importance of their voice and expertise in the therapeutic process can be helpful in increasing family engagement (Hickey et al., 2023; Waid & Kelly, 2020). Similar results can be achieved by increasing mental health literacy. This can include improving family understanding about the full range of normative development for young children, the process and expectations for treatment, and the array of other services and supports available to families tailored to the unique needs of young children (Liverpool et al., 2021). Further, activities aimed at increasing the scheduling convenience and spatial accessibility of services through adjusting service hours and locations; providing appointment reminders, case management, or care coordination; and the use of therapeutic contracting can increase service attendance and adherence to treatment (Becker et al., 2015).

Conducting strengths and needs assessments, eliciting change talk, using rehearsal, modeling, and therapeutic behavioral and verbal reinforcement and rapport building can target attitudinal factors (a family's emotional investment in and commitment to mental healthcare). This can increase cognitive preparation and adherence to treatment (Lindsey et al., 2014). Providing parent peer support services—individually or through support networks or small groups—and providing exercises to increase parent/caregiver coping can address the socialization dimension of family engagement and result in greater care satisfaction (Lindsey et al., 2014).

Many efforts have been dedicated to understanding the organization- and provider-level interventions that can enhance family engagement, but many interventions reported in the research are limited to family consultation or involvement in shared decision-making and rarely address family partnership (Becker et al., 2018; Hickey et al., 2023; Waid & Kelly, 2020). Recall that family partnerships, in contrast to family engagement, are collaborative relationships between care providers and/or their organizations and their patients and families (Carman et al., 2013). These collaborations are aimed at promoting and supporting consumer influence on their healthcare decisions, individually, programmatically, and collectively upon the healthcare system (Coulter, 2011). As such, family partnership may also target the attitudinal dimension of engagement by providing formal channels for families to voice their questions, concerns, and desires for treatment for their child through shared decision-making, partnership, and engagement in policy development. In particular, the inclusion of caregivers as part of the service provider team can reduce social stigma and normalize mental illness and help seeking for other families with young children, can provide those families with knowledge about the resources available for their children, and increase families' confidence in the ability of such resources to help (Waid & Kelly, 2020).

Further, little attention has been paid to the systemic structures and policies that reduce barriers to family engagement, which support organizational or provider interventions to consult or involve families in treatment, or that promote full family partnership in decision-making (Hansen et al., 2021b; Waid & Kelly, 2020). Federal and state policies can play a critical role in supporting provider, organizational, and service system structures and processes that increase all dimensions of family engagement in mental health services for families with young children (Fostering Healthy Mental, Emotional, and Behavioral Development in Children and Youth, 2019).

Many structural- or policy-level interventions can address the facilitative dimension of parent engagement by integrating behavioral health services into primary pediatric care (Burkhart et al., 2020; Waid & Kelly, 2020), locating mental health services within childcare settings (Gilliam et al., 2016) or elementary schools (Sanchez et al., 2018), reducing cost and insurance barriers through mandating insurance coverage parity for mental health and medical care, and expanding access to public health coverage (which provides more coverage for comprehensive behavioral healthcare; So et al., 2019). Financing arrangements (including reimbursement rates and dictates regarding the mental health services that can be covered through public funding) and requirements for provider licensing, accreditation, and enrollment can increase access to services by driving the types of services available and the number of providers who provide those services (Graaf & Snowden, 2021). Funding and administrative decisions about infrastructure can facilitate interorganizational communication and coordination that reduce gaps in care and enhance referrals, care coordination, communication, and transition processes across organizations and service sectors (Hernandez et al., 2016). Finally, financing, governance, and oversight policies can be tied to system operation mandates for early screening and intervention, timely delivery of care, and processes for engaging family perspectives in service planning at the community, organizational, and policy level (Nelson et al., 2022; So et al., 2019). Given the critical role that policy can play in facilitating family engagement and family partnership, attention to the children's mental health policy context is warranted.

The System of Care

Today, many states' administrative decisions about policies that organize and finance community mental health services for children are based on the system of care philosophy (Hernandez et al., 2016). The Children's Mental Health System of Care emerged in the early 1980s in response to a critical report from The Children's Defense Fund, titled *Unclaimed Children: The Failure of Public Responsibility to Children and Adolescents in Need of Mental Health Services.* The report outlined the challenges faced by children with complex mental health needs. It advocated for a holistic policy that would center the needs, values, and perspectives of children and their families. It proposed that children with significant mental health needs should be served through a coordinated system of care to increase their access to less restrictive and more appropriate mental healthcare. The publication of this report, and the state and federal response to it, spurred the creation of the first national policy targeting the needs of children with complex mental health needs and their families. In this landmark federal policy, passed in 1984, congress allocated funding for the National Institute of Mental Health to establish the Child and Adolescent Service System Program (CASSP). This initiative is known today as the Children's Mental Health Initiative (CMHI), and it is administered through the Substance Abuse and Mental Health Services Administration (SAMHSA).

The system of care philosophy is meant to guide the organization of mental health services and interorganizational collaboration, communication, and coordination of programs serving children with complex mental health needs—including young and very young children. Though the average age of this population is 12 to 13 years (Graaf et al., 2023), many young children also present with complex behavioral health needs (Ibeziako et al., 2022). Program evaluations—which have included children and youth with mental health needs of ages ranging from 2 to

21 years of age—have demonstrated that children served in systems of care demonstrate better classroom, home, and community functioning (Stroul et al., 2012). Families report reduced caregiver strain, greater social support, enhanced problem-solving and behavior management practices, and reductions in reliance on formal helping systems (Larson et al., 2022; Stroul et al., 2012). A set of rigorous mental health system studies in the 1990s, examining outcomes for children ages 5 to 17 years, demonstrated families and children served in systems of care demonstrated higher levels of engagement; they were more satisfied with care, stayed in services longer, received needed care more quickly, were more aware of what services were available to help them, and received more individualized treatment in less restrictive settings (Bickman et al., 2004). Perhaps, due to these positive outcomes, the system of care policy continues today as the CMHI, and it has funded the development of systems of care in all 50 states; increasing services for young children will enhance the reach of the CMHI.

Today, the system of care is conceptualized as resting on three key components: (1) a comprehensive array of services and supports for children and families, (2) a community and organizational infrastructure to seamlessly coordinate care across child-serving sectors, and (3) a philosophy to guide the manner in which services are delivered to children and their families (Stroul et al., 2021). Its purpose has been expanded to serve a broader population beyond children with the most complex needs, including children with emerging or mild and moderate needs. As children's mental health needs become more complex, more services and supports are provided, and those with the most significant needs receive larger doses of services for longer periods of time (Stroul et al., 2021). The system of care guidelines also now call for the use of intensive care coordination, trauma-informed care, mobile crisis care, and peer support services. It has been expanded conceptually to encompass public health, care integration, and mental health equity values by including attention to universal mental health promotion, prevention, screening, and early intervention for the whole child population through pediatric care integration and school-based mental healthcare (Stroul et al., 2021).

System of Care Philosophy and Policies' Promotion of Family Engagement

Within the system of care framework, the conceptualization of family engagement is well aligned with that in health services research—which defines family engagement as the promotion and support of patient and family voice in their healthcare decisions and in shaping the healthcare system. A core value of the original Children's Mental Health System of Care model—which continues today as the system of care framework has evolved—is that care should be centered around the needs of the child and their family (Stroul & Friedman, 1986). One of the guiding principles, too, states that families should be full participants in all aspects of planning and delivery of services. As such, the system of care dictates not just family engagement but family partnership and family-driven care (Stroul et al., 2021).

System of care philosophies also reflect the family engagement definitions used in children's mental health research—which promotes family engagement as children and families' use of and active participation and sustainment in mental health services. The policies organized around the system of care philosophy address key family engagement outcomes and stages in the process—the early recognition of mental health problems in children, access to services, and active participation in mental health treatment (McKay & Bannon, 2004) and target the attitudinal, behavioral, and social dimensions of family engagement (Lindsey et al., 2014). Through financing and associated regulation and oversight arrangements, policies rooted in system of care values and principles can drive processes for partnering with families in planning services for infants, toddlers, and young children at the individual, organizational, and policy level (Nelson et al., 2022; So et al., 2019). Because family engagement and partnership are baked into the core values and guiding principles of the system of care, the Child and Adolescent Service System Program (CASSP) (the Children's Mental Health Initiative [CMHI] today)—which funds the development and expansion of systems of care across the United States—laid critical groundwork that has guided state child mental health policymaking for the last 40 years to maximize family and child engagement in mental healthcare (Hernandez et al., 2016; Lourie & Hernandez, 2003). System of care policies support many facets of family engagement in mental health care, including identification of mental health need and the facilitative, behavioral, attitudinal, and social dimensions of engagement.

Identification of Mental Health Need and Promoting Mental Health Service Use The system of care principles facilitate the first step in family engagement—identification of mental health needs in children—by dictating that a well-functioning system should be employing a public health approach. This approach includes the provision of services and supports that promote mental health and prevent the development of mental illness or behavioral problems. Public mental health also provides structures and processes to identify and intervene early in children's mental health needs and the needs of families (Stroul et al., 2021). This can be achieved through community-based settings such as childcare, preschool, and elementary school settings. However, despite the call for early identification and intervention in child mental health needs since the development of the system of care principles in 1986, state mental health administrators feel that current efforts in their state are insufficient and that public investments in the infrastructure needed to advance these goals are inadequate (Hernandez et al., 2016). Efforts continue to expand mental health screening and service delivery through schools (Enos, 2023; McCabe et al., 2021) via provision of public funding for school-based mental healthcare (Graaf & Snowden, 2020) and interorganizational cooperation (Cummings et al., 2022). As a result of these efforts, a large portion of children access mental health services through their school (Ali et al., 2019; Duong et al., 2021) which positively impacts their mental health outcomes (Sanchez et al., 2018).

In particular, early identification of mental health needs in young children can be achieved through screenings in preschools and childcare settings (Gilliam et al., 2016), through elementary schools (Splett et al., 2018) and pediatric healthcare settings (Kuhlthau et al., 2011). Connections to mental health services from these avenues can be critical in achieving access to care (Hansen et al., 2021a, b), and in many states, these services can be covered through private insurance, public mental health grant funds, and Medicaid (Graaf & Snowden, 2019). However, gaps in funding for care—particularly for young children with complex needs—still exist in many states (Graaf & Snowden, 2020). Infants and their mothers around the world face a myriad of health and mental health concerns (Ndwiga et al., 2022). If these concerns are left untreated, mothers, as well as other caregivers, may experience emotional distress and infant development can be negatively affected (Parfitt et al., 2014). Therefore, ensuring that parents and caregivers are referred to system of care services may optimize child development.

Updates to the system of care guiding principles also emphasize the integration of mental healthcare into pediatric health settings—which can be critical to enhancing rates of early detection and treatment for behavioral health needs and facilitating and coordinating access to initial and ongoing services (Lipkin et al., 2020). Integrated pediatric health and mental healthcare can also address attitudinal dimensions of family engagement by reducing the stigma associated with behavioral healthcare by delivering it in a less stigmatizing medical setting (Campo et al., 2018). However, like efforts aimed at population-wide early identification and treatment, comprehensive integration of pediatric medical and behavioral healthcare nationwide remains an unrealized goal; approximately less than 2% of children are reported to have received mental healthcare through pediatric settings (Duong et al., 2021).

Facilitative Dimensions: Access to a Full Continuum of Mental Health Services and Supports for the Child and Their Family From its first inception to today, the system of care guiding principles specify that systems of care should include a comprehensive array of services and supports for children with mental health needs and their families (Stroul et al., 2010, 2021; Stroul & Friedman, 1986). This principle facilitates identification of need and access to services by dictating that a broad selection of services (both formal and informal) must be made available—including screening and early intervention services. By specifying the provision of peer support services to parents, this principle also uniquely addresses the social dimension of family engagement. Peer support services can be provided one on one or in a group setting by parents/primary caregivers who have lived experience of managing child behavioral health concerns and navigating service systems (Acri et al., 2017). Parent peer support providers can attend care planning meetings, provide coaching in coping or advocacy skills, offer support during crises, and aid in navigating complicated systems. These services have been shown to increase family understanding of mental health (Acri et al., 2017), reduce caregiver stress (Nayak et al., 2022), and increase access to and participation in services (Nayak et al., 2022).

Public mental health policy has also evolved to support the system of care guidelines by funding a wide array of other highly specialized services. Due to federal mandates for state Medicaid programs to provide and Early and Periodic Screening, Diagnosis, and Treatment (EPSDT) to all child beneficiaries (often referred to as the EPSDT mandate), many state Medicaid programs fund a diverse selection of specialized behavioral health services that are essential to a system of care (Hernandez et al., 2016). In states in which Medicaid has not provided funding for such services, families have changed Medicaid policy by filing lawsuits under the EPSDT mandate, asserting that states are not complying with the federal mandate to provide all needed treatment for behavioral health diagnoses (Snowden et al., 2008). In other states, these services are funded through HCBS Medicaid programs for children with significant mental health needs (Graaf & Snowden, 2017) or through dedicated programs funded through state allocations—sometimes through the child welfare or juvenile justice systems (Graaf & Snowden, 2019).

Access to Community-Based Care Numerous and expansive policies have proliferated under the system of care philosophy. Many are aimed at expanding the variety, accessibility, and capacity of mental health services (Graaf & Snowden, 2017, 2019, 2020) and reducing financial and availability barriers to family engagement in mental health services. However, in the 1982 Children's Defense fund report, critiques of the public mental health system included that children were being served in inpatient or residential psychiatric settings when their needs could be met through home- or community-based services (Knitzer & Olson, 1982). As a result, the system of care principles prioritize that services should be provided in the least restrictive setting possible for the needs of the child (Stroul et al., 2010, 2021; Stroul & Friedman, 1986). This principle, and its perpetuation through federal Children's Mental Health Initiative (CMHI) Collaborative Agreements (better known as System of Care grants) to communities, tribes, and states nationwide over the last three decades—combined with lawsuits filed under the Americans with Disabilities Act (Olmstead v. LC, 1999)—have increased the availability of home- and community-based mental services (HCBS) for children with mental health needs. Many states have also established more stringent gatekeeping processes and higher clinical thresholds for inpatient or residential care admission (Herbell & Banks, 2020), redirecting funding from residential psychiatric services into home- and community-based services (Graaf & Snowden, 2021).

Interorganizational and Care Coordination Emphasis on systems of care principles increases attention in public mental health systems to the interorganizational collaboration within their community (Hernandez et al., 2016). Many state systems facilitate cooperation through coordination of activities and funding between agencies and service sectors at the state level (Graaf & Snowden, 2021; Hernandez et al., 2016). The outcomes from such efforts have been reviewed positively by providers and families and have been demonstrated to result in earlier identification of mental health needs (He et al., 2015) and greater access to more individualized and appropriate mental healthcare (Cooper et al., 2016). The provision of intensive care coordination, which is also a key feature of system of care principles, has also been found to be pivotal in facilitating access to mental healthcare and other support services (Lindly et al., 2020; Waid et al., 2021). Extending a systems of care philosophy to health and mental healthcare of infants, toddlers, and preschoolers with complex health and mental health needs may promote child development and ease the burden for family practitioners, who may be "de facto" systems of care coordinators (Zanello et al., 2017).

Attitudinal and Behavioral Dimensions: Partnership with Families The system of care guiding principles include several points that also address the attitudinal and behavioral dimensions of family engagement by supporting full family partnership. System of care guidance specifies that services be trauma informed, culturally competent, and developmentally appropriate—all of which can increase the likelihood that families will initiate and sustain participation in services (Moore, 2018) by reducing attitudinal barriers to mental health engagement. These elements of service integrate with a core value of the system of care: that service planning, delivery, and evaluation should be delivered in full partnership with families and be driven by children and their families (Stroul et al., 2021).

System of care guidelines include directives at the provider and organizational level that service plans and delivery of care must be individualized, strengths based, and developed and implemented in full partnership with the family (Stroul et al., 2021). By planning and implementing individualized and strengths-based care in this manner, many attitudinal dimensions of family engagement are activated through activities demonstrated to be effective in promoting child and family service attendance, adherence, and cooperation with treatment processes, as well as cognitive preparation for service engagement. These include assessment of child and family strengths (Lindsey et al., 2014), peer pairing to support parents (Hoagwood, 2005), psychoeducation about services, eliciting change discussion, expectation setting (Becker et al., 2015), relationship and rapport building (Bjønness et al., 2020), and support networking (Lindsey et al., 2014; Nayak et al., 2022). Further, shared decision-making—another term for planning care in partnership with children and families (Fitzpatrick et al., 2023)—is demonstrated to result in greater satisfaction with treatment decisions (Langer et al., 2022), increased knowledge of services and presenting problems (Wyatt et al., 2015), lower dropout rates (Swift et al., 2018), and greater therapeutic gains (Edbrooke-Childs et al., 2016). The provision of system-level guidelines that mandate family engagement and partnership, especially when funding mechanisms are tied to compliance with them—such as through the federal CMHI Collaborative Agreements (i.e., System of Care grants) or through oversight arrangements tied to state funding (Graaf & Snowden, 2017)—has been demonstrated to play a key role in promoting shared decision-making in clinical practice settings (Scholl et al., 2018).

The latest system of care guidelines specify that wraparound is the most evidence-based approach to care planning in partnership with families. Emerging in the 1980s as a model for serving children and adolescents with complex mental health needs at high risk for institutionalization (Winters & Metz, 2009), wraparound is a strengths-based "...collaborative process for developing and implementing individualized care plans for children with severe disorders" (Walker & Bruns, 2006, p. 1580). The process relies on the preferences and perspectives of the child and their family in determining their needs and setting appropriate goals to be included in the plan of care. Engaging natural support systems in the family's environment to participate in the goals and activities of the treatment plan is also emphasized (Bruns et al., 2010).

The evidence base for wraparound, though still emerging, is positive. Meta-analyses of wraparound evaluations, which compare the treatment group with a control group, found an overall moderate positive effect for wraparound participants, based on improvements in functioning in mental health outcomes (Olson et al., 2021). Further, when compared to intensive care management, children and families participating in wraparound had higher rates of home- and community-based service participation (Bruns et al., 2015). Perhaps, based on these outcomes, the use of wraparound has been integrated sustainably into many public mental health systems for children through the development of Medicaid reimbursement for the service (Graaf & Snowden, 2017) and state allocation of funding specifically for wraparound care for high-need behavioral health populations (Graaf & Snowden, 2021).

Family Advocacy. The system of care guiding principles include additional support for family partnership by specifying that family leaders and advocates be full partners at the system level in policy and governance development, and in service design, implementation, and evaluation in their communities and states. The principles also specify that the system of care will collaborate and coordinate with advocacy and peer-led organizations to promote effective advocacy efforts that protect and promote the rights of young children with mental health needs (Stroul et al., 2021). Many states actively partner with family-led support organizations to educate and advocate for policy, legislation, funding, and programmatic efforts at the state level (Cooper & Aratani, 2015; Hoagwood et al., 2008). States rely on these advocate partners to identify community needs, report on child and family system experiences, and advise on ways for states to increase access to services (Hernandez et al., 2016). Some states employ family liaisons in formal policymaking roles (Cooper & Aratani, 2015), and many advocacy organizations receive federal and state funding to support their efforts (Hoagwood et al., 2008). Further, federal and state policies often mandate that public mental health organizations engage local or organizational-level advisory boards comprised of families engaged in behavioral healthcare to provide feedback and oversight to mental health organizations and the services they provide (Certified Community Behavioral Health Clinics, 2021).

Family Engagement in Systems of Care: Social Justice and Health Equity

Harper et al. (2014) propose that children's mental health research and practices have developed two parallel traditions. They refer to these models as systems of care and expert-driven care. Expert-driven care, rooted in a medical model of behavioral healthcare, focuses on clinical assessment for the purpose of diagnosis and symptom treatment and services provided are recommended by the "expertly" trained professional. In this context, care can be seen as oppressive, as it minimizes the preferences, cultural nuances, and lived experience of children and their families, largely excludes the perspectives of key stakeholders, and provides a limited pathway for self-determination. The system of care tradition diverges from expert-driven care by using a treatment team approach to care, integrated with advocacy, in which the "expertly" trained professionals' perspectives are weighed equally with that of nonprofessional and family team members (Harper et al., 2014).

By centering child preferences and family voice, and prioritizing cultural competency, developmentally appropriate and inclusive care, the system of care values and guiding principles lay a foundation for advancing equity and justice in accessing and navigating mental healthcare for all children and their families. In systems of care, treatment planning is driven by child and families' strengths, needs, goals, and values, which creates an anti-oppressive service space that supports self-determination and shared decision-making, centering the child and families' expertise rooted in their lived experiences. Theoretically, when practiced with fidelity, full family partnerships are inherently inclusive of diversity because the amplification and integration of the unique experiences of all types of children and families are embedded into treatment planning and service delivery (Stubbe, 2020). The prioritization of these processes promotes culturally responsive and competent service delivery, as it provides a formal channel for families to communicate the preferences, needs, values, and priorities that matter in their culture or are needed to accommodate the special needs of their child or their family (Stubbe, 2020). Further, the shared decision-making at the center of the system of care approach has been demonstrated to be especially important to increasing health knowledge and satisfaction with care for participants with marginal or oppressed identities or experiences (Durand et al., 2014).

Limitations in Current Family Engagement Knowledge and Practice in Systems of Care

Systems of care for children with significant mental health needs were studied relatively vigorously in peer-reviewed research in the late 1980s and through the 1990s but research in dropped off in the early 2000s (Larson et al., 2022). As a result, many gaps in knowledge exist about systems of care that must be addressed in future research efforts. Early studies firmly established that children and families served in a system of care have higher levels of engagement—when defining engagement as access to and participation in mental health services (Bickman et al., 2004). Less is known about the impact of system of care policies and practices on family partnership. When adhering to the guiding principles of individualized, family-driven care planning, some evidence demonstrates that participants report more individualized care plans, higher levels of satisfaction with the process, and improved child mental health outcomes (Slaton et al., 2012). However, the role of child- and family-centered care planning in families' experience of partnership has been examined minimally and remains an area ripe for future investigations (Larson et al., 2022).

Further, though federal funding has provided support for the development and expansion of systems of care across the United States for over three decades, and federal agencies provide program and funding reports about system of care grantees, little peer-reviewed research reports on the breadth and health of existing systems of care for young children with mental health needs (Larson et al., 2022). Formal estimates are needed to understand the number of young children with mental health needs who have access to a system of care, how well those systems of care are functioning or are sustained over time, the extent to which they operate with fidelity to the guiding principles or core values, and what barriers or challenges exist for communities or organizations in fully implementing a system of care approach. The population-level impacts of system of care implementation and participation are also unknown and merit scholarly attention. Since the implementation of these policies, and as systems of care have proliferated across the nation, whether unmet mental health need for families and children has declined or if racial, income, geographic and insurance-based disparities in unmet mental health need have narrowed is unknown. Such research efforts are hindered by the lack of longitudinal nationally representative datasets identifying children with mental health needs and their service experiences (Ghandour et al., 2018).

Increasingly, health researchers are using community-engaged research approaches to advance the practice relevance of research evidence in addressing the needs of marginalized and historically oppressed populations—including individuals with complex mental health needs (Rhodes et al., 2018a, b). Further, research funders, such as the Patient-Centered Outcomes Research Institute (PCORI), are more frequently explicitly prioritizing studies that actively engage the populations being studied (Maurer et al., 2022). We recommend that children's behavioral health services' researchers leverage the sophisticated participatory research methods and well-aligned funding sources now available to researchers to advance family engagement with systems of care research activities.

Family Engagement in Systems of Care in Practice

Today, many state and local administrative decisions about community mental health for children are based on the system of care framework. This framework calls for full partnership with families at all levels—individual, programmatic, organizational, and in policy and funding decisions (Hernandez et al., 2016). However, the extent to which state or community systems have achieved full partnership with families at all levels is currently unknown. A 2011 published assessment of system of care implementation nationwide suggested that system of care grantees were only achieving moderate levels of family partnership (Kutash et al., 2011), and a recent local assessment of a system of care suggests that the level of family-driven care continues at similar levels (Karikari et al., 2020).

Limitations in widespread adoption of family partnership in systems of care could be overcome through mandates for family partnership and investment of resources. Funding is needed to build organizational and family capacity to partner in mental health policy and service planning (Farrelly et al., 2016). Organizations may benefit from expert guidance on how to deal with differences in perspectives between providers, children (as developmentally appropriate), and caregivers; how to communicate using less clinical or technical language; and how to convey respect and openness to ideas and comments shared by parents and children (Farrelly et al., 2016). Families may more effectively partner with organizations and policy leaders if provided training around the inner workings of mental health systems and the competing priorities faced by organizations and policymakers (Cooper & Aratani, 2015). Family-run organizations (FROs) have the expertise to provide this training as well as a network of families who may be willing and interested in participating—as a full and equal member—in service delivery or on advisory councils, in policy work groups, and in service redesign projects (Hoagwood et al., 2008). However, FROs need resources to support the time required to develop and deliver trainings and support the development of community partnerships.

Funding is also needed for building capacity and expanding the use of family peer support providers (FPSP) in systems of care—the employment of parents/caregivers (and young children) with lived experience to provide information, emotional, and navigational support to child and caregiver mental health service users (Gopalan et al., 2017a, b). FPSP may be an effective strategy for bridging gaps between families and providers—modeling collaboration, perspective taking, and teamwork for the benefit of the child and family. Building this workforce requires an acknowledgment of the important and professional role of the FPSPs, demonstrated through equity in pay and benefits, equality among provider colleagues both within and outside of the organization that employs them, and support for ongoing professional development and advancement. FPSP exists in all states and many states offer Medicaid reimbursement for these services; however, the pay and reimbursement rates remain comparatively low (Schober & Baxter, 2019), and the service is often only accessible to specific populations or areas (Graaf & Snowden, 2017).

Further, to expand the resources available to systems of care to effectively engage in family partnership, states need to prioritize children's mental healthcare in the allocation of federal community mental health block grants (Hernandez et al., 2016). These grants provide funding that is not tied to service delivery, unlike Medicaid funding, and thus allow for the use of funds to develop infrastructure or provider services that are not billable under Medicaid (Graaf & Snowden, 2021). Many states report inadequate state funding allocations to children's mental healthcare, as a result of state administrators and policymakers prioritizing adult mental health (Hernandez et al., 2016). Inserting federal requirements around the percentage of block grant funding that states must dedicate to children's mental health and family-run organizations may provide additional resources to support family partnership.

Finally, families may be discouraged from partnering fully with mental health service providers, organizations, and policymakers due to the stigma that continues to be attached to the use of mental healthcare (Waid & Kelly, 2020). Community efforts at stigma reduction can reduce these pressures (Maunder & White, 2019), but family partnership efforts must acknowledge this and take intentional steps to remove stigma in seeking services and speaking out on behalf of children with mental health needs and their families. Further, because experience of mental health stigma varies across regional and cultural groups (Snowden et al., 2022), engaging families that reflect the full range of racial, ethnic, geographic, gender, or cultural identities of the children and caregivers who use mental health services can be especially challenging (Moore, 2018). Organizations seeking to partner with families should collaborate with cultural centers, local churches, or regional or special interest groups in their community to build relationships, learn how to be culturally responsive, and establish connections with potential family leaders who can become involved at different levels within the organization.

Conclusion

Family partnership is a fundamental value in the Children's Mental Health System of Care, but knowledge regarding the health and sustainability of these systems and the extent to which family partnership is fully implemented within them is limited—particularly for families with very young children. Greater investment is needed to build the knowledge base about the current state of Children's Mental Health Systems of Care nationwide and organizational interventions that can enhance capacity for family partnership for caregivers, young children, providers, and administrators.

References

Acri, M., Hooley, C. D., Richardson, N., & Moaba, L. B. (2017). Peer models in mental health for caregivers and families. *Community Mental Health Journal, 53*(2), 241–249. https://doi.org/10.1007/s10597-016-0040-4

Ali, M. M., West, K., Teich, J. L., Lynch, S., Mutter, R., & Dubenitz, J. (2019). Utilization of mental health services in educational setting by adolescents in the United States. *Journal of School Health, 89*(5), 393–401. https://doi.org/10.1111/josh.12753

Becker, K. D., Lee, B. R., Daleiden, E. L., Lindsey, M., Brandt, N. E., & Chorpita, B. F. (2015). The common elements of engagement in children's mental health services: Which elements for which outcomes? *Journal of Clinical Child & Adolescent Psychology, 44*(1), 30–43. https://doi.org/10.1080/15374416.2013.814543

Becker, K. D., Boustani, M., Gellatly, R., & Chorpita, B. F. (2018). Forty years of engagement research in children's mental health services: Multidimensional measurement and practice elements. *Journal of Clinical Child & Adolescent Psychology, 47*(1), 1–23. https://doi.org/10.1080/15374416.2017.1326121

Bickman, L., Breda, C. S., Foster, E. M., Guthrie, P. R., Heflinger, C. A., Lambert, E. W., & Summerfelt, W. T. (2004). *Evaluating managed mental health services: The Fort Bragg experiment* (Softcover reprint of the original 1st ed. 1995 edition). Springer.

Bjønness, S., Grønnestad, T., & Storm, M. (2020). I'm not a diagnosis: Adolescents' perspectives on user participation and shared decision-making in mental healthcare. *Scandinavian Journal of Child and Adolescent Psychiatry and Psychology, 8*, 139–148. https://doi.org/10.21307/sjcapp-2020-014

Bruns, E. J., Walker, J. S., Zabel, M., Matarese, M., Estep, K., Harburger, D., Mosby, M., & Pires, S. A. (2010). Intervening in the lives of youth with complex behavioral health challenges and their families: The role of the wraparound process. *American Journal of Community Psychology, 46*(3–4), 314–331. https://doi.org/10.1007/s10464-010-9346-5

Bruns, E. J., Pullmann, M. D., Sather, A., Brinson, R. D., & Ramey, M. (2015). Effectiveness of wraparound versus case management for children and adolescents: Results of a randomized study. *Administration and Policy in Mental Health and Mental Health Services Research, 42*(3), 309–322. https://doi.org/10.1007/s10488-014-0571-3

Burkhart, K., Asogwa, K., Muzaffar, N., & Gabriel, M. (2020). Pediatric integrated care models: A systematic review. *Clinical Pediatrics, 59*(2), 148–153. https://doi.org/10.1177/0009922819890004

Campo, J. V., Geist, R., & Kolko, D. J. (2018). Integration of pediatric behavioral health services in primary care: Improving access and outcomes with collaborative care. *Canadian Journal of Psychiatry. Revue Canadienne De Psychiatrie, 63*(7), 432–438. https://doi.org/10.1177/0706743717751668

Carman, K. L., Dardess, P., Maurer, M., Sofaer, S., Adams, K., Bechtel, C., & Sweeney, J. (2013). Patient And family engagement: A framework for understanding the elements and developing interventions and policies. *Health Affairs, 32*(2), 223–231. https://doi.org/10.1377/hlthaff.2012.1133

Certified Community Behavioral Health Clinics (CCBHCs). (2021). *Substance abuse and mental health services administration*. https://www.samhsa.gov/certified-community-behavioral-health-clinics

Cooper, J. L., & Aratani, Y. (2015). Children's mental health policies in the United States: Perspectives from advocates and state leaders. *Health Expectations: An International Journal of Public Participation in Health Care and Health Policy, 18*(6), 2213–2222. https://doi.org/10.1111/hex.12191

Cooper, M., Evans, Y., & Pybis, J. (2016). Interagency collaboration in children and young people's mental health: A systematic review of outcomes, facilitating factors and inhibiting factors. *Child: Care, Health and Development, 42*(3), 325–342. https://doi.org/10.1111/cch.12322

Coulter, A. (2011). *Engaging patients in healthcare*. McGraw-Hill Education. http://ebookcentral.proquest.com/lib/utarl/detail.action?docID=771414

Cummings, J. R., Zhang, Y. X., Wilk, A. S., & Marcus, S. C. (2022). Mental health clinic administrators' perspectives on the impact of clinic-school partnerships on youth mental health services continuity and quality. *School Mental Health, 14*(4), 1086–1097. https://doi.org/10.1007/s12310-022-09531-4

Duong, M. T., Bruns, E. J., Lee, K., Cox, S., Coifman, J., Mayworm, A., & Lyon, A. R. (2021). Rates of mental health service utilization by children and adolescents in schools and other common service settings: A systematic review and meta-analysis. *Administration and Policy in Mental Health, 48*(3), 420–439. https://doi.org/10.1007/s10488-020-01080-9

Durand, M.-A., Carpenter, L., Dolan, H., Bravo, P., Mann, M., Bunn, F., & Elwyn, G. (2014). Do interventions designed to support shared decision-making reduce health inequalities? A systematic review and meta-analysis. *PLoS One, 9*(4), e94670. https://doi.org/10.1371/journal.pone.0094670

Edbrooke-Childs, J., Jacob, J., Argent, R., Patalay, P., Deighton, J., & Wolpert, M. (2016). The relationship between child- and parent-reported shared decision making and child-, parent-, and clinician-reported treatment outcome in routinely collected child mental health services data. *Clinical Child Psychology and Psychiatry, 21*(2), 324–338. https://doi.org/10.1177/1359104515591226

Enos, G. (2023). Backers of school-based mental health don't see pushback as a barrier. *Mental Health Weekly, 33*(1), 1–8. https://doi.org/10.1002/mhw.33488

Farrelly, S., Lester, H., Rose, D., Birchwood, M., Marshall, M., Waheed, W., Henderson, R. C., Szmukler, G., & Thornicroft, G. (2016). Barriers to shared decision making in mental health care: Qualitative study of the Joint Crisis Plan for psychosis. *Health Expectations, 19*(2), 448–458. https://doi.org/10.1111/hex.12368

Fitzpatrick, O. M., Holcomb, J. M., Weisz, J. R., & Langer, D. A. (2023). Shared decision-making as a tool for navigating multi-stakeholder discrepancies in youth psychotherapy. *Journal of Clinical Child and Adolescent Psychology, 52*(1), 95–107. https://doi.org/10.1080/15374416.2022.2127105

Fostering Healthy Mental, Emotional, and Behavioral Development in Children and Youth: A National Agenda. (2019). National Academies Press. 10.17226/25201

Ghandour, R. M., Jones, J. R., Lebrun-Harris, L. A., Minnaert, J., Blumberg, S. J., Fields, J., Bethell, C., & Kogan, M. D. (2018). The design and implementation of the 2016 National Survey of Children's Health. *Maternal and Child Health Journal, 22*(8), 1093–1102. https://doi.org/10.1007/s10995-018-2526-x

Gilliam, W. S., Maupin, A. N., & Reyes, C. R. (2016). Early childhood mental health consultation: Results of a statewide random-controlled evaluation. *Journal of the American Academy of Child & Adolescent Psychiatry, 55*(9), 754–761. https://doi.org/10.1016/j.jaac.2016.06.006

Gopalan, G., Horen, M. J., Bruns, E., Corey, M., Meteyer, S., Pardue, M., Lane, T., & Matarese, M. (2017a). Caregiver perceptions of parent peer support services within the Wraparound service delivery model. *Journal of Child and Family Studies, 26*(7), 1923–1935. https://doi.org/10.1007/s10826-017-0704-x

Gopalan, G., Lee, S. J., Harris, R., Acri, M. C., & Munson, M. R. (2017b). Utilization of peers in services for youth with emotional and behavioral challenges: A scoping review. *Journal of Adolescence, 55*, 88–115. https://doi.org/10.1016/j.adolescence.2016.12.011

Graaf, G., & Snowden, L. (2017). The role of Medicaid home and community-based service policies in organizing and financing care for children with severe emotional disturbance. *Children and Youth Services Review, 81*, 272–283. https://doi.org/10.1016/j.childyouth.2017.08.007

Graaf, G., & Snowden, L. (2019). State approaches to funding home and community-based mental health care for non-Medicaid youth: Alternatives to Medicaid waivers. *Administration and Policy in Mental Health and Mental Health Services Research, 46*(4), 530–541. https://doi.org/10.1007/s10488-019-00933-2

Graaf, G., & Snowden, L. (2020). Medicaid waiver adoption for youth with complex behavioral health care needs: An analysis of state decision-making. *Journal of Disability Policy Studies, 31*(2), 87–98. https://doi.org/10.1177/1044207319897058

Graaf, G., & Snowden, L. (2021). State strategies for enhancing access and quality in systems of care for youth with complex behavioral health needs. *Administration and Policy in Mental Health and Mental Health Services Research, 48*(2), 185–200. https://doi.org/10.1007/s10488-020-01061-y

Graaf, G., Whitfield, E., & Snowden, L. (2023, OnlineFirst). 1915(c). Medicaid waivers for children with severe emotional disturbance: Participant characteristics, enrollment, and out-of-home service use. *Journal of Disability Policy Studies,* 0(0). https://doi.org/10.1177/10442073231157347

Gutman, T., Hanson, C. S., Bernays, S., Craig, J. C., Sinha, A., Dart, A., Eddy, A. A., Gipson, D. S., Bockenhauer, D., Yap, H.-K., Groothoff, J., Zappitelli, M., Webb, N. J. A., Alexander, S. I., Goldstein, S. L., Furth, S., Samuel, S., Blydt-Hansen, T., Dionne, J., et al. (2018). Child and parental perspectives on communication and decision making in pediatric CKD: A focus group study. *American Journal of Kidney Diseases, 72*(4), 547–559. https://doi.org/10.1053/j.ajkd.2018.05.005

Hansen, A. S., Telléus, G. K., & Lauritsen, M. B. (2021a). Changes in referral patterns to outpatient child and adolescent psychiatric services from 2005–2018. *Nordic Journal of Psychiatry, 75*(6), 437–446. https://doi.org/10.1080/08039488.2021.1880636

Hansen, A. S., Telléus, G. K., Mohr-Jensen, C., & Lauritsen, M. B. (2021b). Parent-perceived barriers to accessing services for their child's mental health problems. *Child and Adolescent Psychiatry and Mental Health, 15*, 1–11. https://doi.org/10.1186/s13034-021-00357-7

Harper, G., Sargent, J., & Fernando, P. (2014). Helping troubled children: Divergent discourses. *Journal of the American Academy of Child and Adolescent Psychiatry, 53*(5), 491–493. https://doi.org/10.1016/j.jaac.2014.01.014

He, A. S., Lim, C. S., Lecklitner, G., Olson, A., & Traube, D. E. (2015). Interagency collaboration and identifying mental health needs in child welfare: Findings from Los Angeles County. *Children and Youth Services Review, 53*, 39–43. https://doi.org/10.1016/j.childyouth.2015.03.013

Herbell, K., & Banks, A. J. (2020). "Fighting tooth and nail": Barriers to accessing adolescent mental health treatment from mothers perspectives. *Administration and Policy in Mental Health and Mental Health Services Research, 47*(6), 935–945. https://doi.org/10.1007/s10488-020-01026-1

Hernandez, M., Armstrong, M., Green, A. L., & Johnson, M. H. (2016). National survey of state children's mental health directors: Current status and future directions. *The Journal of Behavioral Health Services & Research, 47*, 935–945. https://doi.org/10.1007/s11414-016-9514-y

Hickey, L., Harms, L., Evans, J., Noakes, T., Lee, H., McSwan, A. A., Bean, H., Hope, J., Allison, L., Price, S., & Harris, N. (2023). Improving access to mental health interventions for children from birth to five years: A scoping review. *Child and Adolescent Mental Health*, 12. https://doi.org/10.1111/camh.12652

Hoagwood, K. E. (2005). Family-based services in children's mental health: A research review and synthesis. *Journal of Child Psychology and Psychiatry, and Allied Disciplines, 46*(7), 690–713. https://doi.org/10.1111/j.1469-7610.2005.01451.x

Hoagwood, K. E., Green, E., Kelleher, K., Schoenwald, S., Rolls-Reutz, J., Landsverk, J., Glisson, C., & Mayberg, S. (2008). Family advocacy, support and education in children's mental health: Results of a national survey. *Administration and Policy in Mental Health and Mental Health Services Research, 35*(1–2), 73–83. https://doi.org/10.1007/s10488-007-0149-4

Ibeziako, P., Kaufman, K., Scheer, K. N., & Sideridis, G. (2022). Pediatric mental health presentations and boarding: First year of the COVID-19 pandemic. *Hospital Pediatrics, 12*(9), 751–760. https://doi.org/10.1542/hpeds.2022-006555

Karikari, I., Walton, B., Bishop, C., Moynihan, S., & Evans, P. (2020). State-community system of care development: An exploratory longitudinal review. *The Journal of Behavioral Health Services & Research, 48*(2), 240–258. https://doi.org/10.1007/s11414-020-09702-8

Knitzer, J., & Olson, L. (1982). *Unclaimed children: The failure of public responsibility to children and adolescents in need of mental health services*. Children's Defense Fund. http://eric.ed.gov/?id=ED223346

Kuhlthau, K., Jellinek, M., White, G., VanCleave, J., Simons, J., & Murphy, M. (2011). Increases in behavioral health screening in pediatric care for Massachusetts Medicaid patients. *Archives of Pediatrics & Adolescent Medicine, 165*(7), 660–664. https://doi.org/10.1001/archpediatrics.2011.18

Kutash, K., Greenbaum, P. E., Wang, W., Boothroyd, R. A., & Friedman, R. M. (2011). Levels of system of care implementation: A national study. *Journal of Behavioral Health Services & Research, 38*(3), 342–357. https://doi.org/10.1007/s11414-011-9242-2

Langer, D. A., Holly, L. E., Wills, C. E., Tompson, M. C., & Chorpita, B. F. (2022). Shared decision-making for youth psychotherapy: A preliminary randomized clinical trial on facilitating personalized treatment. *Journal of Consulting and Clinical Psychology, 90*(1), 29–38. https://doi.org/10.1037/ccp0000702

Larson, J., Kazura, A., Fortuna, L., French, W. P., Hodas, G. R., Metz, P., McGinty, K., Bellonci, C., Lee, T., Lohr, W. D., Sharma, P., Zachik, A., Varma, C., Kamarauche, A., Adade, O. A., Bender, E., Brown, K. A., Concepcion, M., Naylor, M. W., et al. (2022). Clinical update: Child and adolescent behavioral health care in community systems of care. *Journal of the American Academy of Child & Adolescent Psychiatry, 62*(4). https://doi.org/10.1016/j.jaac.2022.06.001

Lindly, O. J., Martin, A. J., & Lally, K. (2020). A profile of care coordination, missed school days, and unmet needs among Oregon children with special health care needs with behavioral and mental health conditions. *Community Mental Health Journal, 56*(8), 1571–1580. https://doi.org/10.1007/s10597-020-00609-4

Lindsey, M. A., Brandt, N. E., Becker, K. D., Lee, B. R., Barth, R. P., Daleiden, E. L., & Chorpita, B. F. (2014). Identifying the common elements of treatment engagement interventions in children's mental health services. *Clinical Child and Family Psychology Review, 17*(3), 283–298. https://doi.org/10.1007/s10567-013-0163-x

Lipkin, P. H., Macias, M. M., Council on Children with Disabilities, S. O. D. A. B. P, Norwood, K. W., Jr., Brei, T. J., Davidson, L. F., Davis, B. E., Ellerbeck, K. A., Houtrow, A. J., Hyman, S. L., Kuo, D. Z., Noritz, G. H., Yin, L., Murphy, N. A., Levy, S. E., Weitzman, C. C., Bauer, N. S., Childers, D. O., Jr., Levine, J. M., et al. (2020). Promoting optimal development: Identifying infants and young children with developmental disorders through developmental surveillance and screening. *Pediatrics, 145*(1), e20193449. https://doi.org/10.1542/peds.2019-3449

Liverpool, S., Pereira, B., Hayes, D., Wolpert, M., & Edbrooke-Childs, J. (2021). A scoping review and assessment of essential elements of shared decision-making of parent-involved interventions in child and adolescent mental health. *European Child & Adolescent Psychiatry, 30*(9), 1319–1338. https://doi.org/10.1007/s00787-020-01530-7

Lourie, I. S., & Hernandez, M. (2003). A historical perspective on national child mental health policy. *Journal of Emotional and Behavioral Disorders, 11*(1), 5–9. https://doi.org/10.1177/106342660301100102

Maunder, R. D., & White, F. A. (2019). Intergroup contact and mental health stigma: A comparative effectiveness meta-analysis. *Clinical Psychology Review, 72*, 101749. https://doi.org/10.1016/j.cpr.2019.101749

Maurer, M., Mangrum, R., Hilliard-Boone, T., Amolegbe, A., Carman, K. L., Forsythe, L., Mosbacher, R., Lesch, J. K., & Woodward, K. (2022). Understanding the influence and impact of stakeholder engagement in patient-centered outcomes research: A qualitative study. *Journal of General Internal Medicine, 37*(Suppl 1), 6–13. https://doi.org/10.1007/s11606-021-07104-w

McCabe, E. M., Jameson, B. E., & Strauss, S. M. (2021). Mental health screenings: Practices and patterns of these and other health screenings in U.S. School Sistricts. *Journal of School Nursing*, 10598405211056648. https://doi.org/10.1177/10598405211056647

McKay, M. M., & Bannon, W. M., Jr. (2004). Engaging families in child mental health services. *Child and Adolescent Psychiatric Clinics, 13*(4), 905–921. https://doi.org/10.1016/j.chc.2004.04.001

Moore, K. L. (2018). Mental health service engagement among underserved minority adolescents and young adults: A systematic review. *Journal of Racial and Ethnic Health Disparities, 5*(5), 1063–1076. https://doi.org/10.1007/s40615-017-0455-9

Nayak, S. S., Tobias, C., Wolfe, J., Roper, K., Méndez-Peñate, L., Moulin, C., Arty, M., Scoglio, A. A. J., Kelleher, A., Rue, J., Brigham, M., Bradshaw, T., Byars, N., Camacho, A., Douglas, S., & Molnar, B. E. (2022). Engaging and supporting young children and their families in early childhood mental health services: The role of the family partner. *Community Mental Health Journal, 58*(1), 87–98. https://doi.org/10.1007/s10597-021-00796-8

Ndwiga, C., Warren, C. E., Okondo, C., Abuya, T., & Sripad, P. (2022). Experience of care of hospitalized newborns and young children and their parents: A scoping review. *PLoS One, 17*(8), e0272912. https://doi.org/10.1371/journal.pone.0272912

Nelson, K. L., Powell, B. J., Langellier, B., Lê-Scherban, F., Shattuck, P., Hoagwood, K., & Purtle, J. (2022). State policies that impact the design of children's mental health services: A modified Delphi study. *Administration and Policy in Mental Health and Mental Health Services Research, 49*(5), 834–847. https://doi.org/10.1007/s10488-022-01201-6

Olmstead v. LC, 527 US 581 (Supreme Court 1999).

Olson, J. R., Benjamin, P. H., Azman, A. A., Kellogg, M. A., Pullmann, M. D., Suter, J. C., & Bruns, E. J. (2021). Systematic review and meta-analysis: Effectiveness of wraparound care coordination for children and adolescents. *Journal of the American Academy of Child and Adolescent Psychiatry, 60*(11), 1353–1366. https://doi.org/10.1016/j.jaac.2021.02.022

Parfitt, Y., Pike, A., & Ayers, S. (2014). Infant developmental outcomes: A family systems perspective. *Infant and Child Development, 23*(4), 353–373. https://doi.org/10.1002/icd.1830

Rhodes, S. D., Tanner, A. E., Mann-Jackson, L., Alonzo, J., Horridge, D. N., Van Dam, C. N., Trent, S., Bell, J., Simán, F. M., Vissman, A. T., Nall, J., & Andrade, M. (2018a). Community-engaged research as an approach to expedite advances in HIV prevention, care, and treatment: A call to action. *AIDS Education and Prevention, 30*(3), 243–253. https://doi.org/10.1521/aeap.2018.30.3.243

Rhodes, S. D., Tanner, A. E., Mann-Jackson, L., Alonzo, J., Simán, F. M., Song, E. Y., Bell, J., Irby, M. B., Vissman, A. T., & Aronson, R. E. (2018b). Promoting community and population health in public health and medicine: A stepwise guide to initiating and conducting community-engaged research. *Journal of Health Disparities Research and Practice, 11*(3), 16–31.

Sanchez, A. L., Cornacchio, D., Poznanski, B., Golik, A. M., Chou, T., & Comer, J. S. (2018). The effectiveness of school-based mental health services for elementary-aged children: A meta-analysis. *Journal of the American Academy of Child and Adolescent Psychiatry, 57*(3), 153–165. https://doi.org/10.1016/j.jaac.2017.11.022

Schober, M., & Baxter, K. (2019). *Medicaid funding for family and youth peer support programs in the United States* (The Institute for Innovation and Implementation). University of Maryland, School of Social Work.

Scholl, I., LaRussa, A., Hahlweg, P., Kobrin, S., & Elwyn, G. (2018). Organizational- and system-level characteristics that influence implementation of shared decision-making and strategies to address them – A scoping review. *Implementation Science, 13*(1), 1–22. https://doi.org/10.1186/s13012-018-0731-z

Segers, E. W., Ketelaar, M., Taddio, A., de Man, M. A. C. P., Schoonhoven, L., van de Putte, E. M., & van den Hoogen, A. (2022). Exploring key elements of approaches that support children's' preferences during painful and stressful medical procedures: A scoping review. *Journal of Pediatric Nursing, 62*, e16–e24. https://doi.org/10.1016/j.pedn.2021.06.018

Slaton, A. E., Cecil, C. W., Lambert, L. E., King, T., & Pearson, M. M. (2012). What a difference family-driven makes: Stories of success and lessons learned. *American Journal of Community Psychology, 49*(3–4), 538–545. https://doi.org/10.1007/s10464-011-9449-7

Snowden, L. R., Masland, M., Wallace, N., Fawley-King, K., & Cuellar, A. E. (2008). Increasing California children's Medicaid-financed mental health treatment by vigorously implementing Medicaid's Early Periodic Screening, Diagnosis, and Treatment (EPSDT) Program. *Medical Care, 46*(6), 558–564. https://doi.org/10.1097/MLR.0b013e3181648e82

Snowden, L., Graaf, G., Keyes, L., & Ryan, A. (2022). Stigma and mental health in ethnic minority populations. In D. Vogel & N. Wade (Eds.), *The Cambridge handbook of stigma and mental health* (pp. 222–240). Cambridge University Press.

So, M., McCord, R. F., & Kaminski, J. W. (2019). Policy levers to promote access to and utilization of children's mental health services: A systematic review. *Administration and Policy in Mental Health and Mental Health Services Research, 46*(3), 334–351. https://doi.org/10.1007/s10488-018-00916-9

Splett, J. W., Trainor, K. M., Raborn, A., Halliday-Boykins, C. A., Garzona, M. E., Dongo, M. D., & Weist, M. D. (2018). Comparison of universal mental health screening to students already receiving intervention in a multitiered system of support. *Behavioral Disorders, 43*(3), 344–356. https://doi.org/10.1177/0198742918761339

Stroul, B. A., & Friedman, R. M. (1986). *A system of care for severely emotionally disturbed children & youth.* CASSP Technical Assistance Center, Georgetown University Child Development Center. http://eric.ed.gov/?id=ED330167

Stroul, B. A., Blau, G. M., & Friedman, R. A. (2010). *Updating the system of care concept and philosophy*. Georgetown University Center for Child and Human Development, National Technical Assistance Center for Children's Mental Health.

Stroul, B., Goldman, S. K., Pires, S. A., & Manteuffel, B. A. (2012). *Expanding the system of care approach: Improving the lives of children, youth, and families*. Georgetown University Center for Child and Human Development, National Technical Assistance Center for Children's Mental Health.

Stroul, B. A., Blau, G. M., & Larsen, J. (2021). *The evolution of the system of care approach*. The Institute for Innovation and Implementation, School of Social Work, University of Maryland. https://nttacmentalhealth.org/resource/the-evolution-of-the-system-of-care-approach-for-children-youth-and-young-adults-with-mental-health-conditions-and-their-families/

Stubbe, D. E. (2020). Practicing cultural competence and cultural humility in the care of diverse patients. *FOCUS, 18*(1), 49–51. https://doi.org/10.1176/appi.focus.20190041

Swift, J. K., Callahan, J. L., Cooper, M., & Parkin, S. R. (2018). The impact of accommodating client preference in psychotherapy: A meta-analysis. *Journal of Clinical Psychology, 74*(11), 1924–1937. https://doi.org/10.1002/jclp.22680

Waid, J., & Kelly, M. (2020). Supporting family engagement with child and adolescent mental health services: A scoping review. *Health & Social Care in the Community, 28*(5), 1333–1342. https://doi.org/10.1111/hsc.12947

Waid, J., Halpin, K., & Donaldson, R. (2021). Mental health service navigation: A scoping review of programmatic features and research evidence. *Social Work in Mental Health, 19*(1), 60–79. https://doi.org/10.1080/15332985.2020.1870646

Walker, J. S., & Bruns, E. J. (2006). Building on practice-based evidence: Using expert perspectives to define the wraparound process. *Psychiatric Services, 57*(11), 1579–1585. https://doi.org/10.1176/ps.2006.57.11.1579

Winters, N. C., & Metz, W. P. (2009). The wraparound approach in systems of care. *Psychiatric Clinics of North America, 32*(1), 135–151. https://doi.org/10.1016/j.psc.2008.11.007

Wyatt, K. D., List, B., Brinkman, W. B., Prutsky Lopez, G., Asi, N., Erwin, P., Wang, Z., Domecq Garces, J. P., Montori, V. M., & LeBlanc, A. (2015). Shared decision making in pediatrics: A systematic review and meta-analysis. *Academic Pediatrics, 15*(6), 573–583. https://doi.org/10.1016/j.acap.2015.03.011

Zanello, E., Calugi, S., Sanders, L. M., Lenzi, J., Faldella, G., Rucci, P., & Fantini, M. P. (2017). Care coordination for children with special health care needs: A cohort study. *Italian Journal of Pediatrics, 43*(1), 1–6. https://doi.org/10.1186/s13052-017-0342-3

Chapter 9
Equity in Engaging Families in Mental Health Interventions for Young Children

Victoria O. Nguyen and Brenda Jones Harden

The first decades of the twenty-first century have been marked by multiple societal crises, including the COVID pandemic, racial/ethnic strife, political polarization, as well as a crisis in child and youth mental health. Scholars, policymakers, and practitioners have issued a clarion call for strategies to address the decline in the mental health status of children and youth in the United States, including for young children (Bitsko et al., 2022; Office of the Surgeon General, 2021). In particular, interventions designed to improve child mental health are critical for children from low-income and minoritized backgrounds, who are at higher risk for a range of adverse outcomes, including mental health challenges (Alegria et al., 2015; Dodge, 2018; Shivers et al., 2022; Yoshikawa et al., 2012). Such outcomes are partially attributable to the disparities children from these populations experience in the context of service delivery systems. For example, these children and their families are less likely to receive quality mental health services (Butler & Rodgers, 2019; Rodgers et al., 2022). Further, they have decreased engagement in school-based, clinic-based, and community-based mental health settings (Alegria et al., 2010; Atkins et al., 2017).

As Iruka et al. (2022) articulate in their discussion of the engagement of diverse families in early childhood programs, family engagement has a key role in promoting the outcomes of children from underserved families. Thus, an important strategy for counteracting mental health disparities and associated outcomes is to increase the engagement of families from low-income and minoritized backgrounds into mental health services for their children. The goal of this chapter is to explore best practices for how this may be achieved. We begin by summarizing the empirical literature on disparities in the prevalence of mental health disorders and access to

---

V. O. Nguyen · B. J. Harden (✉)
School of Social Work, Columbia University, New York, NY, USA
e-mail: von2102@columbia.edu; bjh2180@columbia.edu

L. Nabors, J. D. Bartlett (eds.), *Family Engagement in Mental Health Interventions for Young Children*, Springer Series on Child and Family Studies,
https://doi.org/10.1007/978-3-031-47917-5_9

mental health services for young children from low-income and minoritized backgrounds. Although the literature is sparse, we review the research on challenges to engaging families from low-income and minoritized backgrounds in mental health services writ large and those for their young children specifically. Finally, we offer some conceptual approaches to increasing the engagement of families from these backgrounds into mental health services for their young children, with exemplars of programs that are grounded in these approaches.

Disparities in the Prevalence of Mental Health Disorders

Research has consistently documented elevated rates of mental health disorders of children from low-income and minoritized backgrounds. Mental health disparities begin in early childhood and may be exacerbated across childhood and adolescence (Alegria et al., 2015). Based on a systematic review, Reiss (2013) suggested that children from low-income backgrounds were two to three times more likely to have mental health problems when compared to children from backgrounds considered middle class. Further, Cree et al. (2018) provide national data that young children from low-income families, when compared to those from middle-income families, have a higher likelihood of receiving a diagnosis of a mental or behavioral disorder. Rates of mental health disorders are particularly high for children who experience chronic poverty and extreme poverty (Acri et al., 2017; Lee & Zhang, 2022). The influence of poverty may vary by disorder. For example, Reiss (2013) found that poverty is more related to externalizing than internalizing disorders. Further, research has pointed to delayed diagnosis of autism spectrum disorder (ASD) for children from low-income backgrounds (Durkin et al., 2017). Moreover, Ramphal et al. (2020) found links between postnatal socioeconomic status, brain function (connectivity), and elevated scores on externalizing problems in children at 2 years of age.

Given the overlap between low socioeconomic (SES) status and minoritized status in the United States, SES disparities often translate into racial/ethnic disparities. Some studies have documented that when SES is controlled, the racial-ethnic disparities in child mental health may not be as pronounced, suggesting the higher rates of poverty among minoritized children may explain their higher rates of mental health disorders (Jones Harden & Slopen, 2022). In contrast, Yoshikawa et al. (2012) argue that poverty's influence on child mental health may be exacerbated for specific racial/ethnic groups. Alegria et al. (2015) assert that race/ethnicity has a unique impact on mental health disparities beyond what can be explained by poverty. In both reviews, the authors underscore the import of examining racial disparities above and beyond the disparities attributed to poverty.

There is substantial evidence that children from minoritized backgrounds are more likely to display mental health challenges (Alegria et al., 2010, 2015; Rodgers et al., 2022). Although many of these studies are of older children, early childhood may be critical for the emergence of these disparities due to the pernicious impact of early adversity on children (Alegria et al., 2015; Bethell et al., 2019; Sameroff & Seifer, 2021). For example, research suggests that young children from minoritized backgrounds are more likely to be diagnosed (perhaps over diagnosed) with attentional and behavioral disorders (Ballentine, 2019; Coker et al., 2016).

Variability in racial/ethnic disparities has been found depending on which disorder and which minority group are examined. Huang et al. (2012) found that Asian American children have higher rates of internalizing disorders and interpersonal relationship challenges than white children. Merikangas et al. (2010) also found higher rates of mood disorders among Latin American children when compared to white children. Sarche et al. (2011) documented higher rates of substance use, internalizing behaviors, and externalizing behaviors among Native American children than children of all other racial/ethnic groups.

Disparities in Mental Health Services Access and Utilization

A health service disparity pertains to the differences in treatment and/or access that is not attributable to differences between the health status and preferences of different groups (McGuire et al., 2006). As such, there is substantial research documenting disparities in mental health services for low-income and racial/ethnic minority groups in the United States (Alegria et al., 2015; McGuire et al., 2006). These disparities are particularly harmful for young children's development, including their mental health.

With respect to socioeconomic disparities, children from low-income backgrounds tend to experience delayed diagnosis of mental health problems (Ghandour et al., 2019). They also have a lower likelihood of receiving treatment from mental health professionals and to receive treatment that is evidence based (Ghandour et al., 2019). Further, they are more likely to be prescribed psychotropic medication (Ghandour et al., 2019), to use emergency and inpatient services, and to experience coercive mental health referrals (Chow et al., 2003). In their examination of mental health services for young children, Cree et al. (2018) found that children residing in low-income families were less likely to receive appropriate care for mental or behavioral disorders, when compared to children from higher-income backgrounds.

Of particular relevance to this chapter, Santiago et al. (2013) identified multiple reasons for the lack of mental health services for children from low-income backgrounds which pertained to family engagement. For example, logistical challenges created barriers to utilization, such as competing responsibilities, the lack of childcare and transportation, as well as the inability to pay for mental health treatment. Parental perceptions of mental health care also negatively affected their children's utilization of mental health services, such as their mistrust of mental health professionals and concerns about child protection involvement, as well as the perceived stigma around mental health care. Finally, systemic challenges were identified, including mental health professionals' lack of training and comfort addressing the needs of families from low-income backgrounds and decreased resources to conduct intensive outreach to families and to address their concrete needs (Santiago et al., 2013). Parental perceptions of stigma may also prevent them from discussing their children's behaviors and mental health concerns with pediatricians, further limiting their access to mental health services (Pidano et al., 2020).

There is also evidence that individuals from minoritized backgrounds are less likely to receive appropriate mental health treatment (Chow et al., 2003). They tend to receive inpatient and emergency treatment as opposed to outpatient mental health services, are more likely to have their treatment prematurely terminated, and are less likely to have insurance to cover their treatment (Chow et al., 2003). Further, they often approach their mental health needs through the lens of religious and cultural beliefs, which decreases their engagement with mental health professionals (Chow et al., 2003). Multiple studies have attributed the absence of linguistically matched and culturally sensitive mental health professionals to extant disparities for minoritized groups (Avila & Bramlett, 2013; Chow et al., 2003). The availability of mental health professionals in the communities where minoritized populations reside was important for the mental health utilization of African American and Latin American families (Lê Cook et al., 2013).

Although the research is limited, some studies have documented disparities in mental health service utilization for children and youth from minoritized backgrounds though they have greater need in this arena (Alegria et al., 2015). Further, African American and Latin American children and youth are less likely to receive mental health services in other child service delivery systems, such as schools and child welfare agencies (Butler & Rodgers, 2019).

Alegria et al. (2015) argue for an examination of the interaction of SES and race/ethnicity in studies of mental health service utilization. Chow et al. (2003) documented that minoritized groups in low poverty areas were more likely to use emergency and inpatient mental health services. Thus, it is critical to employ strategies to engage families living in poverty and those who represent minoritized groups in efforts to increase mental health service utilization for young children.

Challenges to Engaging Families in Mental Health Services

Engaging families in evidence-based and evidence-informed mental health prevention and interventions for young children is critical to promote their safety, health, and well-being. Although not explicitly targeting young children, a growing body of research supports the notion of meaningful family engagement, where mental health professionals sustain genuine relationships with families for effective child mental health interventions and services (Haine-Schlagel & Walsh, 2015). The literature also develops a compelling case that enhancing family engagement is foundational for increasing the utilization of child mental health services (Waid & Kelly, 2020). Family engagement requires a comprehensive and concerted effort involving mental health professionals such as psychologists, social workers, psychiatrists, pediatricians, teachers, and community-based health educators. Through collaborative partnerships with families, professionals can encourage children's learning and development and support families in the care they need when and where they need it most. For example, partnerships with families have been created to improve child mental health in the context of Head Start classrooms via parent and teacher training around promotion of social competence and reduction of behavior problems (Webster-Stratton et al., 2001).

Family engagement in mental health services is often hindered by barriers deeply rooted in social and structural obstacles that underlie health inequities. Specifically, perceptions and structural constraints (Reardon et al., 2017) are common themes noted by parents and caretakers in multiple studies addressing challenges to services and treatment. Structural barriers are limitations such as an inability to pay for services, time demands, scheduling conflicts, lack of coordination among services, shortages of services and professionals available for their children, and lack of transportation (Garvey et al., 2006; Stevens et al. 2006). Further, structural barriers specific to young children include the lack of professionals specializing in early childhood mental health and of collaboration between early childhood service delivery systems, such as early intervention, early care and education, and early childhood mental health (Conroy & Brown, 2004). As a result of all these structural barriers, many families drop out prematurely, with many receiving less than half of the intervention (Gomby, 2000).

Social barriers include a lack of trust in or negative experience with mental health professionals (Gross et al., 2001), uncertainty as to when to seek care (Huang et al., 2005), and fear of the stigma associated with accessing care (González, 2005). These social obstacles play a role in a lack of service engagement and, together with inequitable distribution of opportunities and resources, produce and reproduce mental health inequalities. Self-efficacy theory (Bandura & Adams, 1977) posits that families' perceptions about the treatment process, outcomes, setting, and professionals may influence the level of engagement. Families drop out prematurely when their expectations do not match the professionals' expectations (Morrissey-Kane & Prinz, 1999). Identifying barriers to equity in services and understanding how they shape behavior is critical to eliminating them.

Substantial research comparing mental health services across populations yields compelling evidence of disparities in access and use. First, parents from different populations may vary in their concerns about whether children need a mental health assessment and subsequent treatment. For example, findings from a large survey revealed that African American, Asian American, and Latin American parents were less likely to perceive their children's emotional or behavioral problems as being mental health concerns (Alegria et al., 2010). Further, families from racial and minority backgrounds are more likely to delay help-seeking, experience-amplified barriers when attempting to access services, and are more likely to receive poorer-quality mental health care (Viale-Val et al., 1984). Evidence also exists that families at greater risk for poor mental health outcomes, including low-income urban families, are more likely to drop out of services (Snell-Johns et al., 2004). The structural barriers that families experience, including the lack of childcare, engagement with other early childhood systems, and the concrete resources that families with young children need, contribute to their attrition from mental health services (Conroy & Brown, 2004; McKay & Bannon, 2004).

Families from low-income and minoritized backgrounds have had many negative experiences with the health-care system that also deter their engagement in mental health care. For example, families from minoritized backgrounds are more likely to distrust mental health treatment than are white parents (Alegria et al., 2015). They also are more likely to attach stigma to mental health service usage (Alegria et al., 2015). Finally, they are more likely to expect inadequate, unhelpful, or culturally insensitive mental health care (Alegria et al., 2015).

These findings highlight the significance of fostering family engagement in mental health services and interventions. Engaging families requires innovative thinking that embraces broader approaches to address social, economic, and environmental factors influencing engagement and retention. With this broad perspective, mental health professionals can better collaborate with caregivers and families to build more integrated and sustained approaches that reduce long-standing disparities in mental health treatment. To this end, we explore in the following sections five potential strategies to promote equity in engaging families in children's mental health services: (1) capitalizing on sociocultural models of mental health service delivery, (2) culturally adapting mental health interventions, (3) placing families at the center of services, (4) directly addressing obstacles to treatment, and 5) bringing services closer to families' communities.

Sociocultural Perspective on Engaging Families in Mental Health Services

In response to the challenges of engaging families from low-income and minoritized backgrounds in mental health services, research has increasingly turned to sociocultural views of disparities in the access and utilization of mental health services (e.g., García Coll & Garrido, 2000). Although numerous theories fall into the broad sociocultural perspective, they share an underlying awareness of how behaviors are affected by social, economic, and environmental factors. Culture, race, and ethnicity are situated prominently in sociocultural perspectives, with an emphasis on how cultural processes affect children's outcomes as well as their experiences, such as discrimination (García Coll et al., 1996).

Several models grounded in sociocultural perspectives aim to facilitate family engagement and address barriers to seeking or participating in care. For example, the Sociocultural Framework for Health Service Disparities (Alegría et al., 2010) focuses on factors related to treatment, service access, and utilization across the child, caregiver, and provider levels. This framework emphasizes racial and ethnic disparities in services and offers an explanation for why individuals from minoritized groups commence mental health care with higher levels of illness severity.

In this framework, cultural processes (e.g., traditions, values, beliefs, societal perceptions of culture) are implicated in the access to, quality of, and outcomes of mental health care for individuals from specific racial/ethnic groups, which lead to racial/ethnic mental health disparities (Alegria et al., 2010).

This framework highlights multiple social determinants of families' disengagement or underutilization of mental health services, including housing and neighborhood conditions, socioeconomic status, low educational attainment, limited language proficiency, and racism and discrimination (Paradies et al., 2015). In several studies, challenging circumstances such as single-parent status, socioeconomic disadvantage, parent psychopathology, parent strain, ethnic minority status, and low-resource neighborhoods predict lower rates of engagement in clinical services (Snell-Johns et al., 2004) and quality of participation in prevention programs (Nix et al., 2009).

Embracing Cultural Competency in Integrated Services to Engage Families

Given the convincing evidence for sociocultural barriers to mental health care at multiple levels, culturally competent care is a cornerstone for eliminating disparities in mental health. Building on this premise, the research emphasizes the need for mental health professionals to understand diverse social and cultural contexts when attempting to identify the influence of attitudes on service use and engagement (McCabe, 2002; Iruka et al., 2022). Further, evidence-based mental health interventions should be adapted to be socioculturally relevant to families from low-income and minoritized families (Nation et al., 2003). These adaptations should be grounded in the conceptual and empirical literature on relevant populations as well as feedback from practitioners and community members reflecting these populations (Whitbeck, 2006).

An example of sociocultural adaptation of an intervention for young children and their families is a parenting program called Guiandos a Niños Activos (GANA; McCabe & Yeh, 2009), a culturally adapted form of parent-child interaction therapy (PCIT; Lieneman et al., 2017). The GANA intervention embodies values of cultural competency to assure quality care to Mexican American families seeking to address child-externalizing symptoms such as disruptive, hyperactive, and aggressive behaviors. The results showed that the culturally tailored intervention was as effective as the original PCIT on most outcomes (McCabe & Yeh, 2009) and was more effective regarding child internalizing symptoms (McCabe et al., 2012). The intervention developers attributed the success of GANA to their adaption of the protocols and treatment formats to address diverse clinical comorbidities and different diagnostic presentations specific to the Mexican American culture. Further adaptations of PCIT also increased treatment accessibility, by developing and testing PCIT for Native American populations (Bigfoot & Funderburk, 2011), home-based PCIT (Gurwitch et al., 2020), internet-delivered PCIT (Comer et al., 2017), and group-based PCIT (Niec et al., 2016).

Sociocultural mismatches regarding the expectations of treatment are important factors to consider when working with minoritized populations. For example, McCabe (2002), during implementation and evaluation of interventions for preschool children from minoritized backgrounds, documented the relation between parental perceptions of treatment and disengagement and premature termination of services. Specifically, their cultural beliefs about resolving child behavior problems through increasing discipline were often inconsistent with the treatment process. Similarly, Miller and Prinz (2003) found that mismatches in families' pretreatment expectations on the type and structure of treatment led families to drop out of services. The authors underscored the value of assessing family expectations at the outset and showing responsiveness by providing strategies that addressed their expectations. Overall, understanding each family's expectations, identifying common goals, utilizing mutually acceptable strategies, and validating their sociocultural beliefs can increase engagement of families from low-income and minoritized backgrounds.

Finally, it is critical that individual and organizational providers of mental health services to children and families from low-income and minoritized backgrounds work toward a high level of cultural competence. According to Hernandez et al. (2009), the provision of culturally competent mental health services to children and families requires attention to the community context (e.g., the neighborhood context), cultural characteristics of local populations (e.g., cultural child-rearing beliefs of various minoritized groups), organizational infrastructure (e.g., consistency between values of service organizations and participants), and direct service support (e.g., focusing on availability, access, and utilization of mental health services by populations targeted). Training mental health professionals on cultural competence, including a focus on racism and discrimination, is an important strategy that has been found to enhance their ability to engage and provide services to specific cultural groups (Chu et al., 2022). Recent efforts in the early childhood mental health arena have also attempted to address equity in service delivery and access. For example, Candelaria et al. (2021) have described the work in Maryland's Infant and Early Childhood Mental Health Consultation program to advance racial equity by holding a racial equity retreat, using small-group facilitators to address issues of equity, and establishing an equity leadership group. By embracing cultural competency, mental health professionals can engage with families to increase access to and utilization of mental health services, enhance collaboration, improve health outcomes, increase the efficiency and competency of clinical and support staff, and improve family satisfaction and engagement with services (Anderson et al., 2003).

Placing the Family at the Center for Engagement

Family systems theory offers a framework for understanding how families influence the mental health of children (Kerr & Bowen, 1988). Research has documented that the challenges that some families experience, such as poverty, affect parenting behaviors and ultimately their children's outcomes (Fraser, 2006; Knitzer & Cohen, 2007). Theory and research underscore the importance of placing the family at the center of children's mental health services. Thus, a whole-family approach to children's mental health services, especially for young children, has been found to be most effective (e.g., Kristie Brandt et al., 2013; Zeanah, 2018). Interventions grounded in this approach often address children's mental health through dyadic approaches in which the child and parent (and other caregivers) are simultaneously involved in the treatment. Thus, family engagement extends beyond assuring that the child attends therapy sessions to parents being integral participants in the therapeutic process.

An exemplar of this approach is the Engaging Moms Program (2003), a family-based intervention developed as a manualized approach to engaging low-income Black mothers of substance-exposed infants in drug abuse treatment programs. For mothers assigned to the intervention, engagement specialists utilized family therapy techniques such as family genograms to elicit family members' assistance to engage mothers in treatment programs and to promote bonding with mental health professionals in the beginning stages of treatment (Dakof et al. 2003). To help mothers achieve positive change, the intervention provided integrated individual and family sessions with the mother and her family, including individual sessions with the mother, individual sessions with her family/partner, and family and couples' sessions (Dakof et al., 2003). Although the intervention did not lead to more optimized outcomes in critical factors such as overall psychological stress for families, it led to greater enrollment and completion of at least 4 weeks of treatment and demonstrated success in initial family engagement.

Addressing Family Obstacles to Treatment

Motivational interviewing (MI) principles represent a promising approach that mental health professionals may apply to engage families and caregivers in mental health services. Motivational interviewing involves clinical techniques designed to address concerns that families may have about the treatment process (Miller & Rollnick, 2002). Through MI techniques, mental health professionals can communicate empathy, avoid conflict, highlight the discrepancy between present behavior and desired outcomes, elicit self-motivational statements, and collaborate on behavior change plans, hypothesized to reduce resistance, and strengthen the commitment to treatment (Miller & Rollnick 2002).

MI has been used in many interventions with parents and their young children. Grote et al. (2007, 2010) tested a multicomponent engagement intervention incorporating motivational interviewing, ethnographic interviewing, and support services in a treatment program for low-income, depressed new and expectant mothers. In a pretreatment engagement session, mental health professionals used ethnographic interviewing to elicit the mother's "story" and explore the mother's values and cultural perspective on treatment. Motivational interviewing was also adapted to address engagement challenges. Mental health professionals reviewed expectations for treatment, offered treatment options, addressed social and structural barriers to participation (e.g., stigma, lack of interpersonal support, cultural perceptions), and enhanced treatment using MI clinical tools. Professionals also offered supplemental referrals and resources to connect mothers to address daily stressors. The intervention showed a positive effect, with 67% of mothers completing treatment, demonstrating that multiple models such as MI, EI, and family support can be a solution when unified with an integrated approach that includes treatment, provider care, and resources tailored to the family's needs (Grote et al., 2010).

Additionally, Family Check-Up (FCU; Dishion & Stormshak, 2007) and its adapted version for improving health behaviors in primary care, the Family Check-Up 4 Health (FCU4Health; Smith et al., 2018), are brief and family-centered interventions targeting young children that use MI to improve engagement. In one study that examined the relation of MI to parent engagement, Berkel et al. (2021) found that using MI at the first session was related to the caregivers' active engagement during the sessions, attendance at follow-up parenting sessions, and improvements in motivation to address goals related to child health and behavior. Thus, there is emerging research that suggests that MI may increase engagement by collaborating with parents to address potential barriers to their participation in mental health services for their young children.

Given parents' identification of the lack of concrete resources as a barrier to their engagement with mental health services for their children, it is important to identify and implement strategies that reduce these concrete barriers. For example, the Wraparound Demonstration Waiver Program has assisted parents to obtain insurance, including Medicaid, and offered sliding fee scales, in order to pay for their children's mental health services (Blizzard et al., 2017). In other programs, transportation vouchers and childcare for siblings have been provided (e.g., Gopalan et al., 2014). Some programs offer case management services as a complement to mental health intervention (e.g., Lowell et al., 2011). Case managers assist parents with a variety of resource challenges, including food, shelter, clothing, and more psychosocial factors that call for other therapeutic interventions. The explicit needs of families with young children should be addressed, such as childcare, early intervention, and nutritional supports such as the Supplemental Food Program for Women, Infants, and Children (Conroy & Brown, 2004; Klawetter et al., 2021; Kurz, 2008). The provision or identification of these concrete resources for families not only addresses their basic needs but increases their willingness to engage in the mental health services that are delivered by these professionals (Azzi-Lessing, 2010).

Bringing Care for Families Closer to the Community

For families in challenging contexts, mental health services often remain out of reach (Alegria et al., 2015). As Waid and Kelly (2020) document, integrating mental health care into other community-based services is the most effective way of enhancing family engagement in child mental health services. Equity in family engagement requires that treatment and care are available and accessible to those who need it, which can often support engagement and retention. Thus, mental health intervention that is integrated into community-based service delivery, home visitation, and early childhood education holds promise for reaching more families, thus improving their engagement in mental health services for their children.

Community-Based Services Parents of young children have articulated that the lack of availability of mental health services, which are in their communities and reflect their community cultures, is a major barrier for their children's participation in mental health services (Alegria et al., 2010). Thus, mental health services should be integrated into respected and valued community-based settings to increase engagement. For example, there is evidence that providing mental health care at community-based health clinics improves access to care (Bonilla et al., 2021). A programmatic exemplar is the Community Parent Education Program (COPE), a parent-training prevention program for families of preschoolers. It is delivered in a multiple-family group format to improve participation due to the social isolation faced by some families with young children with behavior and mental problems (Cunningham et al., 1995). The authors examined whether small-group sessions with 5–7 families held in local community centers (during the evening) led to greater engagement and retention than individual clinic-based family sessions. Cunningham et al. (1995) found that families traditionally less likely to participate in preventive parenting programs, including immigrant, ESL, and parents of children with greater aggression, were more likely to enroll in group-based services. Of greater importance, mental health professionals shared personalized interactions in which they identified and addressed families' sources of barriers to treatment, including a lack of understanding about treatment processes and hopelessness due to perceived past failures in previous treatment. Families engaged in treatment more often when professionals acknowledged and addressed barriers, such as scheduling, transportation, and financial concerns. Other interventions that have been implemented for families with young children from low-income and other high-risk backgrounds utilizing this multifamily group format include the Incredible Years (Webster-Stratton et al., 2001) and Circle of Security (Cassidy et al., 2017).

Home Visiting The federal Maternal, Infant, and Early Childhood Home Visiting program (MIECHV; Health Resources and Services Administration, 2023) has led to a proliferation of home-based interventions that have improved child and family functioning for low-income families. Home visiting models vary in duration, curriculum, and orientation; however, their foundations for success include integrating cultural competency and responsiveness, which are critical for sustained engagement. Evaluations of these programs have revealed benefits for families that are linked to positive mental health of children, as well as directly for young children's social-emotional development (see Sama-Miller et al., 2017, for a review). The federal impact of evaluation of MIECHV (Michalopoulos et al., 2019) documented reductions in parental mental health challenges, as well as fewer child behavior problems.

In regard to evaluations of specific programs, improved parental mental health, enhanced parenting, and reduced child maltreatment have been documented as a result of multiple programs, including Attachment and Biobehavioral Catch-up (Dozier & Barnard, 2019), Early Head Start (Chazan-Cohen et al., 2007; Green et al., 2014a, b), Family Connects (Dodge & Goodman, 2019), Healthy Families America (HFA; Lee et al., 2018), Promoting First Relationships (Oxford et al., 2016), and Safe Care (Chaffin et al., 2012). Further, several programs have resulted in reductions in toddlers' and preschool children's social, emotional, and behavioral problems, including Attachment and Biobehavioral Catch-up (Jones Harden et al., 2021), Early Head Start (Chazan-Cohen et al., 2007), Family Check-Up (Sitnick et al., 2015), and Nurse Family Partnership (Olds, 2006).

In addition to these preventive home-based interventions, those that are more therapeutic in nature have also led to improved children's mental health outcomes. For example, participation in child-parent psychotherapy (CPP) has resulted in decreased parental mental health challenges, higher levels of infant secure attachment, and reductions in children's behavior problems and symptoms of trauma exposure (Lieberman & Van Horn, 2008; Lowell et al., 2011). Therapeutic interventions with a goal of reducing child behavior problems through enhancing parents' skills at managing child behaviors have been effective, such as parent-child interaction therapy (PCIT; Lieneman et al., 2017; Thomas et al., 2017) and the parent management component of Triple P (Prinz et al., 2009; Sanders et al., 2014).

It is important to note that many of these home-based programs were targeted to low-income families, thus grounded in approaches to increase the engagement of these populations. However, research has not directly investigated whether such programs indeed create more equitable access to supports for low-income families. Further, few studies explicitly focused on improving the disparities in the engagement of families from diverse racial/ethnic backgrounds, although the MIECHV evaluation suggests that families of a wide range of backgrounds benefit from these programs (Michalopoulos et al., 2019). Evaluators of Family Connects (FC) specifically tackled these two conundrums in the home visiting literature. In a recent implementation study, Mersky et al. (2022) provided preliminary evidence that because FC is a universal program that engages families from high-risk and low-risk backgrounds, it promotes more equity among families because all families receive services relative to their needs. Further, Dodge et al. (2022) investigated racial/ethnic disparities across a range of FC impact studies. They found reductions in disparities between African American and their non-Hispanic white counterparts in multiple domains of parent functioning related to child mental health, including maternal anxiety and depression, father nonsupport, utilization of infant emergency medical care, and incidence of child maltreatment investigations. Overall, these recent findings with respect to the Family Connects home visiting program underscore the import of scaling up more universal approaches as a way of averting the stigma that families may feel when they need to access mental health services.

Early Childhood Education and Intervention Many early childhood (EC) programs are comprehensive in nature and address children's academic school readiness, as well as their health and mental health (Azzi-Lessing, 2010). These programs often utilize broad frameworks, such as the Pyramid Model (Fox & Hemmeter, 2009), which identify strategies to address all children's social-emotional needs and to support children with more intensive mental health needs. As such, young children are engaged in a variety of universal programs to address their social-emotional development, including interventions emanating from the social-emotional learning arena (e.g., PATHS curriculum; Domitrovich et al., 2007; Stanley, 2019). Further, they may benefit from more intensive interventions, particularly those designed to decrease children's behavior problems, such as BEST in CLASS (Conroy et al., 2015; Sutherland et al., 2020) and Learning to Objectively Observe Kids (LOOK; Downer et al., 2018). Parents are often willing to engage their children in such programs due to the lack of stigma and because the children receive the services in the EC setting. Clearly, there is a need to expand these models, so they are available in the range of EC programs that children attend.

Infant and Early Childhood Mental Health Consultation (IECMHC) programs are comprehensive approaches that are gaining momentum across the United States. IECMHC programs support the overall early care and education programs, the staff, and classrooms, as well as parents and children, with a goal of enhancing children's social-emotional functioning (Ash et al., 2017). IECMH consultants collaborate with program administrators to establish policies and procedures that facilitate a positive social-emotional climate and children's social-emotional competence. At the classroom level, consultants support teachers to effectively manage their classrooms via utilizing positive behavior supports. To address the needs of children with problem behavior and other mental health challenges, consultants collaborate with the young child's teacher and parents to identify classroom, home, and therapeutic supports for these children. Emerging research has documented that IECMHC programs are effective at the child, teacher, and classroom level, including improved child social-emotional competence and reduced behavior problems, improved teacher-child relationships, and enhanced classroom climate (Center for Excellence for Infant and Early Childhood Mental Health Consultation, 2020; Reyes & Gilliam, 2021). Shivers et al. (2022) documented a strong decrease in teacher-child conflict for African American children and a marginal reduction in African American boys' expulsion rate as a result of IECMH consultation.

Because of the recognition that many health, academic, and mental health disparities begin in early childhood, there has been a call for the creation of an early childhood system of care that would address young children's needs across a variety of developmental domains and potentially reduce the disparities in their outcomes over the course of childhood and even into adulthood (e.g., Dodge, 2018). Building on this systemic approach, the federal Project LAUNCH (i.e., Linking Actions for Unmet Needs in Children's Health) was initiated with an overarching goal of promoting the mental health and wellness of children from birth to age eight. Project LAUNCH has been administered in several communities, undertaking a multi-pronged approach to addressing young children's mental health needs, including screening and assessment, behavioral health in primary care, mental health consultation in early care and education programs and schools, enhanced home visiting, and family strengthening. It is also designed to reduce socioeconomic and racial/ethnic disparities by implementing strategies to improve access, engagement, and outcomes among young children from low-income and minoritized environments. Preliminary findings suggest that Project LAUNCH has conferred benefits on professionals, parents, and children, including parents' positive perceptions of the program, as well as improving their parenting skills and children's development as a result of program participation (Molnar et al., 2018).

A growing body of research has demonstrated that mental health intervention can be integrated within services that are more accessible to families, including community-based services, home visitation, and early childhood education (Goodman et al., 2019). Mental health interventions in these settings promote family engagement in services early in children's development, thereby fostering a more positive attitude toward these services over the trajectory of childhood. Further, such an approach underscores the advantage of universal interventions, which reduce the stigma that families experience when they utilize mental health services (Dodge, 2018). Providing short-term mental health treatment to children and families can prevent issues from escalating and can support accessible care, which is especially critical, given the challenges families face in accessing mental health support through the system as it is currently structured.

Concluding Remarks

Advancing the full inclusion of young children and their families across all social identities and backgrounds with access to mental health services will take sustained efforts far beyond those of mental health professionals alone. Professionals, however, have a unique opportunity and obligation to advance equity in their services and interventions. This chapter examined the social and structural barriers that impede equity in care, adaptations to improve care, and the accumulating evidence on interventions that focus on family engagement. Many of these ideas are summarized in Fig. 9.1. Implementing such family engagement strategies will result in improved utilization of mental health services for young children from low-income and minoritized backgrounds and ultimately enhance their mental health outcomes.

Brief interventions in which mental health professionals embodied cultural competency in addressing families' structural (e.g., schedules, transportation) and social (e.g., members' resistance) obstacles in early sessions have demonstrated effectiveness in longer-term participation. Access and delivery of appropriate services are

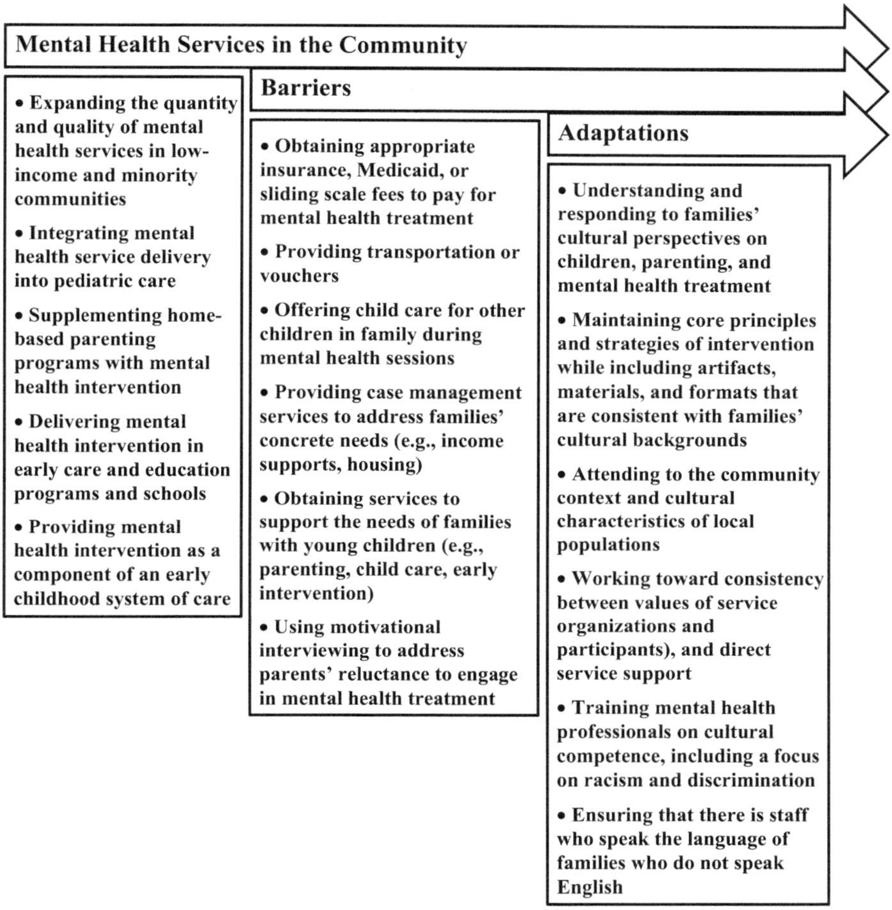

Fig. 9.1 Ideas for socioculturally appropriate mental health services in the community, barriers to address, and adaptations for consideration

achievable by offering multiple modalities such as group-based care, home visits, and community-based care. Collaborating on family engagement with the whole-family system and integrating treatment or services with approaches such as motivational interviewing (MI) and case management allows professionals to address family reluctance to engage in mental health service in concrete ways.

Although the modalities varied across the studies reviewed in this chapter, meeting family expectations and addressing their concerns, cultural needs, and social and structural barriers were common factors in family engagement. Equity in engaging families includes genuine efforts to understand each family's beliefs, values, priorities, goals, and aspirations. A collaborative approach to addressing challenges conveys understanding and respect for families, strengthening the bond between the mental health provider and the family. While current research has yielded important findings, evidence remains limited. Research is needed in mental health equity to include young children and their families across all social identities and backgrounds. Family engagement practices should be a focus of mental health research and program evaluation, helping families and professionals to collaborate and create a nurturing environment where young children can thrive. As mental health challenges among young people are becoming more pervasive, especially among those from low-income and minoritized backgrounds, there is not only an opportunity but an obligation for professionals and families to collaborate and sustain efforts for the mental health and well-being of all young children.

References

Acri, M. C., Bornheimer, L. A., Jessell, L., Chomancuzuk, A. H., Adler, J. G., Gopalan, G., & McKay, M. M. (2017). The intersection of extreme poverty and familial mental health in the United States. *Social Work in Mental Health, 15*(6), 677–689. https://doi.org/10.1080/15332985.2017.1319893

Alegria, M., Pescosolido, B. A., Williams, S., & Canino, G. (2010). Culture, race/ethnicity and disparities: Fleshing out the socio-cultural framework for health services disparities. In *Handbook of the sociology of health, illness, and healing: A blueprint for the 21st century* (pp. 363–382). Springer.

Alegria, M., Green, J. G., McLaughlin, K. A., & Loder, S. (2015). *Disparities in child and adolescent mental health and mental health services in the US* (p. 26). William T. Grant Foundation.

Anderson, L. M., Scrimshaw, S. C., Fullilove, M. T., Fielding, J. E., Normand, J., & Task Force on Community Preventive Services. (2003). Culturally competent healthcare systems. A systematic review. *American Journal of Preventive Medicine, 24*(3 Suppl), 68–79. https://doi.org/10.1016/S0749-3797(02)00657-8

Ash, T., Bowling, A., Davison, K., & Garcia, J. (2017). Physical activity interventions for children with social, emotional, and behavioral disabilities – A systematic review. *Journal of Developmental and Behavioral Pediatrics, 38*(6), 431–445. https://doi.org/10.1097/DBP.0000000000000452

Atkins, M. S., Cappella, E., Shernoff, E. S., Mehta, T. G., & Gustafson, E. L. (2017). Schooling and children's mental health: Realigning resources to reduce disparities and advance public health. *Annual Review of Clinical Psychology, 13*, 123–147. https://doi.org/10.1146/annurev-clinpsy-032816-045234

Avila, R. M., & Bramlett, M. D. (2013). Language and immigrant status effects on disparities in Hispanic children's health status and access to health care. *Maternal and Child Health Journal, 17*(3), 415–423. https://doi.org/10.1007/s10995-012-0988-9

Azzi-Lessing, L. (2010). Meeting the mental health needs of poor and vulnerable children in early care and education programs. *Early Childhood Research & Practice, 12*(1), 1–14. https://eric.ed.gov/?id=EJ889716

Ballentine, K. L. (2019). Understanding racial differences in diagnosing ODD versus ADHD using critical race theory. *Families in Society, 100*(3), 282–292. https://doi.org/10.1177/1044389419842

Bandura, A., & Adams, N. E. (1977). Analysis of self-efficacy theory of behavioral change. *Cognitive Therapy and Research, 1*(4), 287–310. https://doi.org/10.1007/BF01663995

Berkel, C., Mauricio, A. M., Rudo-Stern, J., Dishion, T. J., & Smith, J. D. (2021). Motivational interviewing and caregiver engagement in the family check-up 4 health. *Prevention Science, 22*, 737–746. https://doi.org/10.1007/s11121-020-01112-8

Bethell, C., Jones, J., Gombojav, N., Linkenbach, J., & Sege, R. (2019). Positive childhood experiences and adult mental and relational health in a statewide sample: Associations across adverse childhood experiences levels. *JAMA Pediatrics, 173*(11), e193007. https://doi.org/10.1001/jamapediatrics.2019.3007

Bigfoot, D. S., & Funderburk, B. W. (2011). Honoring children, making relatives: The cultural translation of parent-child interaction therapy for American Indian and Alaska native families. *Journal of Psychoactive Drugs, 43*(4), 309–318. https://doi.org/10.1080/02791072.2011.628924

Bitsko, R. H., Claussen, A. H., Lichstein, J., Black, L. I., Jones, S. E., Danielson, M. L., Hoenig, J. M., Davis Jack, S. P., Brody, D. J., Gyawali, S., Maenner, M. J., Warner, M., Holland, K. M., Perou, R., Crosby, A. E., Blumberg, S. J., Avenevoli, S., Kaminski, J. W., Ghandour, R. M., & Contributor. (2022). Mental health surveillance among children – United States, 2013–2019. *MMWR Supplements, 71*(2), 1–42. https://doi.org/10.15585/mmwr.su7102a1

Blizzard, A. M., Glos, L. J., Stephan, S. H., Medoff, D., & Slade, E. P. (2017). Impacts of a Medicaid wraparound model demonstration program on youth specialty mental health services use. *Journal of Behavioral Health Services & Research, 44*, 373–385. https://doi.org/10.1007/s11414-016-9520-0

Bonilla, A. G., Pourat, N., Chuang, E., Ettner, S., Zima, B., Chen, X., ... & Sripipatana, A. (2021). *Mental health staffing at HRSA-funded health centers may improve access to care. Psychiatric Services, 72*(9), 1018-1025.

Butler, A. M., & Rodgers, C. R. R. (2019). Developing a policy brief on child mental health disparities to promote strategies for advancing equity among racial/ethnic minority youth. *Ethnicity & Disease, 29*(Suppl 2), 421–426. https://doi.org/10.18865/ed.29.S2.421

Candelaria, M., Latta, L., Afkinich, J., Wasserman, K. S., Kane, A., Shivers, E. M., & Gal-Szabo, D. (2021). Maryland's infant and early childhood mental health consultation equity efforts. *Journal of Ethnic & Cultural Diversity in Social Work*. https://doi.org/10.1080/15313204.2021.2001403

Cassidy, J., Brett, B. E., Gross, J. T., Stern, J. A., Martin, D. R., Mohr, J. J., & Woodhouse, S. S. (2017). Circle of security-parenting: A randomized controlled trial in Head Start. *Development and Psychopathology, 29*(2), 651–673. https://doi.org/10.1017/S0954579417000244

Center for Excellence for Infant and Early Childhood Mental Health Consultation. (2020). Retrieved from https://www.samhsa.gov/early-childhood-mental-health-programs/center-of-excellence-iecmh

Chaffin, M., Hecht, D., Bard, D., Silovsky, J. F., & Beasley, W. H. (2012). A statewide trial of the SafeCare homebased services model with parents in Child Protective Services. *Pediatrics, 129*(3), 509–515.

Chazan-Cohen, R., Ayoub, C., Pan, B. A., Roggman, L., Raikes, H., McKelvey, L., et al. (2007). It takes time: Impacts of Early Head Start that lead to reductions in maternal depression two years later. *Infant Mental Health Journal, 28*(2), 151–170. https://doi.org/10.1002/imhj.20127

Chow, J. C., Jaffee, K., & Snowden, L. (2003). Racial/ethnic disparities in the use of mental health services in poverty areas. *American Journal of Public Health, 93*(5), 792–797. https://doi.org/10.2105/ajph.93.5.792

Chu, W., Wippold, G., & Becker, K. D. (2022). A systematic review of cultural competence trainings for mental health providers. *Professional Psychology: Research and Practice, 53*(4), 362.

Coker, T. R., Elliott, M. N., Toomey, S. L., Schwebel, D. C., Cuccaro, P., Tortolero Emery, S., Davies, S. L., Visser, S. N., & Schuster, M. A. (2016). Racial and ethnic disparities in ADHD diagnosis and treatment. *Pediatrics, 138*(3), e20160407. https://doi.org/10.1542/peds.2016-0407

Comer, J. S., Furr, J. M., Miguel, E. M., Cooper-Vince, C. E., Carpenter, A. L., Elkins, R. M., Kerns, C. E., Cornacchio, D., Chou, T., Coxe, S., DeSerisy, M., Sanchez, A. L., Golik, A., Martin, J., Myers, K. M., & Chase, R. (2017). Remotely delivering real-time parent training to the home: An initial randomized trial of Internet-delivered parent-child interaction therapy (I-PCIT). *Journal of Consulting and Clinical Psychology, 85*(9), 909–917. https://doi.org/10.1037/ccp0000230

Conroy, M. A., & Brown, W. H. (2004). Early identification, prevention, and early intervention with young children at risk for emotional or behavioral disorders: Issues, trends, and a call for action. *Behavioral Disorders, 29*(3), 224–236. https://doi.org/10.1177/019874290402900303

Conroy, M. A., Sutherland, K. S., Algina, J., Wilson, R., Martinez, J., & Whalon, K. (2015). Measuring teacher implementation of the BEST in CLASS intervention program and corollary child outcomes. *Journal of Emotional and Behavioral Disorders, 23*(3), 144–155. https://doi.org/10.1177/1063426614532949

Cree, R. A., Bitsko, R. H., Robinson, L. R., Holbrook, J. R., Danielson, M. L., Smith, C., Kaminski, J. W., Kenney, M. K., & Peacock, G. (2018). Health care, family, and community factors associated with mental, behavioral, and developmental disorders and poverty among children aged 2–8 years – United States, 2016. *MMWR. Morbidity and Mortality Weekly Report, 67*(50), 1377–1383. https://doi.org/10.15585/mmwr.mm6750a1

Cunningham, C. E., Bremner, R., & Boyle, M. (1995). Large group community-based parenting programs for families of preschoolers at risk for disruptive behaviour disorders: Utilization, cost effectiveness, and outcome. *Journal of Child Psychology and Psychiatry, and Allied Disciplines, 36*(7), 1141–1159. https://doi.org/10.1111/j.1469-7610.1995.tb01362.x

Dakof, G. A., Quille, T. J., Tejeda, M. J., Alberga, L. R., Bandstra, E., & Szapocznik, J. (2003). Enrolling and retaining mothers of substance-exposed infants in drug abuse treatment. *Journal of Consulting and Clinical Psychology, 71*(4), 764–772. https://doi.org/10.1037/0022-006x.71.4.764

Dishion, T. J., & Stormshak, E. A. (2007). *Intervening in children's lives: An ecological, family centered approach to mental health care*. American Psychological Association.

Dodge, K. A. (2018). Toward population impact from early childhood psychological interventions. *American Psychologist, 73*(9), 1117–1129. https://doi.org/10.1037/amp0000393

Dodge, K. A., & Goodman, W. B. (2019). Universal reach at birth: Family connects. *The Future of Children, 29*(1), 41–60. https://www.jstor.org/stable/26639555

Dodge, K. A., Goodman, W. B., Bai, Y., Best, D. L., Rehder, P., & Hill, S. (2022). Impact of a universal perinatal home-visiting program on reduction in race disparities in maternal and child health: Two randomised controlled trials and a field quasi-experiment. *Lancet Regional Health–Americas, 15*, 100356. https://doi.org/10.1016/j.lana.2022.100356

Domitrovich, C. E., Cortes, R. C., & Greenberg, M. T. (2007). Improving young children's social and emotional competence: A randomized trial of the preschool "PATHS" curriculum. *Journal of Primary Prevention, 28*(2), 67–91. https://doi.org/10.1007/s10935-007-0081-0

Downer, J. T., Williford, A. P., Bulotsky-Shearer, R. J., Vitiello, V. E., Bouza, J., Reilly, S., & Lhospital, A. (2018). Using data-driven, video-based early childhood consultation with teachers to reduce children's challenging behaviors and improve engagement in preschool classrooms. *School Mental Health, 10*, 226–242. https://doi.org/10.1007/s12310-017-9237-0

Dozier, M., & Bernard, K. (2019). *Coaching parents of vulnerable infants: The attachment and biobehavioral catchup approach.* Guilford Publications.

Durkin, M. S., Maenner, M. J., Baio, J., Christensen, D., Daniels, J., Fitzgerald, R., Imm, P., Lee, L. C., Schieve, L. A., Van Naarden Braun, K., Wingate, M. S., & Yeargin-Allsopp, M. (2017). Autism spectrum disorder among US children (2002–2010): Socioeconomic, racial, and ethnic disparities. *American Journal of Public Health, 107*(11), 1818–1826. https://doi.org/10.2105/AJPH.2017.304032

Fox, L., & Hemmeter, M. L. (2009). A programwide model for supporting social emotional development and addressing challenging behavior in early childhood settings. In W. Sailor, G. Dunlop, G. Sugai, & R. Horner (Eds.), *Handbook of positive behavior support* (pp. 177–202). Springer. https://doi.org/10.1007/978-0-387-09632-2_8

Fraser, M. E. (2006). Child mental health policy: Promise without fulfillment? In J. M. Jenson & M. W. Fraser (Eds.), *Social policy for children and families: A risk and resilience perspective* (pp. 93–130). Sage.

García Coll, C., & Garrido, M. (2000). Minorities in the United States: Sociocultural context for mental health and developmental psychopathology. In A. J. Sameroff, M. Lewis, & S. M. Miller

(Eds.), *Handbook of developmental psychopathology* (pp. 177–195). Kluwer Academic Publishers. https://doi.org/10.1007/978-1-4615-4163-9_10

García Coll, C., Lamberty, G., Jenkins, R., McAdoo, H. P., Crnic, K., Wasik, B. H., & Garcia, H. V. (1996). An integrative model for the study of developmental competencies in minority children. *Child Development, 67*(5), 1891–1914. https://doi.org/10.2307/1131600

Garvey, C., Julion, W., Fogg, L., Kratovil, A., & Gross, D. (2006). Measuring participation in a prevention trial with parents of young children. *Research in Nursing & Health, 29*(3), 212–222. https://doi.org/10.1002/nur.20127

Ghandour, R. M., Sherman, L. J., Vladutiu, C. J., Ali, M. M., Lynch, S. E., Bitsko, R. H., & Blumberg, S. J. (2019). Prevalence and treatment of depression, anxiety, and conduct problems in US children. *Journal of Pediatrics, 206*, 256–267. https://doi.org/10.1016/j.jpeds.2018.09.021

Gomby, D. S. (2000). Promise and limitations of home visitation. *JAMA, 284*(11), 1430–1431. https://doi.org/10.1001/jama.284.11.1430

González, M. J. (2005). Access to mental health services: The struggle of poverty affected urban children of color. *Child & Adolescent Social Work Journal, 22*(3–4), 245–256. https://doi.org/10.1007/s10560-005-0036-3

Goodman, W. B., O'Donnell, K., Murphy, R. A., & Dodge, K. A. (2019). Moving beyond program to population impact: Toward a universal early childhood system of care. *Journal of Family Theory & Review, 11*(1), 112–126. https://doi.org/10.1111/jftr.12302

Gopalan, G., Acri, M., Lalayants, M., Hooley, C., & Einbinder, E. (2014). Child welfare involved caregiver perceptions of family support in child mental health treatment. *Journal of Family Strengths, 14*(1), 1–25. Downloaded from https://www.ncbi.nlm.nih.gov/pmc/articles/PMC4351812/pdf/nihms-664148.pdf

Green, B. L., Ayoub, C., Bartlett, J. D., Von Ende, A., Furrer, C., Chazan-Cohen, R., Vallotton, C., & Klevens, J. (2014a). The effect of Early Head Start on child welfare system involvement: A first look at longitudinal child maltreatment outcomes. *Children and Youth Services Review, 42*, 127–135. https://doi.org/10.1016/j.childyouth.2014.03.044

Green, B. L., Tarte, J. M., Harrison, P. M., Nygren, M., & Sanders, M. B. (2014b). Results from a randomized trial of the healthy families Oregon accredited statewide program: Early program impacts on parenting. *Children and Youth Services Review, 44*, 288–298. https://doi.org/10.1016/j.childyouth.2014.06.006

Gross, D., Julion, W., & Fogg, L. (2001). What motivates participation and dropout among low-income urban families of color in a prevention intervention? *Family Relations: An Interdisciplinary Journal of Applied Family Studies, 50*(3), 246–254. https://doi.org/10.1111/j.1741-3729.2001.00246.x

Grote, N. K., Zuckoff, A., Swartz, H., Bledsoe, S. E., & Geibel, S. (2007). Engaging women who are depressed and economically disadvantaged in mental health treatment. *Social Work, 52*(4), 295–308. https://doi.org/10.1093/sw/52.4.295

Grote, N. K., Bridge, J. A., Gavin, A. R., Melville, J. L., Iyengar, S., & Katon, W. J. (2010). A meta-analysis of depression during pregnancy and the risk of preterm birth, low birth weight, and intrauterine growth restriction. *Archives of General Psychiatry, 67*(10), 1012–1024. https://doi.org/10.1001/archgenpsychiatry.2010.111

Gurwitch, R. H., Salem, H., Nelson, M. M., & Comer, J. S. (2020). Leveraging parent-child interaction therapy and telehealth capacities to address the unique needs of young children during the COVID-19 public health crisis. *Psychological Trauma: Theory, Research, Practice and Policy, 12*(S1), S82–S84. https://doi.org/10.1037/tra0000863

Haine-Schlagel, R., & Walsh, N. E. (2015). A review of parent participation engagement in child and family mental health treatment. *Clinical Child and Family Psychology Review, 18*(2), 133–150. https://doi.org/10.1007/s10567-015-0182-x

Health Resources and Services Administration. (2023). *The Maternal, Infant, and Early Childhood Home Visiting Program Brief.* Retrieved on 5/2023 from https://mchb.hrsa.gov/sites/default/files/mchb/about-us/program-brief.pdf

Hernandez, M., Nesman, T., Mowery, D., Acevedo-Polakovich, I. D., & Callejas, L. M. (2009). Cultural competence: A literature review and conceptual model for mental health services. *Psychiatric Services (Washington, DC), 60*(8), 1046–1050. https://doi.org/10.1176/ps.2009.60.8.1046

Huang, L., Stroul, B., Friedman, R., Mrazek, P., Friesen, B., Pires, S., & Mayberg, S. (2005). Transforming mental health care for children and their families. *American Psychologist, 60*(6), 615–627. https://doi.org/10.1037/0003-066X.60.6.615

Huang, K. Y., Calzada, E., Cheng, S., & Brotman, L. M. (2012). Physical and mental health disparities among young children of Asian immigrants. *Journal of Pediatrics, 160*(2), 331–336.e1. https://doi.org/10.1016/j.jpeds.2011.08.005

Iruka, I. U., Cabrera, N., & Páez, M. (2022). Supporting and engaging with diverse families during the early years: Emerging approaches that matter for children and families. *Early Childhood Research Quarterly, 60*, 390–393.

Jones Harden, B., & Slopen, N. (2022). Inequitable experiences and outcomes in young children: Addressing racial and social-economic disparities in physical and mental health. *Annual Review of Developmental Psychology, 4*, 133–159. https://doi.org/10.1146/annurev-devpsych-121020-031515

Jones Harden, B., Martoccio, T. L., & Berlin, L. J. (2021). Maternal psychological risk moderates the impacts of attachment-based intervention on mother-toddler mutuality and toddler behavior problems: A randomized controlled trial. *Prevention Science*, 1–12. https://doi.org/10.1007/s11121-021-01281-0

Kerr, M. E., & Bowen, M. (1988). *Family evaluation: An approach based on Bowen theory*. W. W. Norton & Company.

Klawetter, S., Glaze, K., Sward, A., & Frankel, K. A. (2021). Warm connections: Integration of infant mental health services into WIC. *Community Mental Health Journal, 57*(6), 1130–1141. https://doi.org/10.1007/s10597-020-00744-y

Knitzer, J., & Cohen, E. (2007). Promoting resilience in young children and families at the highest risk: The challenge for early childhood mental health. In D. F. Perry, R. K. Kaufmann, & J. Knitzer (Eds.), *Social and emotional health in early childhood: Building bridges between services and systems* (pp. 335–359). Paul H. Brookes Publishing Co.

Kristie Brandt, C. N. M., Perry, B. D., Stephen Seligman, D. M. H., & Tronick, E. (Eds.). (2013). *Infant and early childhood mental health: Core concepts and clinical practice*. American Psychiatric Publishing. https://doi.org/10.1176/appi.books.9781585625291

Kurz, B. (2008). Depression and mental-health service utilization among women in WIC. *Journal of Ethnic & Cultural Diversity in Social Work, 14*(3–4), 81–102. https://doi.org/10.1300/J051v14n03_05

Lê Cook, B., Barry, C. L., & Busch, S. H. (2013). Racial/ethnic disparity trends in children's mental health care access and expenditures from 2002 to 2007. *Health Services Research, 48*(1), 129–149. https://doi.org/10.1111/j.1475-6773.2012.01439.x

Lee, K., & Zhang, L. (2022). Cumulative effects of poverty on children's social-emotional development: Absolute poverty and relative poverty. *Community Mental Health Journal, 58*(5), 930–943. https://doi.org/10.1007/s10597-021-00901-x

Lee, E., Kirkland, K., Miranda-Julian, C., & Greene, R. (2018). Reducing maltreatment recurrence through home visitation: A promising intervention for child welfare involved families. *Child Abuse & Neglect, 86*, 55–66. https://doi.org/10.1016/j.chiabu.2018.09.004

Lieberman, A. F., & Van Horn, P. (2008). *Psychotherapy with infants and young children: Repairing the effects of stress and trauma on early attachment*. The Guilford Press.

Lieneman, C. C., Brabson, L. A., Highlander, A., Wallace, N. M., & McNeil, C. B. (2017). Parent–child interaction therapy: Current perspectives. *Psychology Research and Behavior Management, 10*, Article 239–256. https://doi.org/10.2147/PRBM.S91200

Lowell, D. I., Carter, A. S., Godoy, L., Paulicin, B., & Briggs-Gowan, M. J. (2011). A randomized controlled trial of child FIRST: A comprehensive home-based intervention translat-

ing research into early childhood practice. *Child Development, 82*(1), 193–208. https://doi.org/10.1111/j.1467-8624.2010.01550.x
McCabe, K. M. (2002). Factors that predict premature termination among Mexican-American children in outpatient psychotherapy. *Journal of Child and Family Studies, 11*, 347–359. https://doi.org/10.1023/A:1016876224388
McCabe, K., & Yeh, M. (2009). Parent-child interaction therapy for Mexican Americans: A randomized clinical trial. *Journal of Clinical Child and Adolescent Psychology, 38*(5), 753–759. https://doi.org/10.1080/15374410903103544
McCabe, K., Yeh, M., Lau, A., & Argote, C. B. (2012). Parent-child interaction therapy for Mexican Americans: Results of a pilot randomized clinical trial at follow-up. *Behavior Therapy, 43*(3), 606–618. https://doi.org/10.1016/j.beth.2011.11.001
McGuire, T. G., Alegria, M., Cook, B. L., Wells, K. B., & Zaslavsky, A. M. (2006). Implementing the Institute of Medicine definition of disparities: An application to mental health care. *Health Services Research, 41*(5), 1979–2005. https://doi.org/10.1111/j.1475-6773.2006.00583.x
McKay, M. M., & Bannon, W. M., Jr. (2004). Engaging families in child mental health services. *Child and Adolescent Psychiatric Clinics, 13*(4), 905–921. https://doi.org/10.1016/j.chc.2004.04.001
Merikangas, K. R., He, J. P., Brody, D., Fisher, P. W., Bourdon, K., & Koretz, D. S. (2010). Prevalence and treatment of mental disorders among US children in the 2001–2004 NHANES. *Pediatrics, 125*(1), 75–81. https://doi.org/10.1542/peds.2008-2598
Mersky, J. P., Janczewski, C. E., Lee, C. P., & Yasin, T. (2022). Impact of home visiting programs on parenting stress in low-income women: Findings from a community-based trial at an urban health department. *Children and Youth Services Review, 142*, 106638. https://doi.org/10.1016/j.childyouth.2022.106638
Michalopoulos, C., Faucetta, K., Hill, C. J., Portilla, X. A., Burrell, L., Lee, H., et al. (2019). Impacts on family outcomes of evidence-based early childhood home visiting: Results from the mother and infant home visiting program evaluation. *Research, and Evaluation, Administration for Children and Families, US Department of Health and Human Services, 7*.
Miller, W. R., & Rollnick, S. (2002). *Motivational interviewing: Preparing people for change*. Guilford Press.
Molnar, B. E., Lees, K. E., Roper, K., Byars, N., Méndez-Peñate, L., Moulin, C., McMullen, W., Wolfe, J., & Allen, D. (2018). Enhancing early childhood mental health primary care services: Evaluation of MA project LAUNCH. *Maternal and Child Health Journal, 22*(10), 1502–1510. https://doi.org/10.1007/s10995-018-2548-4
Morrissey-Kane, E., & Prinz, R. J. (1999). Engagement in child and adolescent treatment: The role of parental cognitions and attributions. *Clinical Child and Family Psychology Review, 2*(3), 183–198. https://doi.org/10.1023/a:1021807106455
Nation, M., Crusto, C., Wandersman, A., Kumpfer, K. L., Seybolt, D., Morrissey-Kane, E., & Davino, K. (2003). What works in prevention. Principles of effective prevention programs. *American Psychologist, 58*(6–7), 449–456. https://doi.org/10.1037/0003-066x.58.6-7.449
Niec, L. N., Barnett, M. L., Prewett, M. S., & Shanley Chatham, J. R. (2016). Group parent-child interaction therapy: A randomized control trial for the treatment of conduct problems in young children. *Journal of Consulting and Clinical Psychology, 84*(8), 682–698. https://doi.org/10.1037/a0040218
Nix, R. L., Bierman, K. L., McMahon, R. J., & Conduct Problems Prevention Research Group. (2009). How attendance and quality of participation affect treatment response to parent management training. *Journal of Consulting and Clinical Psychology, 77*(3), 429–438. https://doi.org/10.1037/a0015028
Office of the Surgeon General (OSG). (2021). *Protecting youth mental health: The U.S. Surgeon General's Advisory*. US Department of Health and Human Services.
Olds, D. L. (2006). The nurse-family partnership: An evidence-based preventive intervention. *Infant Mental Health Journal, 27*(1), 5–25. https://doi.org/10.1002/imhj.20077

Oxford, M. L., Spieker, S. J., Lohr, M. J., & Fleming, C. B. (2016). Promoting First Relationships®: Randomized trial of a 10-week home visiting program with families referred to child protective services. *Child Maltreatment, 21*(4), 267–277.

Paradies, Y., Ben, J., Denson, N., Elias, A., Priest, N., Pieterse, A., Gupta, A., Kelaher, M., & Gee, G. (2015). Racism as a determinant of health: A systematic review and meta-analysis. *PLoS One, 10*(9), e0138511. https://doi.org/10.1371/journal.pone.0138511

Pidano, A. E., Segool, N. K., Delgado, N., Forness, K., Hagen, K., Gurganus, E. A., Honigfeld, L., Hess, C., Hicks, A., & Morgan, C. (2020). Parent perceptions of pediatric primary care providers' mental health–related communication and practices. *Journal of Pediatric Health Care, 34*(5), e49–e58. https://doi.org/10.1016/j.pedhc.2020.04.009

Prinz, R. J., Sanders, M. R., Shapiro, C. J., Whitaker, D. J., & Lutzker, J. R. (2009). Population-based prevention of child maltreatment: The U.S. triple p system population trial. *Prevention Science, 10*(1), 1–12. https://doi.org/10.1007/s11121-009-0123-3

Ramphal, B., Whalen, D. J., Kenley, J. K., Yu, Q., Smyser, C. D., Rogers, C. E., & Sylvester, C. M. (2020). Brain connectivity and socioeconomic status at birth and externalizing symptoms at age 2 years. *Developmental Cognitive Neuroscience, 45*, 100811. https://doi.org/10.1016/j.dcn.2020.100811

Reardon, T., Harvey, K., Baranowska, M., O'Brien, D., Smith, L., & Creswell, C. (2017). What do parents perceive are the barriers and facilitators to accessing psychological treatment for mental health problems in children and adolescents? A systematic review of qualitative and quantitative studies. *European Child & Adolescent Psychiatry, 26*(6), 623–647. https://doi.org/10.1007/s00787-016-0930-6

Reiss, F. (2013). Socioeconomic inequalities and mental health problems in children and adolescents: A systematic review. *Social Science & Medicine, 90*, 24–31. https://doi.org/10.1016/j.socscimed.2013.04.026

Reyes, C. R., & Gilliam, W. S. (2021). Addressing challenging behaviors in challenging environments: Findings from Ohio's early childhood mental health consultation system. *Development and Psychopathology, 33*(2), 634–646. https://doi.org/10.1017/S0954579420001790

Rodgers, C. R. R., Flores, M. W., Bassey, O., Augenblick, J. M., & Cook, B. L. (2022). Racial/ethnic disparity trends in children's mental health care access and expenditures from 2010–2017: Disparities remain despite sweeping policy reform. *Journal of the American Academy of Child and Adolescent Psychiatry, 61*(7), 915–925. https://doi.org/10.1016/j.jaac.2021.09.420

Sama-Miller, E., Akers, L., Mraz-Esposito, A., Coughlin, R., & Zukiewicz, M. (2017). *Home visiting evidence of effectiveness review: Executive summary*. Mathematica Policy Research. https://www.acf.hhs.gov/opre/report/home-visiting-evidence-effectiveness-review-executive-summary-brief-september-2017

Sameroff, A. J., & Seifer, R. (2021). Accumulation of environmental risk and child mental health. In *Children of poverty* (pp. 233–258). Routledge.

Sanders, M. R., Kirby, J. N., Tellegen, C. L., & Day, J. J. (2014). The triple P-positive parenting program: A systematic review and meta-analysis of a multi-level system of parenting support. *Clinical Psychology Review, 34*(4), 337–357. https://doi.org/10.1016/j.cpr.2014.04.003

Santiago, C. D., Kaltman, S., & Miranda, J. (2013). Poverty and mental health: How do low-income adults and children fare in psychotherapy? *Journal of Clinical Psychology, 69*(2), 115–126. https://doi.org/10.1002/jclp.21951

Sarche, M. C., Spicer, P., Farrell, P., & Fitzgerald, H. E. (Eds.). (2011). *American Indian and Alaska native children and mental health: Development, context, prevention, and treatment*. Praeger/ABC-CLIO.

Shivers, E. M., Farago, F., & Gal-Szabo, D. E. (2022). The role of infant and early childhood mental health consultation in reducing racial and gender relational and discipline disparities between black and white preschoolers. *Psychology in the Schools, 59*(10), 1965–1983. https://doi.org/10.1002/pits.22573

Sitnick, S. L., Shaw, D. S., Gill, A., Dishion, T., Winter, C., Waller, R., Gardner, F., & Wilson, M. (2015). Parenting and the family check-up: Changes in observed parent-child interaction following early childhood intervention. *Journal of Clinical Child and Adolescent Psychology, 44*(6), 970–984. https://doi.org/10.1080/15374416.2014.940623

Smith, J. D., Berkel, C., Rudo-Stern, J., Montaño, Z., St George, S. M., Prado, G., Mauricio, A. M., Chiapa, A., Bruening, M. M., & Dishion, T. J. (2018). The Family Check-Up 4 Health (FCU4Health): Applying implementation science frameworks to the process of adapting an evidence-based parenting program for prevention of pediatric obesity and excess weight gain in primary care. *Frontiers in Public Health, 6*, 293. https://doi.org/10.3389/fpubh.2018.00293

Snell-Johns, J., Mendez, J. L., & Smith, B. H. (2004). Evidence-based solutions for overcoming access barriers, decreasing attrition, and promoting change with underserved families. *Journal of Family Psychology, 18*(1), 19–35. https://doi.org/10.1037/0893-3200.18.1.19

Stanley, L. (2019). Is the preschool PATHS curriculum effective? A review. *Journal of Evidence-Based Social Work, 16*(2), 130–143. https://doi.org/10.1080/23761407.2018.1558141

Stevens, J., Kelleher, K. J., Ward-Estes, J., & Hayes, J. (2006). Perceived barriers to treatment and psychotherapy attendance in child community mental health centers. *Community Mental Health Journal, 42*(5), 449–458. https://doi.org/10.1007/s10597-006-9048-5

Sutherland, K. S., Conroy, M. A., & Granger, K. (2020). BEST in CLASS: A tier-2 program for children with and at-risk for emotional/behavioral disorders. In T. W. Farmer, M. A. Conroy, E. M. Z. Farmer, & K. Sutherland (Eds.), *Handbook of research on emotional and behavioral disorders* (pp. 214–227). Routledge.

Thomas, R., Abell, B., Webb, H. J., Avdagic, E., & Zimmer-Gembeck, M. J. (2017). Parent-child interaction therapy: A meta-analysis. *Pediatrics, 140*(3), e20170352. https://doi.org/10.1542/peds.2017-0352

Viale-Val, G., Rosenthal, R. H., Curtiss, G., & Marohn, R. C. (1984). Dropout from adolescent psychotherapy: A preliminary study. *Journal of the American Academy of Child Psychiatry, 23*(5), 562–568.

Waid, J., & Kelly, M. (2020). Supporting family engagement with child and adolescent mental health services: A scoping review. *Health & Social Care in the Community, 28*(5), 1333–1342. https://doi.org/10.1111/hsc.12947

Webster-Stratton, C., Reid, M. J., & Hammond, M. (2001). Preventing conduct problems, promoting social competence: A parent and teacher training partnership in head start. *Journal of Clinical Child Psychology, 30*(3), 283–302. https://doi.org/10.1207/S15374424JCCP3003_2

Whitbeck, L. B. (2006). Some guiding assumptions and a theoretical model for developing culturally specific preventions with native American people. *Journal of Community Psychology, 34*(2), 183–192. https://doi.org/10.1002/jcop.20094

Yoshikawa, H., Aber, J. L., & Beardslee, W. R. (2012). The effects of poverty on the mental, emotional, and behavioral health of children and youth: Implications for prevention. *The American Psychologist, 67*(4), 272–284. https://doi.org/10.1037/a0028015

Zeanah, C. H. (Ed.). (2018). *Handbook of infant mental health*. Guilford Publications.

Chapter 10
Future Directions

Jessica Dym Bartlett and Laura Nabors

Many infant and early childhood mental health treatments are effective and offer a good return on our investments (Oppenheim & Bartlett, 2023), but children do not reap the full benefits of treatment when their families are not engaged in and committed to the process (Waid & Kelly, 2020). As we reviewed the information in our book, we noted that there is a broad-brush stroke portrait of family engagement. Similar to Halgunseth (2009), who focused on school engagement, we define family engagement in mental health services for young children broadly. As such, family engagement involves connection, advocacy, and shared decision-making. In order to allow connection, family advocacy should be encouraged, and family input for formulating diagnoses and making decisions about treatment planning and implementation should be a standard of care for mental health practitioners. Treatment planning and intervention should encompass the classroom/school, the agency and program, the home setting, and other entities working with the family to improve their overall well-being, including but not limited to mental health. Moreover, interventions can extend to family and service contexts that are most important and culturally relevant to the child and family, including school, early childhood education, and community services settings. To extend family engagement throughout the child's treatment – beginning with the very first contact with a family – an atmosphere of collaboration, with parents and family as partners and team members, promotes strong family engagement. To enhance collaboration, mental health professionals can borrow tenants from social work, psychology, and other social sciences by fostering an atmosphere of "meeting them where they are" when

J. D. Bartlett
Thriving Together, LLC, West Newton, MA, USA

L. Nabors (✉)
University of Cincinnati, Cincinnati, OH, USA
e-mail: naborsla@ucmail.uc.edu

L. Nabors, J. D. Bartlett (eds.), *Family Engagement in Mental Health Interventions for Young Children*, Springer Series on Child and Family Studies,
https://doi.org/10.1007/978-3-031-47917-5_10

engaging parents and other caregivers and family members in all aspects of treatment planning, engagement, and assessment of progress. This approach necessarily involves a deep appreciation for and responsiveness to family race, ethnicity, socioeconomic conditions, beliefs, worldviews, and values, as well as the cultural reference group(s) for the child and family members (Halgunseth, 2009).

Accordingly, in recent years, program, state, territory, tribal, and federal leaders have begun to make the important distinction between *family involvement* and *family engagement*. Family involvement comprises traditional methods of interacting with families in service settings, including focusing primarily on presenting problems, providing information on parenting and child development, sharing updates on the child's progress in treatment, inviting families to program-led events, and other means of interacting with families that reinforce current program and organizational values and practices. Although these strategies may be well intended, they often lead to a top-down, deficits-based approach that limits a family's voice and choice in their treatment. The absence of shared power and focus on family deficits also undermines a family's confidence, self-efficacy, and trust in the treatment process, particularly among historically minoritized families (Baquedano-Lopez et al., 2013; Ishimaru et al., 2019; Robles-Ramamurthy et al., 2022).

King et al. (2014) assert that there are many definitions of family engagement in the mental health literature and many different ways to assess or measure engagement, which leads to different theoretical orientations and a myriad of findings addressing factors related to engagement in children's mental health services. We agree that this is true, but in taking a strengths-based, trauma-informed stance (King et al., 2014; Substance Abuse and Mental Health Service Administration [SAMHSA], 2014), we view the term family engagement as expanding early approaches to include a wider array of approaches to partnering with families in their child's mental health care. The efforts of providers, and the capability for outreach of the mental health organization and policy, play a vital role in engaging families (Jose et al., 2020). For example, when discussing engagement in school processes, Williams and Baber (2007) highlight the critical nature of trust when engaging African American families. The chapters in this book, which summarize extant literature across young children's developmental stages, race and ethnicity, socioeconomic status, and service settings, clearly show that trust and respect are critical aspects of strong provider-family relationships and the foundation for effective family engagement in mental health services for young children.

Establishing Trust and Collaboration Are Critical to Family Engagement

Family engagement emphasizes shared power between the mental health provider/program and family by positioning the provider as a facilitator rather than leader of treatment. That is, "the goal of family engagement is not to serve clients but to gain partners" (Ferlazzo, 2011, pp. 10–11). Thus, family engagement requires a fundamental shift in the field away from traditional mental health treatment aimed at ameliorating problems toward a strengths-based approach in which treatment goals, activities, and desired outcomes are codeveloped with families, and services are responsive to the racial and ethnic background, gender identity, sexual orientation, assets, and challenges of each family member and the family system. Family engagement also highlights the importance of partnering with families to overcome barriers to accessing treatment, whether due to challenges meeting concrete needs (e.g., health insurance, childcare, transportation), stigma, lack of alignment between family culture and the treatment modality, or personal and cultural beliefs and values that prevent parents and other caregivers from seeking help for their child. As defined by the US Department of Health and Human Services (2018):

> Family engagement is an interactive process through which program staff and families, family members, and their children build positive and goal-oriented relationships. It is a shared responsibility of families and professionals that requires mutual respect for the roles and strengths each has to offer. Family engagement means doing with – not doing to or for – families. At the program level, family engagement involves parents' engagement with their children and with staff as they work together toward the goals that families choose for themselves and their children. It also involves families and staff working toward goals to improve the program…staff work together with families, other professionals, and community partners in ways that promote equity, inclusiveness, and cultural and linguistic responsiveness. (p. 2)

In a scoping review of key literature, King et al. (2014) reported that mental health providers must also support each family's self-efficacy in the treatment process. Maybery et al. (2021) identified seven practices associated with motivating and engaging families: "(1) identify and acknowledge family and carers; (2) engage and communicate with family and carers; (3) involve family and carers in planning/collaboration in consumer's treatment; (4) assess vulnerable family member or carer's needs; (5) provide or offer ongoing support to family and carers; (6) provide psychoeducation to family and carers; and (7) provide or recommend referrals for family and carers" (p. 4). These seven practices show overlap with the steps mentioned by Turnbull et al. (2021) for establishing a trust between the provider and parents or family. In Chapter 4, Malone and her colleagues highlighted Turnbull's principles of respect, fairness (equity), communication, advocacy, and commitment as provider behaviors which are cornerstones for establishing trust in the therapeutic relationship between provider and family. In fact, we believe that combining the aforementioned behaviors with the seven steps for engaging families establishes a family-centered care environment which will promote positive outcomes for the child and promote well-being at the family level.

As Staudt's (2007) framework for family engagement suggests, the attitudes held by providers and their organizations are as consequential as their behaviors. For example, valuing parents, other primary caregivers, and family members (i.e., carers) for what they are – the most important influences in their child's life – is at the heart of family engagement. Relatedly, a provider's expressed interest in and respect for each family's cultural beliefs, values, goals, strengths, and needs is an essential step in making a successful connection or forming a "therapeutic alliance" (Ardito & Rabellino, 2011). Making a commitment to involving and, more than that, engaging them in care through shared decision-making with providers is another key step in engagement. Collaboration to determine the course of interventions is a feature of the shared decision-making that will help tailor interventions to child needs and what parents and family members can do to support the intervention. Providing sufficient, clear, linguistically and culturally appropriate information so that parents and families can make educated choices about their child's treatment and advocate for their needs is another pillar of family engagement.

This relationship-based approach differs considerably from traditional approaches to parent education, in which the "expert" provider offers information and advice to parents, who may be treated as if they are empty vessels awaiting direction rather than as the true experts on their child. Of course, no single intervention can fully address young children's mental health needs, and thus, providing referrals and connecting families to community resources are part of the logistics that can help families overcome barriers and further connect families and mental health providers. All of these beliefs and attitudes must also be aligned with a trauma-informed approach in which the principles upheld include safety; trustworthiness and transparency; peer support; collaboration and mutuality; empowerment, voice, and choice; and cultural, historical, and gender issues (SAMHSA, 2014).

This is a tall task for many reasons, not the least of which is that mental health providers are usually committed to family engagement approaches that reflect the policy and culture of the mental health organization in which they work, for better or worse. The organization itself must be flexible and committed to learning about families from backgrounds that are both similar to and different from their own, ongoing communication with caregivers, and sharing power in decision-making. Other provider qualities include receptivity to feedback, transparency in providing information about child progress and functioning, empathy for the needs and barriers faced by families and the child, and being friendly and approachable should family members have concerns (Jacques & Villegas, 2018).

Connection and Communication to Foster Family Engagement in Mental Health Services

There are many studies examining engagement, and we encourage readers to review research and find what fits for meeting families where they are for their specific services, given the culture of the families they serve. For those in primary care, it may be that a "navigator" will help families to enter the web of mental health services. Godoy et al. (2019) reflected that many children do not receive needed mental health services. They recommended finding a way "in" to services from primary care, proposing that a family navigator could assist parents in traversing the complex and overloaded mental health system. The family navigator is well positioned to address the perceived barriers (e.g., stigma about mental health services, financial concerns) the family has to seeking care and then engaging in the child's therapy and then help the family make appointments and wade through long "wait times" for a child to access a mental health provider and make a first appointment. Similarly, family service workers and infant and early childhood mental health consultants in two-generational programs such as Head Start/Early Head Start serve a key role in helping families navigate the complex and challenging landscape of services related to infant and early childhood mental health. For instance, they link families to community-based resources, refer them to mental health and other services, and support families in crisis (Warren et al., 2023).

Langley et al. (2013) conducted research using focus groups to understand parent perspectives on ways to engage them in trauma-related mental health services offered at schools. Critical factors included education about services and their potential outcomes for youth. Also, providers need to be aware of and committed to communication with parents throughout the course of service provision. Communication also was a critical factor in Halgunseth's (2009) perspectives on key factors defining engagement. Understanding family culture and needs can improve communication and guide providers so that they can provide education that counts and can be absorbed by families (Halgunseth, 2009). Considering family needs and concerns and their values can assist providers in meeting the families' needs and in meeting the care needs of the service user, which we define as meeting them where they are.

As highlighted by Hornstein, in his chapter on fathers (in this volume), establishing connections, care, and trust improves engagement of fathers in treatment, and fathers are essential to child development in many ways, such as providing social support through sensitive and critical play with the child (Grossmann et al., 2002). Fathers also teach the child structure and social rules as they provide discipline and transmit cultural mores to their children even while they are working to actively disrupt gender stereotypes associated with parenting (Miller, 2011; O'Connell, 2005). Dr. Hornstein provides several strategies for enhancing trust to engage fathers, including a commitment to involving fathers, scheduling sessions after work or on weekends, and targeting fathers' ideas for care during treatment (Tully et al., 2017). His treatment recommendations including finding opportunities for fathers to spend quality time engaging with their child at home can also promote the child's functioning and contribute to the success of therapeutic interventions (Ellis et al., 2014).

Understanding what factors facilitate communication in different circumstances for children of different ages also may foster family engagement and positive outcomes for the child. For instance, in terms of engaging families of children with chronic illnesses, Nabors and her colleagues (this volume) mention using a family systems approach (e.g., Balling & McCubbin, 2001) to communication with the family and key players in the child's life. At the same time, it is important to understand the interconnections among family members to match recommendations to the needs of the family members and the child, with these interconnections in mind (Knafl et al., 2017). There are several areas for related future research, including determining what communication works in different contexts and with intervention goals for the child. For instance, if the goal is improving academic performance, then factors enhancing communication between the family, medical team, and teachers, such as having regular meetings to discuss the child's medical and academic progress, become important. Considering the illness type, course, and treatment is important as well. For example, it may be critical to assess academic performance to determine if cognitive changes are influencing the academic performance of young children with different types of cancer with varying treatment courses, who were diagnosed at different ages, who are experiencing late effects related to chemotherapy treatments (Armstrong et al., 1999; Erdmann et al., 2021).

On the other hand, aspects of communication that influence adherence to medical recommendations, such as interventions to improve parent health literacy, may be critical to engaging families, especially when parents are having difficulty understanding instructions provided by the medical team (DiMatteo, 2004). Adherence to medical recommendations could also be impacted by misreading interconnections among family members – if a child has diabetes and must test herself, which involves needle sticks, and has a fear of needles shared by her mother, it may not be advantageous to ask her mother to help with these checks, especially if her father is comfortable with taking on this role and has a strong connection with his child to help him soothe her fears. At the same time, health and mental health professionals need to consider the developmental stage of the child (Berk & Meyers, 2016). In the case of the youngster with diabetes, coaching might be very different for a young preschooler, using the "Tell, Show, Do" method, which involves telling the child about the procedure, demonstrating it, and then conducting the procedure (Dahlquist, 1997). Conversely, a child in early elementary school may benefit from learning relaxation skills and could discuss the procedure with her father, and he would not necessarily have to demonstrate the procedure to the child (dos Santos Felix et al., 2019). Health and mental health professionals need to be aware of factors impacting communication to engage families and children. The same factors could influence teachers' recommendations – family interconnections determine who the child turns to for advice on homework or for listening about how to improve classroom behaviors. Conducting research to increase knowledge about factors impacting communication and family engagement will advance the field, spurring better connections to engage families and children in clinical practice.

Family Engagement Leads to Successful Outcomes

Family engagement in mental health interventions for young children and their caregivers is critical to successful treatment outcomes in both generations (Walter et al., 2019). Research has firmly established the importance of family engagement in a range of service settings for young children, their families, and the programs with whom they work, including but not limited to behavioral health, early childhood education, schools, Head Start/Early Head Start, early intervention, child welfare, home visiting, medical settings, and parenting/fatherhood programs (Henderson & Mapp, 2002; Ingoldsby, 2010). For example, high-quality family engagement is associated with improved social, behavioral, and emotional functioning for children and their families (Podell & Kendall, 2011) and higher student achievement and fewer child behavior problems in school (Smith et al., 2013; Van Voorhis et al., 2013). In addition, when respectfully and actively engaged, families develop more self-efficacy, confidence, and skills (Green et al., 2007; Hoover-Dempsey et al., 2005) and are better positioned to help providers and programs identify new ways to build safe and welcoming environments (Powell et al., 2010; Reedy & McGrath, 2010). Conversely, low-quality family engagement limits the success of prevention and intervention programs. This is especially concerning given that many infants, toddlers, and preschoolers never receive the mental health care they need, and 20–80% of families drop out of treatment prematurely (Armbruster & Kazdin, 1994; Gomby, 2000; Masi et al., 2003).

One of the many areas in which engagement is critical is the treatment of young children who have experienced trauma as a result of exposure to adversity (Bartlett et al., 2017). By extension, mental health providers and professionals are also treating the indirect trauma the family experiences or intergenerational trauma, which encompasses the family history of trauma (American Psychological Association, n.d.). It is important to engage the family in treatment to understand and address their own trauma and to partner with them to develop the skills they need for working with the young child who reexperiences and reenacts trauma at home (Child Welfare Information Gateway, 2017). Bartlett also points to the importance of considering family socioeconomic status and health disparities when treating children and families for trauma, which disproportionally affects historically marginalized families due to historical and structural racism and discrimination (Bartlett & Sacks, 2019). Encouraging trust may be especially important for engaging families where the experience of trauma impacts parents and the family unit (Nicholson et al., 2022). In her chapter, Bartlett provides examples of evidence-based treatments, such as Parent-Child Interaction Therapy (Eyberg et al., 1995) and Trauma-Focused Cognitive Behavioral Therapy (Cohen & Mannarino, 2015). When parents and families are engaged in two-generational treatments, children can begin to heal, return to their typical levels of functioning, gain motivation, improve school readiness, increase their social and self-regulation skills, and exhibit higher levels of positive, prosocial behaviors (see Dowell & Ogles, 2010 for a review). Parents learn to understand their young child's challenging behavior as symptoms of trauma exposure ("What's wrong with you versus what happened to you?"), along with skills for successfully managing these behaviors at home, which in turn leads to improved child functioning and well-being, as well as improved parent morale and psychological well-being (Child Welfare Information Gateway, 2017).

In their chapter on children with intellectual and developmental disabilities, Malone and colleagues (this volume) discuss the importance of parents as partners on the treatment team. They write that parents and caregivers of children with special needs in early education programs typically are perceived as active contributors and decision-makers – both during initial assessment and treatment planning processes and throughout the child's intervention processes (Division for Early Childhood, 2014). Malone and colleagues promoted the Sunshine Model (Turnbull et al., 2021; Turnbull & Turnbull, 2022), which identifies parents, siblings, and extended family as partners in the child's care, who help to co-construct interventions and care of the child. For instance, their Sunshine Model is fluid in nature, which helps ensure a family-friendly partnership, allowing for critical team players or members to shift over time according to child and family needs (Turnbull & Turnbull, 2022). The notion of parents and all team members as partners, in the different systems of the young child's life, ensures care of the child in multiple contexts that influence development. As the partners, including professionals, work as a team, their partnership is transdisciplinary, and this team can integrate the many services young children with special needs may need, thereby engaging families and team members as key players facilitating the young child's growth and development (Hernandez, 2013).

Successful outcomes are data for change in policy that will lead to large-scale positive change for children and families – which might be considered a community-, state-, and national-level outcome promoting child development and family flourishing. In their chapter (this volume), Graaf and Sweeney provide many useful ideas for policy change, enacted through collaboration with families as partners, which is supported at systems levels. They recommended that policymakers engage families in the policymaking process by reaching out to organizations like the Family-Run Executive Director Leadership Association (FREDLA, https://www.fredla.org/). This is an association of family-run organizations calling for families to be involved as partners in decision-making at the community, state, and national levels (Stroul et al., 2021). This organization has adapted Carman and colleague's model (Carman et al., 2013) for understanding how to engage families in children's mental health services, emphasizing commitment to and communication with families as partners to develop policy and programs that reflect family-driven care models. To achieve successful programs, families would be integrated into the development, implementation, and evaluation teams. Family members would help in determining therapeutic activities, outcomes to measure, and evaluation and dissemination of results of program evaluations. In this way, families would be engaged throughout the process of care for the child and family, making family-centered care the heart of service provision and evaluation of future goals (Carman et al., 2013). Graaf and Sweeney (this volume) proposed key areas for assessing outcomes including (a) assessment of factors related to continuous quality improvement at the program level (e.g., satisfaction with the intervention, change in family quality of life), (b) child-level change (e.g., academic progress, improvement in mental health), (c) family change (e.g., decreased parent stress, improved family living situation or conditions), (d) systems-level outcomes (e.g., reduced inpatient hospitalizations and out-of-home placements for young children, improved academic readiness for preschool-age children), (e) managed care outcomes (improved child mental health outcomes, improved family quality of life), and (f) community outcomes (e.g., reducing health disparities in access to mental health services, reducing cultural disconnects in service provision, changing stigmatized attitudes to accessing mental health services).

Contemporary research on family engagement highlights the critical importance of integrating lived expertise, including both family and community voice, throughout the planning, treatment, and evaluation of interventions to improve the social and emotional development of young children and their caregivers – a key principle of trauma-informed care ("Empowerment, Voice and Choice;" SAMHSA, 2014, p. 11). It is also consistent with Irving Harris Foundation's Diversity-Informed Tenets for Work with Infants, Children, and Families in that high-quality family engagement honors diverse family structures and recognizes the importance of non-traditional "ways of knowing" when developing, implementing, and evaluating which service approaches are best for which families under which conditions (see https://diversityinformedtenets.org/the-tenets/overview/; https://diversityinformedtenets.org/the-tenets/english/). Diversity-informed practice involves respect for culturally nondominant ways of understanding and dealing with problems and focusing on healing within different families and communities. Relatedly, we believe it is positive that outcomes in the aforementioned areas overlap, and this means that evaluators can provide outcome data across settings by assessing child outcomes, changes in perceptions of participating in mental health services, changes in family living conditions, and reducing health disparities in accessing mental health services for young children and their families. Consequently, families having a "voice" in what interventions would work and help the family and child should be related to positive outcomes, producing successful results in terms of family functioning and child mental health and positive developmental trajectories.

Future Directions

Training the Workforce

Bartlett, Nabors, and Chase (this volume) discuss the importance of training the workforce, including teachers and medical and mental health professionals, to engage families of young children and to promote their growth and development. Providing more education, training, and professional development on the treatment of mental health problems in young children is needed both in graduate and continuing education, as well as workforce training, to ensure the availability of well-trained mental health providers who specialize in treating young children and their families (Kim et al., 2021). Professional development and training to improve professionals' abilities to consult with teachers and parents is needed to help service providers and families in schools and homes, as well training focusing on diversity and culture to engage family members in families who are facing health disparities

(Shivers et al., 2022). Examining training on skills to promote family-centered care and improving knowledge of assisting very young children with mental health problems are two areas of focus for training about consulting and meeting the needs of diverse families in hospital or clinic settings (Smith & Sheridan, 2019; Vilaseca et al., 2019). Training providers in need for parents and family members from different cultures, and developing evidence-based interventions for parents from groups that may face health disparities, such as the "Effective Black Parenting Intervention" (Alvy, 2019 see https://www.dcctf.org/aboutebp), which has already been identified as a promising intervention; see https://preventionservices.acf.hhs.gov/programs/460/show), or Mamás y Bebés (Muñoz et al., 2007), which is available in Spanish, will improve the availability of interventions to engage families from different cultures.

When discussing care of children with intellectual and developmental disabilities (IDD), Malone and her colleagues also emphasize other training needs – for understanding how to work with youngsters with IDD and learning to work with children and family members in low-income families. Understanding how to work with young children with IDD and orienting education and care to needs of their families allow professionals to collaborate with families (incorporating a "whole child-family-engaged approach," advocated by the National Head Start Association; https://nhsa.org/whole-child-whole-family/) to develop treatments that fit within the bounds of their resources (Fadus et al., 2019). Nabors and her colleagues echoed the need to develop care that meets family and child needs, as it has the potential to improve health literacy and family adherence to medical recommendations for families and young children who have chronic medical conditions. Furthermore, research pinpointing needs of those in different cultures and at different family income levels, for children with chronic illnesses or developmental disabilities, will provide new knowledge to reach those who can be underrepresented in terms of receiving mental health services. Within a whole child and whole family approach, children with special needs and children who are developing typically can receive services to engage the child and family (https://nhsa.org/whole-child-whole-family/).

Addressing Health Disparities, Access to Services, and Related Policy

Three factors needed to improve care – addressing disparities, improving access to services, and adding and changing policy – are related but uniquely important. Nguyen and Harden (this volume) point to the continuing health disparities in providing mental health services among low-income families and those in minoritized groups (Butler & Rodgers, 2019; Rodgers et al., 2022). Families living in extreme poverty may face the greatest difficulty in accessing mental health services for their children (Lee & Zhang, 2022; Strohschein & Gauthier, 2018). Linking ideas for policy change to overcome health disparities is important and will help build child and family resilience. Moreover, accessing mental health services may boost child functioning in future years and reduce costs of care. For example, Oppenheim and Bartlett reviewed the benefit-cost literature on infant and early childhood mental health treatment and found that an investment of $1 in mental health prevention yields $1.80–$3.30 in savings in healthcare, education, criminal justice, and labor market expenditures. Moreover, the return on investment (ROI) for evidence-based treatments is encouraging – child-parent psychotherapy has an average ROI of $13.82 per child, and parent-child interaction therapy has an average ROI of $15.11 per child (see https://gucchd.georgetown.edu/Docs/iecmh/Cost-Effectiveness%20of%20Infant%20and%20Early%20Childhood%20Mental%20Health%20Treatment.pdf).

Structural changes can improve access to care and some of these are decreasing costs, improving scheduling to include weekend hours, improving service coordination for youth needing multiple services (e.g., occupational therapy and mental health), providing transportation, and training more providers to address care shortages (Bringewatt & Gershoff, 2010; Garvey et al., 2006; Stevens et al., 2006; Thomas & Holzer, 2006).

Graaf and Sweeney (this volume) provided recommendations for practice to engage families in mental health services. At the program level, conducting strengths and needs assessments for families of color and families residing in poverty might assist in directing administrators and mental health providers to programs that meet family needs and capitalize on their strengths. Once the program is selected, mental health professionals and teachers can engage parents by discussing positive changes that can result from interventions and arranging meetings with parents (at convenient times for the family) to model ideas for implementing interventions. Providing reinforcement for parent and family change efforts and successes and building rapport with families by understanding and accepting cultural differences are critical for all families, to acknowledge growth and promote further engagement. Graaf and Sweeney cite Lindsey et al.'s (2014) research as showing that increasing preparation for, investment in, and knowledge of the treatment process can positively impact adherence to intervention steps and process, resulting in positive outcomes for children and their families treatment (Lindsey et al., 2014).

Additionally, if parents have difficulty engaging in mental health services, providing parent peer support groups or advocates – through mentoring networks or small group – may engage parents in the intervention, use it at home, and potentially experience higher levels of satisfaction with mental health services, leading to more positive outcomes at the child and family levels (Gopalan et al., 2017; Lindsey et al., 2014). We also recommend having family and cultural celebrations – to support change efforts – and program-level celebrations to emphasize the value of family engagement and partnerships and to emphasize the importance of partnering with families from diverse backgrounds. Celebrating the value that families bring to services for young children also communicates that providers and programs have prioritized engagement of all families.

Policymakers can be especially influential in helping infant and early childhood mental health providers and programs to address health disparities and improve access to early childhood mental health services. In light of the multiple challenges to family engagement (e.g., mistrust, power imbalances, family stressors and logistical challenges, implicit bias and structural racism), leveraging policy to advance the field is essential to health and mental health equity. First, federal, state, and local policymakers should consider requiring a high level of cultural competence among all providers whose work brings them into contact with young children and their families. Mandated training in Irving Harris Foundation's Diversity-Informed Tenets for Work with Infants, Children, and Families or similar approaches to family engagement grounded in sociocultural perspectives are one potential approach (https://diversityinformedtenets.org/the-tenets/english/). Policy solutions also are needed to address racial, ethnic, and socioeconomic disparities in mental health access and use. Importantly, all policies with the aim of improving young children's mental health and reducing mental health inequities among minoritized families must be grounded in the empirical literature as well as ongoing, meaningful input from populations served. Family engagement might be increased, for example, by offering sliding fee scales for children's mental health (e.g., Blizzard et al., 2017), transportation and childcare vouchers (e.g., Gopalan et al., 2017), and other services to meet the concrete needs of families with young children including childcare, early intervention, and nutritional supports (Klawetter et al., 2021).

One interesting policy approach is to keep a scorecard to assist programs in tracking family engagement outcomes. Karoly et al. (2001) suggested a policy scorecard to track the benefits of early intervention programs. This scorecard is intended to track key program components (or descriptors), costs, and outcomes. It is a mechanism for tracking what is implemented and how it works. Other potential variables to track might include the number of children in served and outcomes for young children in very low-income families or those in minoritized groups to determine if the intervention is reaching those who may be in need of services. Another area to track would be any changes made to disseminate the program effectively and changes needed to hire or train staff (e.g., hiring a mental health provider, teacher training). Thus, our preliminary idea for a scorecard, adapted from and developed after considering two publications by Karoly and colleagues (Karoly et al., 1998, 2001) for the RAND Corporation and Casey Family Programs, is presented in Table 10.1.

A scorecard, such as the one in Table 10.1, can facilitate tracking of program costs and benefits, changes needed to disseminate the program in the setting, and adaptations that will reduce disparities in accessing care for young children from minoritized groups and those who are residing in low-income families. Our list of outcomes to track is preliminary, and leaving a category for other types of outcomes allows programs to record outcomes that are meaningful to their own growth and development. Comparing the results of different interventions on a scorecard allows program administrators and providers to assess which programs work and how they need to be adapted. Conducting program evaluations and research in the areas on the scorecard and, ultimately, conducting randomized-controlled trials and

Table 10.1 Scorecard for tracking program use and impact

Site name			
	Program A	**Program B**	**Program C**
Costs Supplies Personnel Staff effort/time			
Providers *Required/training* Mental health Other			
Program components Type(s) of intervention Number of sessions Critical components			
Dissemination What works What needed to change			
Adaptations for minoritized groups			
Adaptations for low-income families			
Outcomes *Child* Developmental changes Cognitive Academic achievement Physical development Health Mental health *Family* Resilience Functioning Parent satisfaction *Program* Teacher satisfaction Quality of care Child functioning Cost savings *Other outcomes* (a) (b)			

Notes. Other outcomes could include assessment of family engagement, assessment of program quality, assessment of child reading levels, assessment of academic readiness, and assessment of outside funding for selected programs. Adaptations for minoritized groups should be at all the levels cited for low-income families.

comparisons of outcomes for different interventions will add to the literature and provide ideas on how to adapt programs to fit community needs and reach young children in very low-income families or who are in minority groups. To reach this goal, collaboration in evaluation and research across programs may be required, and policy changes, which facilitate collaboration and documentation of program implementation and outcomes, may add information to advance the field. In many instances, policy change may be needed to facilitate the support and mandated change that will foster the value of engagement, making the results of scorecard data that much more meaningful and pragmatic for advancing needs of families.

Future Research

Research on family engagement in infant and early childhood mental health treatment has grown in recent years and expanded operationalization, definition, and implementation of the construct across fields of practice. However, there are a number of areas that warrant further investigation in the future if families are to reap the full benefits of engaging in their children's services. First, mental health services for young children are increasingly integrated into broadly accessible, community-based services, such as early childhood education and home visiting (Goodman et al., 2021), yet rigorous testing of such interventions remains limited. For instance, infant and early childhood mental consultation (IECMHC), which is offered in multiple early childhood settings (e.g., early childhood education, home visiting, primary care, child welfare), has not yet been established as an evidence-based practice, and there is little understanding of what "dose" is needed to produce intended outcomes (Zeanah et al., 2023). Generally speaking, there is a dearth of research on strategies on effective approaches to reducing such inequities through strong family engagement and professional development. Finally, we find it deeply concerning that research continues to be scant on equitable family engagement, culturally targeted and adapted mental health interventions for young children, and specific strategies for reducing racial, ethnic, and socioeconomic disparities in treatment access, engagement, and outcomes. Only with increased attention to these issues from researchers, policymakers, and practitioners will we make significant progress toward all young children and families receiving the care they need.

Conclusions

It is our hope that this book presents timely and actionable information about the evidence based for promoting family engagement in infant and early childhood mental health care, as this fosters positive outcomes for youth and their families. Advancing our understanding of *how* promoting family-engaged interventions leads to program success (i.e., moderators and mediators) will continue to increase our understanding of how using interventions engage the family; promote child, family, and program well-being; and contribute to high quality of care for the young child. We also discussed behaviors related to engagement, highlighting the impact of trust and collaboration in engaging families and facilitating care of the child. Engaging the family and especially the parents of young children makes sense, as this allows parents to continue integrate key components of care at home through the most important relationships in a young child's life. Meeting the needs of families in all types of cultural groups, such as military families, families of different races, and families of children with disabilities or chronic illnesses, remains a critical step in engaging families (FREDLA, 2020, https://www.fredla.org/wp-content/uploads/2020/01/NeedsOfAllFamilies__FINAL_SCR-1.pdf). Continuing to advance research on interventions that engage families and young children is important – understanding how to engage families and address well-being may address health disparities for those from low-income and marginalized groups while contributing to long-term flourishing of the child and family, thereby ultimately changing trajectories to more positive avenues for child and family development.

Finally, infant and early childhood mental health both describes the young child's developing social and emotional development and the multidisciplinary nature of the field. Accordingly, there are opportunities for service providers across fields of practice to play a role in promoting children's psychological well-being, first and foremost by engaging caregivers in the services that promote healing. Zeanah and colleagues (2023) reported that children's mental health is not separable from cultural and family contexts and the factors that influence caregiving. Ultimately, the mental health of our youngest citizens will depend largely on the extent to which there is an ample, well-trained workforce that recognizes the inextricable link between parent/caregiver and child well-being and can successfully engage families from all backgrounds in services to prevent and address mental health challenges that emerge in the earliest years of life.

References

Alvy, K. T. (2019). *Effective Black Parenting Program: Instructor's manual* (3rd ed.). Center for the Improvement of Child Caring.

American Psychological Association. (n.d.). *APA dictionary of psychology: Intergenerational trauma*. https://dictionary.apa.org/intergenerational-trauma

Ardito, R. B., & Rabellino, D. (2011). Therapeutic alliance and outcome of psychotherapy: Historical excursus, measurements, and prospects for research. *Frontiers in Psychology, 18*(2), 1–11. https://doi.org/10.3389/fpsyg.2011.00270

Armbruster, P., & Kazdin, A. E. (1994). Attrition in child psychotherapy. In T. H. Ollendick & R. J. Prinz (Eds.), *Advances in clinical child psychology* (pp. 81–108). Springer.

Armstrong, F. D., Blumberg, M. J., & Toledano, S. R. (1999). Neurobehavioral issues in childhood cancer. *School Psychology Review, 28*(2), 194–203. https://doi.org/10.1080/02796015.1999.12085957

Balling, K., & McCubbin, M. (2001). Hospitalized children with chronic illness: Parental caregiving needs and valuing parental expertise. *Journal of Pediatric Nursing, 16*(2), 110–119. https://doi.org/10.1053/jpdn.2001.23157

Baquedano-Lopez, P., Alexander, R. A., & Hernandez, S. J. (2013). Equity issues in parental and community involvement in schools: What teacher educators need to know. *Review of Educational Research, 37*, 137–139. https://doi.org/10.3102/0091732X12459718

Bartlett, J. D., & Sacks, V. (2019). *Adverse childhood experiences are different than child trauma, and it's critical to understand why*. Child Trends. https://www.childtrends.org

Bartlett, J. D., Smith, S., & Bringewatt, E. (2017). *Helping young children who have experienced trauma: Policies and strategies for early care and education*. Child Trends. https://www.childtrends.org/publications/ecetrauma

Berk, L. E., & Meyers, A. B. (2016). *Infants and children* (8th ed.). Pearson.

Blizzard, A. M., Glos, L. J., Stephan, S. H., Medoff, D., & Slade, E. P. (2017). Impacts of a Medicaid wraparound model demonstration program on youth specialty mental health services use. *Journal of Behavioral Health Services & Research, 44*, 373–385. https://doi.org/10.1007/s11414-016-9520-0

Bringewatt, E. H., & Gershoff, E. T. (2010). Falling through the cracks: Gaps and barriers in the mental health system for America's disadvantaged children. *Children & Youth Services Review, 32*(10), 1291–1299. https://doi.org/10.1016/j.childyouth.2010.04.021

Butler, A. M., & Rodgers, C. R. R. (2019). Developing a policy brief on child mental health disparities to promote strategies for advancing equity among racial/ethnic minority youth. *Ethnicity & Disease, 29*(Suppl 2), 421–426. https://doi.org/10.18865/ed.29.S2.421

Carman, K. L., Dardess, P., Maurer, M., Sofaer, S., Adams, K., Bechtel, C., & Sweeney, J. (2013). Patient and family engagement: A framework for understanding the elements and developing interventions and policies. *Health Affairs, 32*(2), 223–231. https://doi.org/10.1377/hlthaff.2012.113

Child Welfare Information Gateway, Administration on Children, Youth, & Families, Administration for Children & Families, U.S. Department of Health & Human Services. (2017). *The Family Engagement Inventory: A brief cross-disciplinary synthesis*. www.childwelfare.gov/pubPDFs/synthesis.pdf#page=2&zoom=100,-213,716

Cohen, J. A., & Mannarino, A. P. (2015). Trauma-focused Cognitive Behavior Therapy for traumatized children and families. *Child & Adolescent Psychiatric Clinics of North America, 24*(3), 557–570. https://doi.org/10.1016/j.chc.2015.02.005

Dahlquist, L. M. (1997). Decreasing children's distress during medical procedures. *Psychotherapy in Practice, 3*(1), 43–54. https://doi.org/10.1002/(SICI)1520-6572(199721)3:1<43::AID-SESS4>3.0.CO;2-9

DiMatteo, M. R. (2004). The role of effective communication with children and their families in fostering adherence to pediatric regimens. *Patient Education and Counseling, 55*(3), 339–344. https://doi.org/10.1016/j.pec.2003.04.003

Division for Early Childhood. (2014). *DEC recommended practices in early intervention/early childhood special education*. https://www.dec-sped.org/dec-recommended-practices

dos Santos Felix, M. M., Ferreira, M. B. G., da Cruz, L. F., & Barbosa, M. H. (2019). Relaxation therapy with guided imagery for postoperative pain management: An integrative review. *Pain Management Nursing, 20*(1), 3–9. https://doi.org/10.1016/j.pmn.2017.10.014

Dowell, K. A., & Ogles, B. M. (2010). The effects of parent participation on child psychotherapy outcome: A meta-analytic review. *Journal of Clinical Child & Adolescent Psychology, 39*(2), 151–162. https://doi.org/10.1080/15374410903532585

Erdmann, F., Frederiksen, L. E., Bonaventure, A., Mader, L., Hasle, H., Robison, L. L., & Winther, J. F. (2021). Childhood cancer: Survival, treatment modalities, late effects and improvements over time. *Cancer Epidemiology, 71, 101733*. https://doi.org/10.1016/j.canep.2020.101733

Ellis, S., Khan, Y., Harris, V., McWilliams, R., & Converse, D. (2014). *The impact of fathers on children's well-being*. University of Florida/Institute of Food and Agricultural Sciences, Extension Service (FCS3321), Family, Youth, and Community Sciences Department. University of Florida.

Eyberg, S. M., Boggs, S. R., & Algina, J. (1995). Parent-child interaction therapy: A psychosocial model for the treatment of young children with conduct problem behavior and their families. *Psychopharmacology Bulletin, 31*(1), 83–91.

Fadus, M. C., Ginsburg, K. R., Sobowale, K., Halliday-Boykins, C. A., Bryant, B. E., Gray, K. M., & Squeglia, L. M. (2019). Unconscious bias and the diagnosis of Disruptive Behavior Disorders and ADHD in African American and Hispanic youth. *Academic Psychiatry, 44*(1), 95–102. https://doi.org/10.1007/s40596-019-01127-6

Ferlazzo. (2011). Involvement or engagement? *Educational Leadership: Schools, Families, & Communities, 68*(8), 10–14. http://www.ascd.org/publications/educational-leadership/may11/vol68/num08/abstract.aspx
Garvey, C., Julion, W., Fogg, L., Kratovil, A., & Gross, D. (2006). Measuring participation in a prevention trial with parents of young children. *Research in Nursing & Health, 29*, 212–222. https://doi.org/10.1002/nur.20127
Godoy, L., Hodgkinson, S., Robertson, H. A., Sham, E., Druskin, L., Wambach, C. G., Beers, L. S., & Long, M. (2019). Increasing mental health engagement from primary care: The potential role of family navigation. *Pediatrics, 143*(4), e20182418. https://doi.org/10.1542/peds.2018-2418
Goodman, W. B., Dodge, K. A., Bai, Y., Murphy, R. A., & O'Donnell, K. (2021). Effect of a universal postpartum nurse home visiting program on child maltreatment and emergency medical care at 5 years of age: A randomized clinical trial. *JAMA Network Open, 4*(7), e2116024-e2116024. https://doi.org/10.1001/jamanetworkopen.2021.16024
Gomby, D. S. (2000). Promise and limitations of home visitation. *Journal of the American Medical Association, 284(11), 1430–1431.* https://doi.org/10.1001/jama.284.11.1430
Gopalan, G., Horen, M. J., Bruns, E., Corey, M., Meteyer, S., Pardue, M., Lane, T., & Matarese, M. (2017). Caregiver perceptions of parent peer support services within the Wraparound service delivery model. *Journal of Child and Family Studies, 26*(7), 1923–1935. https://doi.org/10.1007/s10826-017-0704-x
Green, C. L., Walker, J. M. T., Hoover-Dempsey, K. V., & Sandler, H. M. (2007). Parents' motivations for involvement in children's education: An empirical test of a theoretical model of parental involvement. *Journal of Educational Psychology, 99*(3), 532–544. https://doi.org/10.1037/0022-0663.99.3.532
Grossmann, K., Grossmann, K. E., Fremmer-Bombik, E., Kindler, H., Scheuerer-Englisch, H., & Zimmermann, A. P. (2002). The uniqueness of the child–father attachment relationship: Fathers' sensitive and challenging play as a pivotal variable in a 16-year longitudinal study. *Social Development, 11*(3), 301–337. https://doi.org/10.1111/1467-9507.00202
Halgunseth, L. (2009). Family engagement, diverse families, and early childhood. *Young Children, 64*(5), 56–58.
Henderson, A. T., & Mapp, K. L. (2002). *A new wave of evidence: The impact of school, family, and community connections on student achievement.* Southwest Educational Development Laboratory.
Hernandez, S. (2013). Collaboration in special education: Its history, evolution, and critical factors necessary for successful implementation. *U.S. China. Education Review, 3*(6), 480–498. https://eric.ed.gov/?id=ED544122
Hoover-Dempsey, K. V., Walker, J. M., & Sandler, H. M. (2005). Parents' motivations for involvement in their children's education. In E. N. Patrikakou, R. P. Weissberg, S. Redding, & H. J. Walberg (Eds.), *School-family partnerships for children's success* (pp. 40–56). Teachers College Press.
Ingoldsby, E. M. (2010). Review of interventions to improve family engagement and retention in parent and child mental health programs. *Journal of Child and Family Studies, 19*(5), 629–645. https://doi.org/10.1007/s10826-009-9350-2
Ishimaru, A. M., Lott, J., Torres, K., & O'Reilly-Diaz, K. (2019). Families in the driver seat: Catalyzing familial transformative agency for equitable collaboration. *Teachers College Record, 121*(11), 1–39. https://doi.org/10.1177/016146811912101108
Jacques, C., & Villegas, A. (2018). Strategies for equitable family engagement. *State Support Network: Partnering for School Improvement.* https://oese.ed.gov/files/2020/10/equitable_family_engag_508.pdf downloaded June 16, 2023
Jose, K., Taylor, C. L., Venn, A., Jones, R., Preen, D., Wyndow, P., & Hansen, E. (2020). How outreach facilitates family engagement with universal early childhood health and education services in Tasmania, Australia: An ethnographic study. *Early Childhood Research Quarterly, 53*, 391–402. https://doi.org/10.1016/j.ecresq.2020.05.006

Karoly, L. A., Greenwood, P. W., Sohler Everingham, S. M., Jill Hoube, J., Kilburn, M. R., Rydell, C. P., Sanders, M., & Chiesa J. (1998). *Early childhood interventions: Benefits, costs, and savings*. RAND Corporation. https://www.rand.org/pubs/research_briefs/RB5014.html

Karoly, L., Kilburn, R., Bigelow, J. H., Caulkins, J. P., & Cannon, J. S. (2001). Assessing costs and benefits of early childhood intervention programs: Overview and applications to the Starting Early Starting Smart Program. Casey Family Programs and RAND Corporation. https://apps.dtic.mil/sti/pdfs/ADA399318.pdf

Kim, S., Crooks, C. V., Bax, K., & Shokoohi, M. (2021). Impact of trauma-informed training and mindfulness-based social–emotional learning program on teacher attitudes and burnout: A mixed-methods study. *School Mental Health, 13*(1), 55–68. https://doi.org/10.1007/s12310-020-09406-6

King, G., Currie, M., & Petersen, P. (2014). Child and parent engagement in the mental health intervention process: A motivational framework. *Child & Adolescent Mental Health, 19*(1), 2–8. https://doi.org/10.1111/camh.12015

Klawetter, S., Glaze, K., Sward, A., & Frankel, K. A. (2021). Warm connections: Integration of infant mental health services into WIC. *Community Mental Health Journal, 57*(6), 1130–1141. https://doi.org/10.1007/s10597-020-00744-y

Knafl, K. A., Havill, N. L., Leeman, J., Fleming, L., Crandell, J. L., & Sandelowski, M. (2017). The nature of family engagement in interventions for children with chronic conditions. *Western Journal of Nursing Research, 39*(5), 690–723. https://doi.org/10.1177/0193945916664700

Langley, A., Santiago, C. D., Rodríguez, A., & Zelaya, J. (2013). Improving implementation of mental health services for trauma in multicultural elementary schools: Stakeholder perspectives on parent and educator engagement. *Journal of Behavioral Health Services & Research, 40*(3), 247–262. https://doi.org/10.1007/s11414-013-9330-6

Lee, K., & Zhang, L. (2022). Cumulative effects of poverty on children's social-emotional development: Absolute poverty and relative poverty. *Community Mental Health Journal, 58*(5), 930–943. https://doi.org/10.1007/s10597-021-00901-x

Lindsey, M. A., Brandt, N. E., Becker, K. D., Lee, B. R., Barth, R. P., Daleiden, E. L., & Chorpita, B. F. (2014). Identifying the common elements of treatment engagement interventions in children's mental health services. *Clinical Child & Family Psychology Review, 17*(3), 283–298. https://doi.org/10.1007/s10567-013-0163-x

Masi, M. V., Miller, R. B., & Olson, M. M. (2003). Differences in dropout rates among individual, couple, and family therapy clients. *Contemporary Family Therapy, 25*(1), 63–75. https://doi.org/10.1023/A:1022558021512

Maybery, D., Jaffe, I. C., Cuff, R., Duncan, Z., Grant, A., Kennelly, M., Ruud, T., Skogoy, B. E., Weimand, B., & Reupert, A. (2021). Mental health service engagement with family and carers: What practices are fundamental? *BMC Health Services Research, 21*(1), 1–11. https://doi.org/10.1186/s12913-021-07104-w

Miller, T. (2011). Falling back into gender? Men's narratives and practices around first-time fatherhood. *Sociology, 45*(6), 1094–1109. https://doi.org/10.1177/0038038511419180

Muñoz, R. F., Le, H. N., Ippen, C. G., Diaz, M. A., Urizar, G. G., Jr., Soto, J., Mendelson, T., Delucchi, K., & Lieberman, A. F. (2007). Prevention of postpartum depression in low-income women: Development of the Mamás y Bebés/Mothers and Babies Course. *Cognitive & Behavioral Practice, 14*(1), 70–83. https://doi.org/10.1016/j.cbpra.2006.04.021

Nicholson, J., Kurtz, J., Rivas, L., Henneman, T., Peterson, E., Bryant, S., & Lin, B. (2022). *Trauma-responsive family engagement in early childhood: Practices for equity and resilience*. Routledge.

O'Connell, M. (2005). *The good father: On men, masculinity, and life in the family*. Scribner.

Oppenheim, J., & Bartlett, J. D. (2023). *Cost-effectiveness of infant and early childhood mental health treatment*. Infant & Early Childhood Mental Health Technical Assistance Center, Substance Abuse and Mental Health Services Administration, Georgetown University Center for Child and Human Development, ZERO TO THREE, and Thriving Together.

Podell, J. L., & Kendall, P. C. (2011). Mothers and fathers in family cognitive-behavioral therapy for anxious youth. *Journal of Child and Family Studies, 20*(2), 182–195. https://doi.org/10.1007/s10826-010-9420-5

Powell, D. R., Son, S. H., File, N., & San Juan, R. R. (2010). Parent-school relationships and children's academic and social outcomes in public school pre-kindergarten. *Journal of School Psychology, 48*(4), 269–292. https://doi.org/10.1016/j.jsp.2010.03.002

Reedy, C. K., & McGrath, W. H. (2010). Can you hear me now? Staff-parent communication in child care centers. *Early Child Development & Care, 180*(3), 347–357. https://doi.org/10.1080/03004430801908418

Robles-Ramamurthy, B., Sandoval, J., Tobon, L., & Fortuna, L. R. (2022). Beyond children's mental health: Cultural considerations to foster Latino child and family mental health. *Child & Adolescent Psychiatric Clinics of North America, 31*(4), 765–778. https://doi.org/10.1016/j.chc.2022.05.005

Rodgers, C. R., Flores, M. W., Bassey, O., Augenblick, J. M., & Lê Cook, B. (2022). Racial/ethnic disparity trends in children's mental health care access and expenditures from 2010-2017: Disparities remain despite sweeping policy reform. *Journal of the American Academy of Child & Adolescent Psychiatry, 61*(7), 915–925.

Shivers, E. M., Farago, F., & Gal-Szabo, D. E. (2022). The role of infant and early childhood mental health consultation in reducing racial and gender relational and discipline disparities between Black and white preschoolers. *Psychology in the Schools, 59*(10), 1965–1983. https://doi.org/10.1002/pits.22573

Smith, T. E., & Sheridan, S. M. (2019). The effects of teacher training on teachers' family-engagement practices, attitudes, and knowledge: A meta-analysis. *Journal of Educational & Psychological Consultation, 29*(2), 128–157. https://doi.org/10.1080/10474412.2018.1460725

Smith, S., Robbins, T., Stagman, S., & Mahur, D. (2013). *Parent engagement from preschool through grade 3: A guide for policymakers.* National Center for Children in Poverty.

Staudt, M. (2007). Treatment engagement with caregivers of at-risk children: Gaps in research and conceptualization. *Journal of Child and Family Studies, 16*(2), 183–196. https://doi.org/10.1007/s10826-006-9077-2

Stevens, J., Kelleher, K. J., Ward-Estes, J., & Hayes, J. (2006). Perceived barriers to treatment and psychotherapy attendance in child community mental health centers. *Community Mental Health Journal, 42*, 449–458. https://doi.org/10.1007/s10597-006-9048-5

Strohschein, L., & Gauthier, A. H. (2018). Poverty dynamics, parenting, and child mental health in Canada. *Society and Mental Health, 8*(3), 231–247. https://doi.org/10.1177/2156869317731603

Stroul, B. A., Blau, G. M., & Larsen, J. (2021). *The evolution of the system of care approach.* The Institute for Innovation and Implementation, School of Social Work, University of Maryland. https://www.cmhnetwork.org/wp-content/uploads/2021/05/The-Evolution-of-the-SOC-Approach-FINAL-5-27-20211.pdf

Substance Abuse and Mental Health Services Administration, SAMHSA. (2014). *SAMHSA's Concept of trauma and guidance for a trauma-informed approach. HHS Publication No. (SMA) 14-4884.* https://store.samhsa.gov/product/SAMHSA-s-Concept-of-Trauma-and-Guidance-for-a-Trauma-Informed-Approach/SMA14-4884

Thomas, C. R., & Holzer, C. E. (2006). The continuing shortage of child and adolescent psychiatrists. *Journal of the American Academy of Child & Adolescent Psychiatry., 45*(9), 1023–1031. https://doi.org/10.1097/01.chi.0000225353.16831

Tully, L., Piotrowska, P. J., Collins, D. A. J., Mairet, K. S., Black, N., Kimonis, E. R., Hawes, D. J., Moul, C., Lenroot, R. K., Frick, P. J., Anderson, V., & Dadds, M. R. (2017). Optimising child outcomes from parenting interventions: Fathers' experiences, preferences and barriers to participation. *BMC Public Health, 17*(1), 550–550. https://doi.org/10.1186/s12889-017-4426-1

Turnbull, A., & Turnbull, R. (2022). Trusting partnerships and belonging for families of students with disabilities. In J. Jones & K. Gallus (Eds.), *Belonging and resilience in individuals with developmental disabilities: Community and family engagement* (pp. 35–47). Springer. https://doi.org/10.1007/978-3-030-81277-5_3

Turnbull, A. P., Turnbull, R. H., Francis, G. L., Burke, M., Kyzar, K., Haines, S. J., Gershwin, T., Shepherd, K. G., Holdren, N., & Singer, G. H. S. (2021). *Families and professionals: Trusting partnerships in general and special education* (8th ed.). Pearson.

U.S. Department of Health and Human Services, Administration for Children and Families, Office of Head Start, National Center on Parent, Family, and Community Engagement. (2018). *Key indicators of high-quality family engagement for Quality Rating Improvement Systems*. https://childcareta.acf.hhs.gov/sites/default/files/public/indicators-final-508.pdf

Van Voorhis, F. L., Maier, M. F., Epstein, J. L., & Lloyd, C. M. (2013). *The impact of family involvement on the education of children ages 3 to 8*. MDRC.

Vilaseca, R. M., Galván-Bovaira, M. J., González-del-Yerro, A., Baqués, N., Oliveira, C., Simó-Pinatella, D., & Giné, C. (2019). Training needs of professionals and the family-centered approach in Spain. *Journal of Early Intervention, 41*(2), 87–104. https://doi.org/10.1177/1053815118810236

Waid, & Kelly. (2020). Supporting family engagement with child and adolescent mental health services: A scoping review. *Health & Social Care in the Community, 28*(5), 1333–1342. https://doi.org/10.1111/hsc.12947

Walter, A. W., Yuan, Y., Morocho, C., & Thekkedath, R. (2019). Facilitators and barriers to family engagement and retention of young children in mental health care: A qualitative study of caregivers' perspectives. *Social Work in Mental Health, 17*(2), 173–196. https://doi.org/10.1080/15332985.2018.1517402

Warren, J., Thomson, D., & LaForett, D. R. (2023). *Head Start family service workers' attitudes, knowledge, and practices are connected to how they link families to two-generational supports*. Child Trends. https://www.childtrends.org/publications/head-start-family-service-workers-attitudes-knowledge-and-practices-are-connected-to-how-they-link-families-to-two-generation-supports

Williams, E. R., & Baber, C. R. (2007). Building trust through culturally reciprocal home-school-community collaboration from the perspective of African-American parents. *Multicultural Perspectives, 9*(2), 3–9. https://doi.org/10.1080/15210960701386228

Zeanah, P. D., Steier, A., Lim, I., Korfmacher, J., & Zeanah, C. H. (2023). Current approaches and future directions for addressing ethics in infant and early childhood mental health. *Infant Mental Health Journal, 44*, 625–637. https://doi.org/10.1002/imhj.22077

Index

L. Nabors, J. D. Bartlett (eds.), *Family Engagement in Mental Health Interventions for Young Children*, Springer Series on Child and Family Studies, https://doi.org/10.1007/978-3-031-47917-5